Healthy Cooking
for the Jewish Home

Healthy Cooking for the Jewish Home

---

200 RECIPES FOR EATING WELL ON HOLIDAYS AND EVERY DAY

Faye Levy

WILLIAM MORROW

An Imprint of HarperCollins*Publishers*

HarperCollins books may be purchased for educational, business,
or sales promotional use. For information please write: Special
Markets Department, HarperCollins Publishers, 10 East 53rd
Street, New York, NY 10022.

FIRST EDITION

Designed by Fritz Metsch

Library of Congress Cataloging-in-Publication Data
Levy, Faye.
Healthy cooking for the Jewish home: 200 recipes for eating well
on holidays and every day / by Faye Levy.
   p. cm.
  ISBN: 978-0-06-078784-4
  ISBN-10: 0-06-078784-8
  1. Cookery, Jewish. 2. Menus. I. Title.

TX724.L4128 2008
641.5'676—dc22   2006047089

08 09 10 11 12 WBC/QWF 10 9 8 7 6 5 4 3 2 1

In loving memory of my dear mother,

Who made the Jewish holidays into healthy, joyful celebrations

Who enjoyed dining and dancing and never got fat!

✿

PAULINE KAHN LURIA

1916–2005

Warsaw—Washington, D.C.—Jerusalem—Los Angeles

Contents

Acknowledgments

First I wish to express my deep gratitude to my mother, Pauline Kahn Luria, whose spirit pervades this book. I owe my background in Jewish cooking most of all to her. She taught me Ashkenazi cooking and kashrut, as well as the importance of health conscious cooking and of exercise. And she passed on to me her joy in celebrating Shabbat and all the Jewish holidays with traditional foods.

I feel so lucky to have received ideas and cooking tips from chefs, caterers, friends, relatives, students of my cooking classes, and even shoppers I met at markets, who eagerly told me how they prepare their favorite dishes.

I owe much of my knowledge of fine cuisine to master chef Fernand Chambrette and pastry chef Albert Jorant, and to the many other teachers at École de Cuisine La Varenne in Paris. What they taught me was the key to understanding how cooking works, and made it possible for me to follow such cooks' directions as "add a bit of this" or "add water until the dough feels good." I am grateful to Anne Willan, founder of the Parisian cooking school, and to prominent Israeli cookbook author Ruth Sirkis, for enabling me to spend fascinating years working on their wonderful cookbooks.

My mother-in-law, Rachel Levy, taught me a most important culinary lesson—the value of spices, as well as how to prepare delicious Yemenite Jewish specialties. I also learned a lot about Israeli–Middle Eastern food, traditional and contemporary, from my sisters-in-law Hedva Cohen, Ety Levy, Nirit Levy, and Mati Kahn, and from my husband's Moroccan cousin Dvora Cohen.

My cousin Mildred Greenberg, Jewish cook par excellence, is full of good ideas for ways to prepare holiday foods that are tasty, healthy, and easy to fix. She always encourages me with her enthusiastic support, as did my dear aunt Sylvia Saks.

I have learned many wonderful Moroccan-Israeli dishes from my friends Valerie and Hayim Alon, who make Shabbat into a feast that is not only delicious but healthy, too. My creative friend Aviva Maoz also gave me many good ideas, as did her sister Ofra Alon, and their Iraqi-born mother, Karmela Arad. My friend, cookbook author Ronnie Venezia, and her mother, Lebanese-born Suzanne Elmaleh, taught me much about Lebanese Jewish cooking. I also gained a lot of information about Israeli cooking from my friend Lior Moore of Givatayim, who founded and runs cuisinemiddleast.com.

Good friends also taught me so much about ethnic foods and ingredients from around the world, which help to enliven healthy cooking. I learned about Asian foods from my dear friends Thai chef Somchit Singchalee, authors Nina Simonds and Linda Burum, about Turkish cuisine from Filiz Hosukoglu of Gaziantep, Turkey, and about Mexican foods from Leticia Ortega.

My friend, chef, and cookbook author Akasha Richmond has always been generous with her many inventive ideas for healthful cooking. I learned a lot about vegetarian cooking from my friends Nancy Eisman of Melissa's Worldwide Produce and cookbook author Dana Jacobi.

I gained ideas for creative kosher cooking from Nili Goldstein, the owner of Magic Carpet, a Los Angeles Yemenite-Israeli restaurant; from chef and kosher caterer Nir Weinblut of Los Angeles; from Nilu Saadian, who gave me information about Persian-Jewish cooking; and from Guta Ben Simhon, chef-owner of La Guta restaurant in Jerusalem.

I thank Dr. Steven G. Pratt, author of *Superfoods,* for answering my nutrition questions. Robert Schueller of Melissa's Worldwide Produce has always found the answers to my numerous queries about fruits and vegetables.

I appreciate the encouragement of my editors, Kim Upton at Tribune Media Services (formerly called the Los Angeles Times Syndicate) and Amanda Borschel-Dan, Atira Winchester, and Liat Collins of the *Jerusalem Post.*

I am so grateful to my agent, Jane Dystel, for her invaluable support. I wish to thank my editor at HarperCollins, Gail Winston, for making the process of producing the book so pleasant. I also appreciate the contributions of assistant editor Sarah Whitman-Salkin, copy editor Sonia Greenbaum, and production editor Ann Cahn.

Most of all, I appreciate the contribution of my virtual co-author—my husband, Yakir Levy, who helped me with every stage of preparing the book and made it such a pleasure to produce, from planning the book to interviewing people about their cooking, to revising what I wrote, and for always being happy to taste, to research, to learn, and to discover new ingredients and dishes.

Introduction

This is a glorious time to be cooking healthy, kosher food. Modern Jewish cuisine has been enhanced and enlivened with the convergence in Israel of healthy traditions of both the Ashkenazi (Eastern and Central European) and Sephardi (Mediterranean and Middle Eastern) cooking styles.

Due to the cultural impact of the state of Israel on Jewish cooking everywhere, and thanks to the influx of Israeli immigrants to the United States, many Americans have become more familiar with Sephardi cuisine. This style of eating is essentially the Mediterranean diet, a popular model in America for healthy living.

Never before has such a wonderful array of foods been available for the Jewish home, both for holidays and everyday meals. Today, kosher ingredients are everywhere—not just in Jewish markets. In mainstream supermarkets, kosher foods are easy to find and ethnic markets offer a variety of interesting specialties. I have used kosher-certified foods from Turkey, Italy, and France. A variety of kosher flatbreads is available, both Middle Eastern and Mexican; new kinds of lavash and many of the innovative tortillas made in interesting flavors and in whole-grain versions are kosher.

For cooks who wish to prepare healthy dinners with a creative touch, it's exciting to discover the excellent selection of kosher foods in many gourmet markets and markets featuring natural, organic foods. Indeed, in many cases, these three types of foods—natural, gourmet, and kosher—have merged. Many professional chefs praise the flavor of kosher poultry, which gets high marks in taste comparisons in food magazines. Delicious cheeses free of animal rennet are enjoyed by kosher and vegetarian cooks, and can also be found in many Middle Eastern markets. Faux meats such as soy pepperoni make possible a great range of dishes that previously could not be prepared by kosher cooks, and often are healthier than the original. Nutritious soy ice cream is a perfect pareve ending for a Shabbat roast chicken dinner.

All of these tasty choices are great news for kosher cooks. Having access to so many more healthy ingredients than before makes it easy to prepare wholesome versions of tried-and-true favorites and to branch out in new culinary directions.

Ashkenazi Jewish food has a reputation with some for being laden with high-fat meat and dairy products, but this is often due to their impressions from eating at delis eager to promote their reputations as "home of the overstuffed sandwich." Those deli menus were originally designed for special occasions and were developed when immigrants were en-thralled by the plentiful rich food of the United States; this is not typical home cooking. I grew up in an Orthodox Ashkenazi home and our meals often consisted of fish as an en-trée, without a great deal of meat or high-fat dairy.

Since so many families, including my own, now have members originating in both Jewish groups, menus in many homes become Jewish fusion, presenting the best elements from east and west, north and south, or what we sometimes call Ashkesephard cooking.

Serving our families such wholesome creations is in keeping with ancient Jewish tradi-tion, when all the Jews lived in the land of Israel. The holidays in the Torah had an agri-cultural basis dating back to the agrarian way of life of the Jews at that time. Passover is the holiday of springtime, Shavuot is the festival of first fruits, and Sukkot is the harvest hol-iday. Emphasizing the natural products of the Holy Land, these holidays have healthy themes that highlight fresh produce. Remembering this biblical spirit is helpful in pro-viding us with an incentive to create meaningful, healthy, delicious, contemporary kosher meals.

I hope you will enjoy reading and cooking from this book and that these recipes will enrich many healthy celebrations.

Le'chaim tovim—to the good life!

Healthy Cooking
for the Jewish Home

What Is Healthy Cooking?

Many people define healthiness in the negative, dwelling upon ingredients that should be avoided. What determines whether a recipe is healthy for me is what good things are in it, not what foods are omitted. Emphasizing wholesome foods is central to my approach to healthy cooking. Planning menus this way is much more fun.

Anyone who knows me knows how much I love to eat! Knowing that a meal is nutritious adds to my pleasure in eating it.

Eating in a healthy manner means enjoying such menus as a colorful salad of baby greens, tomatoes, and a little feta cheese, drizzled with fruity olive oil or luscious hazelnut oil, followed by grilled salmon with fresh asparagus and an aromatic side dish of brown basmati rice with toasted pistachios and dried cranberries. Dessert might include fresh raspberries and blueberries with a touch of honey (see Milk N' Honey First Fruits Salad, page 129) or fine quality dark chocolate.

Naturally, there is a certain amount of compromise involved in creating healthy menus and recipes. Some dishes might be more delicious with more butter, but often you might choose to reduce the amount of fat and to substitute olive oil for better nutrition. Some find keeping kosher to be useful in designing healthy meals because of the discipline involved and due to the prohibition of eating dairy and meat in the same meal, since both are sources of saturated fat.

A helpful guide to planning healthy menus is the *Dietary Guidelines for Americans*, also known as the "Revised Pyramid," published by the United States Department of Health and Human Services and the Department of Agriculture. Depending on a person's weight and activity level, it shows how much to eat of various categories of food. To find the choices that are best for you, see http://www.mypyramid.gov/.

In the nutrition community, there has been plenty of debate regarding the best way to eat, but there is general agreement on one key aspect: we should add more vegetables to our diet. Nobody disputes that vegetables are good for us.

In recent years there has been a lively controversy between the proponents of low-fat

THE BENEFITS OF ORGANIC FOODS

*D*emand for organic foods is booming and they are becoming more and more widely available, as people are becoming more concerned about the importance of preserving the environment and treating animals humanely. The U.S. Department of Agriculture (USDA) recognized the importance of this issue and established federal standards for certifying foods as organic.

Whole Foods Markets, a chain that heavily promotes organic foods, lists many reasons to buy organic. Regarding the question of whether organic foods are more healthful, Whole Foods states its position on this issue on its Web site:

"Organic foods are not necessarily more nutritious, rather organic foods are spared the application of potentially harmful long-lasting insecticides, herbicides, fungicides and fertilizers. . . . Now, the EPA [Environmental Protection Agency] considers 60% of all herbicides, 90% of all fungicides, and 30% of all insecticides as potentially cancer-causing."

Experts disagree vigorously about whether organic foods are healthier and worth the higher price. Some feel that the pesticide residue in foods is low and has not been proven harmful. They claim that the U.S. food supply is one of the safest in the world, and that pesticide residues are not a significant risk compared with other hazards. In the case of children and pregnant women, however, some argue that these amounts could be significant.

Certain studies have demonstrated higher levels of some nutrients in organic foods, but most experts find them inconclusive.

MEAT, EGGS, AND DAIRY PRODUCTS

The USDA has four requirements to define milk as organic: It must come from cows that have not been treated with growth hormone to increase milk production and have not been given antibiotics. Their feed, whether it is grass or grain, must be grown without pesticides, and they must have some access to grazing in a pasture. Certain studies indicate that organic milk is higher in some nutrients.

Organically grown chickens are raised without hormones or antibiotics and have an organically grown diet. Free-range chickens are allowed access to the outdoors.

and low-carb diets. Good nutritionists have learned from both trends. Now there is a general consensus that instead of drastically cutting one or the other, the best solution is to choose good fats and good carbs, as well as good proteins.

This sensible message is welcome news to health-conscious food lovers! When you

In some kosher markets, you can buy organic kosher poultry and meat. The birds are free range, and the cattle are fed with grass and organic grains.

Some studies find that grass-fed cattle produce meat that is lower in saturated fat and slightly higher in some nutrients.

Many markets carry cage-free and organic eggs. There are also eggs from chickens fed a special diet to increase the eggs' omega-3 content and decrease their cholesterol. They have become popular, although some nutritionists feel that people don't eat enough eggs for this to make a significant difference in their diets.

PRODUCE

Food certified as organic must be produced without synthetic fertilizers and pesticides and cannot make use of genetic engineering methods, ionizing radiation, and sewage sludge for fertilization.

Some nutritionists argue that certain conventionally grown produce items contain a much higher amount of pesticide residues than their organic equivalents. They contend that buying organic is important when those residues cannot be washed off or peeled away. Lists of which produce items are most susceptible to containing residues are available online at several sites, including the World's Healthiest Foods and the Organic Consumers Association, and usually include apples, peaches, pears, and strawberries.

THE GOVERNMENT'S ADVICE

The EPA sets limits on how much of a pesticide residue can remain on food. It advises the following practices to reduce the amount of pesticides that people consume:

1. *Wash and scrub all fresh produce thoroughly under running water.*
2. *Peel fruits and vegetables when possible; discard outer leaves of leafy vegetables.*
3. *Trim fat from meat and skin from poultry and fish.*
4. *Eat foods from a variety of sources for a variety of nutrients and less likelihood to consume too much of a single pesticide.*

For more details, see http://www.epa.gov/pesticides/food/tips.htm

don't feel constrained to avoid an entire category of foods, you can prepare delicious meals much more easily.

Good fats come from plant sources rather than animal ones and include nuts, olive oil, nut oils, and vegetable oils instead of butterfat and fatty meats. It's best to avoid hydrogenated fats, found in shortening, margarine, and many packaged crackers, cookies, cakes, and processed foods; fortunately, many of these food products have been reformulated and so you can find versions that are trans-fat free.

Healthy carbohydrates come from whole grains, rather than from highly processed and refined ones, and from legumes and certain vegetables like sweet potatoes. Because whole grains contain fiber, they increase people's feeling of satiety so they feel fuller than they would from an equal amount of calories from refined-flour foods. According to the government guidelines, adults should eat 6 servings of grains a day, at least half from whole grains. A serving is small—28 grams, or 1 ounce, which equals a small slice of bread or ½ cup cooked rice or pasta. This is for an average-size adult who can consume 2,000 calories per day without gaining weight.

The best protein foods come from legumes and nuts for fiber-rich, cholesterol-free protein, from fatty fish for omega-3 fatty acids, and from lean meats such as turkey and low-fat dairy foods. It's best to aim to have a high proportion of your protein from plant-based sources, as they have little or no saturated fat.

Other recommendations in the pyramid guidelines (for those at the 2,000 calories/day level) include eating 2½ cups of vegetables, 2 cups of fruit, and 3 cups of fat-free or low-fat dairy foods a day, and minimizing the amount of sugar, saturated fat, and trans fat. Daily protein totaling 5.5 ounces of meat or equivalents a day can come from lean meat, poultry, or fish; or, as equivalents of 1 ounce of meat, any of the following: 1 egg, ¼ cup cooked dried beans or tofu, 1 tablespoon peanut butter, or ½ ounce nuts or seeds. The guidelines also include advice to exercise 60 to 90 minutes a day.

Moderation isn't exciting, but most agree that it is the key to a wholesome diet. Portion sizes of most foods, including healthy ones, make a difference. It's important not to eat more calories than are expended in the course of the day; otherwise even beneficial foods turn into fat in the body.

According to Dr. Barbara Rolls, author of *The Volumetrics Eating Plan*, in order to lose weight or avoid gaining, it's important to choose "high-satiety food," or food that helps you feel satisfied at the end of a meal yet is not high in calories. She advises choosing foods high in fiber and eating adequate amounts of lean protein but not too much fat. Fiber helps people feel full because it has few calories that the body can use; thus adding fiber helps to reduce the calories of a dish.

The water content of foods is also important. Rolls notes that people tend to eat about the same weight of food every day, and studies show that they feel just as satisfied if they eat casseroles containing water-rich vegetables. With more water, they eat fewer calories for the same size portion. I find that thick vegetable soups satisfy in the same way. So do big salads of raw or cooked vegetables, moistened lightly with a healthy dressing. That's why you'll find lots of recipes for soups and salads in this book, as well as rice and pasta dishes studded generously with vegetables.

The best foods to choose are nutrient dense but not calorie dense. In other words, opt for those that pack a powerful nutritional punch for the amount of calories they contain. Doing so makes each calorie count, in a positive way.

A good way to include such valuable foods on the menu is to make a point of frequently eating certain nutritious foods that are known as "superfoods" or "power foods."

SAFE COOKING TIPS

When using pans with a nonstick coating, be careful not to let them get too hot, as they may give off irritating or poisonous fumes. Never preheat an empty nonstick pan.

If you use aluminum pans, do not use them to cook tomatoes or other acidic foods, as these foods absorb aluminum during cooking.

The Food and Drug Administration advises that you should not let plastic wrap, even if it is microwave safe, directly touch food in the microwave.

When microwaving, be sure to use microwave-safe dishes.

Do not microwave food in take-out containers from restaurants. Such containers might melt or warp.

When storing food in plastic containers, always make sure they were intended for food.

Although "old-fashioned" vitamins and minerals are important, nutrition science now has much more knowledge about substances that are beneficial to the body. Some examples of superfoods are those that are high in cholesterol-reducing soluble fiber, such as oatmeal, barley, broccoli, and apples. Another group of superfoods is vegetables and fruits that are high in phytochemicals, which act as antioxidants to protect the body from disease; examples include deep green leafy vegetables, blueberries, and kiwis. A third category is foods that are rich in heart-healthy omega-3 fatty acids, such as salmon, walnuts, and flax seeds.

This does not mean you should have repetitive menus. On the contrary, variety is the spice of nourishment. As each ingredient contains a different combination of nutrients, the best assurance of getting a good selection of beneficial compounds is eating a broad variety of foods. In the course of a day, the best route is to choose fruits and vegetables of different types—green vegetables, cruciferous vegetables (cabbage family), and citrus

TEN GUIDELINES FOR A HEALTHY DIET

1. *Eat a wide variety of foods.*
2. *Eat plenty of vegetables and fruits, between 5 and 9 servings a day.*
3. *To help feel satisfied on fewer calories, opt for dishes with a high proportion of liquid, such as hearty soups with plenty of vegetables.*
4. *For proteins, give preference to vegetarian proteins, such as legumes and soy foods.*
5. *Eat omega-3 rich fish, such as salmon and tuna.*
6. *Enhance your menus with a modest amount of healthy fats, such as nuts, olives, avocados, olive oil, and nut oils.*
7. *When eating carbs, opt for whole grains and whole-grain bread rather than refined grains and white bread.*
8. *When eating dairy foods, choose those that are low in fat or fat free.*
9. *Rather than indulging in desserts, which tend to be high in sugar and fat, end your meals with fruit most of the time.*
10. *Exercise every day.*

fruits, for example. An easier way to express this is to group fruits and vegetables by colors—those that are green (such as broccoli and kiwi), orange (such as carrots and oranges), red (such as red peppers and watermelon), white (such as onions and garlic), and blue (such as eggplant and plums), all make their own contributions to our diets.

Eating should be a source of delight rather than one of stress. Most nutritionists agree that there are no "bad" foods (except those high in trans fats); it's okay to enjoy favorite foods, even those that are not considered healthy, once in a while.

Rosh Hashanah

SWEET BEGINNINGS FOR A HEALTHY NEW YEAR

❧

The food customs of Rosh Hashanah, the Jewish New Year, are easy to love. Who wouldn't enjoy a holiday in which Jewish mothers take the traditional greeting "Have a good and sweet New Year" so literally that they infuse the menu with sweetness? What could be a more enticing beginning to a meal than the season's crisp apples dipped in honey?

Most of the eating customs of the two-day holiday developed over the millennia by Ashkenazi and Sephardi Jews turn out to be amazingly up to date. Somehow dishes that have been popular for ages are in harmony with the latest nutritional guidelines.

The menu usually begins with fish, an age-old symbol of abundance. Whether it's Ashkenazi gefilte fish or Sephardi-style tilapia in saffron tomato sauce (pages 140 and 13), the lean protein of fish is one of the healthiest ways to start the dinner.

As an expression of thanks for a plentiful harvest, vegetables and fruits play a major role in Rosh Hashanah dinners. On the second day of Rosh Hashanah, a new fruit is tasted and a special blessing is recited expressing joy and thanks. Pomegranates are a popular and particularly healthy choice, since they have a high concentration of nutrients, but there are many other possibilities (see "The Holiday of New Fruit," page 10). Fruit also are prominent in a favorite Ashkenazi main course stew, tzimmes, and often in a Moroccan entrée, tajine.

Many of the time-honored Rosh Hashanah foods happen to be good for us. Eating carrots on the holiday is an Ashkenazi Rosh Hashanah custom; the coin-shaped slices stand for prosperity. But carrots are also a great source of vitamin A. So are the sweet potatoes that appear on many tables as part of the tzimmes.

Sephardi Jews have a special custom highlighting vegetables. They are tasted in a ceremony resembling a mini-Seder. Each symbolizes a wish for the coming year—greens, such as spinach or chard for a bountiful harvest, rice and black-eyed peas for abundance in general, and leeks and beets for protection. Moroccan Jews serve couscous traditionally garnished with winter squash, carrots, turnips, chickpeas, and raisins. All these foods give a healthy boost to the holiday menu.

Certainly apples are healthy, and the honey for dipping them is favored by some nu-

THE HOLIDAY OF NEW FRUIT

*O*ne of my favorite Rosh Hashanah customs is eating a new fruit. The tradition came about to provide a reason to say the Shehecheyanu blessing—which gives thanks for living until now—on the holiday's second day.

So what is a "new" fruit? That's a topic of debate among rabbis and educators. Some say it's a fruit that's just coming into season, or one you haven't eaten since last year. Some people avoid certain seasonal fruit until Rosh Hashanah to be sure it will be "new."

A more relaxed attitude suggests choosing a fruit you haven't eaten for at least 30 days, or simply one you don't eat often. Rabbi Michael Strassfeld, author of The Jewish Holidays, describes this approach: "At the beginning of the second evening meal of Rosh Hashanah, it is customary to eat a 'funny fruit,' which means any fruit we have not eaten in a long time." He suggests kiwis or unusual melons.

So many fruits are available almost year-round that it is hard to find a "new" fruit, wrote Rabbi Yehudah Prero in his Rosh Hashanah article for the Project Genesis Web site, www.torah.org, adding that it depends on your markets. When he lived in Chicago he chose hard-to-find starfruits, fresh dates, or figs.

Writing about the Rosh Hashanah table of her childhood in Italy, Edda Servi Machlin, the author of The Classic Cuisine of the Italian Jews, recalled that there were always fresh figs, pomegranates, and jujubes, also known as Chinese dates.

In some families, the time-honored tradition is to eat an unfamiliar fruit. As more varieties of fruit become available, our idea of what is exotic evolves. Having a fresh pineapple was an event in our home when I was growing up, and we had never heard of avocados or persimmons. These are still the holiday's special fruits on some tables.

The choice is personal. If my Asian pear tree has fruit, for me that's a perfect pick for the holiday table.

tritionists over sugar. Dr. Steven G. Pratt and Kathy Matthews, authors of *Superfoods HealthStyle*, consider honey a "superfood" because it is high in health-promoting antioxidants. Perhaps less surprising, they call apples a superfood too.

Honey also sweetens the most famous Rosh Hashanah specialty—honey cake. I like to make a light but luscious version moistened with applesauce and embellished with almonds and chocolate chips; thus the meal begins and ends with apples and honey.

Recently I got some ideas for interesting holiday fruits from fruit maven Robert Schueller of Melissa's Worldwide Produce. I sampled a huge, luscious Keitt mango that was so sweet that you could almost eat it with its skin. He also introduced me to the tropical monstera deliciosa—*"delicious monster." With its elongated shape and dark green scales, it somewhat resembles an alligator. When the scales fall off, you eat the fruit, which looks and tastes like a hybrid of banana and pineapple.*

The most gorgeous fruit was the shocking pink dragon fruit. When I saw it, I recognized it as the pitaya that I bought a couple of years ago during a stroll in Jerusalem's Mahaneh Yehudah market. Native to Latin America, this cactus fruit, which comes in various colors, has been the subject of Israeli research in developing drought-resistant export crops to grow in the Negev. Some feel its delicately sweet flavor recalls watermelon, cactus pear (sabra), and kiwi. Others feel it resembles melon. To me it tastes a little like all of these.

Emboldened by these experiences, my husband and I went to a Filipino supermarket and bought the world's funniest fruit, the durian. This large, spiky fruit is known for its pungent aroma and thus is suitable for only the most daring diners. But we liked its sweet taste and rich custard texture, and could understand why East Asians dubbed it the "king of fruit" and even make it into ice cream.

Yellow barhi dates are in season just in time for Rosh Hashanah. They are fabulous when yellow and firm and when softened, brown, and honeylike.

All these fruits are worthy candidates for the holiday blessing. So are fresh figs and pomegranates, which, along with dates and grapes, are preferred by many because they are biblical fruits. Aromatic guavas are another good choice. But why stop at one fruit? Why not present a beautiful platter of unusual and best-of-the-season fruits?

The most delicate "new fruits" are best savored as is, so that nothing intrudes on their special flavors. I wouldn't cook pitayas or fresh lychees. Fresh pineapples, figs, dates, and mangoes taste good in simple recipes that don't obscure their character, such as fruit salads, or as a garnish for delicate rice dishes like Rosh Hashanah Fruity Rice (page 18).

Rosh Hashanah Tilapia in Saffron Sauce

Chicken with Dates and Almonds

Lamb Tajine with Prunes, Apricots, and Sweet Vegetables

Veal Tzimmes with Butternut Squash and Matzo Balls

Rosh Hashanah Fruity Rice

Late Summer Fruit Compote

Shehecheyanu Salad

Almond Applesauce Cake with Chocolate Chips and Honey

When I celebrate Rosh Hashanah with a group of Israeli and American neighbors, our menu usually begins with a version of this dish. It is vaguely based on Moroccan-Israeli fish, but for Rosh Hashanah, unlike the rest of the year, it is not made with hot chiles. Sweet peppers, garlic, and spices give the dish a warm, deep flavor: good-quality paprika, turmeric in many families, saffron in some, and a combination of both in others.

Often the fish is moistened lavishly with olive oil. For this lighter rendition, I use less oil, but I choose a fruity extra virgin olive oil for maximum impact. Tilapia, long a popular fish in Israel and now in the United States as well, is a good choice, and so are sea bass and halibut (see "Safe Fish," page 237). For Rosh Hashanah, fish is usually a first course, but this dish can also be served as a delicious main course with basmati rice.

You can make the sauce with red or yellow tomatoes, using either drained, chopped tomatoes or tomato sauce. Red peppers give the most attractive result when matched with yellow tomatoes, or yellow peppers with red tomatoes.

2 to 3 tablespoons extra virgin olive oil
1 small onion, chopped
1 small red or yellow bell pepper, or ½ pasilla
  (poblano) chile (optional), cut into strips
4 garlic cloves, minced
¾ cup red or yellow tomato sauce, or drained,
  chopped canned red or yellow tomatoes
⅛ to ¼ teaspoon saffron threads

⅛ to ¼ teaspoon turmeric
½ teaspoon paprika
½ teaspoon dried oregano
1¼ pounds tilapia fillets
Salt and freshly ground black pepper
⅓ cup cilantro or flat-leaf parsley
Cayenne pepper (optional)

Heat 1 tablespoon oil in a deep sauté pan. Add onion and red pepper, and cook over medium-low heat for 7 minutes or until nearly tender; if pan becomes dry during cooking, add 1 tablespoon water and cover pan. Remove mixture from pan.

Heat another tablespoon oil in pan. Add half the garlic and cook for ½ minute over medium-low heat. Add tomato sauce, ⅔ cup water, saffron, turmeric, paprika, and oregano, and bring to a simmer. Add about half the tilapia fillets, or enough to make one layer. Sprinkle each with salt and pepper to taste. Cover and cook over medium-low heat for 3 minutes per side or until fish just changes color throughout. Remove tilapia gently with a slotted spoon. Cook remaining tilapia and remove it also.

Add remaining garlic to sauce and bring to a simmer. Return onion mixture to pan, heat briefly, and remove from heat. Add cilantro. Taste and adjust seasoning. Add cayenne to taste and a little more oil if desired. Return tilapia to pan. Serve warm or at room temperature.

Makes 5 to 6 appetizer or 3 to 4 main-course servings

This recipe is perfect for Rosh Hashanah, but it was inspired by a completely different occasion—a dinner, cooked by food historian Charles Perry, of specialties from the palaces of fourteenth-century Baghdad.

Perhaps most striking were the entrées that combined meat and fruit. There was a chicken in pomegranate sauce, which had a Bordeaux hue like French coq au vin (chicken in red wine sauce), and an alluring sweetness from pomegranate syrup and ground almonds.

This dish is a lighter version of a delicious entrée of lamb stewed with dates and sweet spices. Using boneless chicken thighs substantially cuts the simmering time, as well as the saturated fat. The fragrant sauce is flavored with cinnamon, ginger, and onion, which turns mellow as it cooks. Instead of using dates, you can make this dish with a combination of dried apricots and raisins; because they sweeten the sauce less than dates, add a little honey as well.

Matching nuts and fruits with savory foods is a technique still favored in the Middle East. Fruit-enhanced main courses, often accented with sweet spices, are popular in the cuisines of Morocco and Persia. With brief simmering, dried fruit softens and acquires a luscious texture. Not only does it dress up the dish and act as an interesting foil for the richness of the meat, but it adds a pleasing flavor to the sauce as well. Serve this festive dish with long-grain rice, preferably aromatic basmati, which is available at well-stocked supermarkets, or brown basmati, which you'll find at natural foods shops.

1¼ to 1½ pounds skinless, boneless chicken thighs
1 large onion, finely chopped
Salt and freshly ground black pepper
1 tablespoon vegetable oil (optional)
1 cup chicken broth
¾ teaspoon ground ginger

Pinch of ground cloves or freshly grated nutmeg (optional)
¼ to ½ teaspoon ground cinnamon
1 cup pitted dates, or ¾ cup dried apricots and ¼ cup raisins
1 to 2 tablespoons honey (optional)
⅓ cup whole blanched almonds, toasted

Cut chicken into about 1 × ½ × ½-inch cubes and put them in a heavy stew pan. Add onion, salt, pepper, and oil (if using). Cover and cook over medium-low heat, stirring occasionally, for 5 minutes. Add broth, ginger, cloves (if using), and ¼ teaspoon cinnamon and bring to a boil. Cover and simmer over low heat for 10 minutes. Add dates and simmer, uncovered, for 10 minutes or until chicken is tender.

Taste and adjust seasoning; add remaining cinnamon and honey, if you like. If you want a thicker sauce, remove chicken and dates with a slotted spoon to a plate and simmer sauce, uncovered, over medium heat for 2 to 3 minutes or until thickened to taste, then return chicken and dates to sauce and heat through. Serve garnished with almonds.

Makes 4 to 6 servings

✹ LAMB TAJINE WITH PRUNES, APRICOTS, AND SWEET VEGETABLES

I like to serve a Moroccan-inspired tajine with fruit to usher in a sweet New Year. This one combines dried fruit and a touch of honey with gentle spices—saffron, ginger, cinnamon, and nutmeg.

The classic tajine contains onions, which melt into the sauce and thicken the stew naturally. To turn it into a whole-meal dish, just add additional vegetables. I opt for sweet ones—carrots, sweet potatoes, and yellow squash. Tasty, time-honored accompaniments are couscous and a garnish of toasted almonds.

Lamb is a favorite meat for tajines and because it is so flavorful, it satisfies when served in smaller portions.

1 tablespoon vegetable oil or mild olive oil

1½ pounds lamb stew meat, trimmed of fat, cut into 1-inch cubes

2 medium onions (about 1 pound), chopped

Large pinch of saffron threads (about ⅛ teaspoon tightly packed, ¼ teaspoon loosely packed)

Salt

½ teaspoon freshly ground black pepper, or more to taste

1½ to 2¼ cups water

2 large carrots, sliced ¼ inch thick

⅓ large orange-fleshed sweet potato (about ½ pound), cut into 1 × 1 × ½-inch dice

1 teaspoon ground ginger

¼ teaspoon ground cinnamon

Freshly grated nutmeg (optional)

¾ cup dried apricots

1 cup pitted prunes

2 yellow crookneck squashes, necks cut into ½-inch slices, bodies cut into 1 × 1 × ½-inch dice

1 tablespoon honey

Heat oil in a stew pan. Add lamb cubes in two batches and brown lightly on all sides over medium-high heat, about 5 minutes. Remove from pan to a plate with a slotted spoon.

Add onions to pan and sauté over medium heat for 5 to 7 minutes or until light brown; if pan becomes dry during sautéing, add 1 tablespoon water and cover pan. Return meat and any juices from plate to pan. Add saffron, salt to taste, ½ teaspoon pepper, and 1½ cups water. Mix well; liquid will not cover lamb. Bring to a boil. Cover and simmer over low heat, stirring occasionally, for 1 hour and 15 minutes or until lamb is tender. Remove lamb cubes with tongs, leaving onions in pan. Skim fat from sauce.

Bring sauce to a simmer. Add carrots and sweet potato. Cover and cook over low heat for 10 minutes. If sauce is too thick, add ⅓ cup hot water. Add ginger, cinnamon, nutmeg (if using), apricots, prunes, and squash. Cover and cook, gently stirring once or twice, for 10 minutes or until vegetables and fruit are tender.

Return lamb cubes to pan and heat through. If sauce is too thick, add 3 to 4 tablespoons hot water. Add honey and stir very gently. Cover and cook over low heat for 5 minutes. Taste, and adjust seasoning for salt, pepper, and nutmeg. Serve hot.

Makes 6 servings

VEAL TZIMMES WITH BUTTERNUT SQUASH AND MATZO BALLS

In my family when I was growing up, tzimmes consisted of cubes of chuck (beef shoulder) stewed with vegetables and dried fruit. In other households, brisket is braised in a large piece and served in slices in the sauce. By using veal and a higher proportion of vegetables to meat, I make this tzimmes lighter than the old-fashioned versions. One traditional element I keep is the prunes, which some now prefer to call dried plums. Our mothers were right! They are very good for you.

Although sweet potatoes are commonly paired with the carrots in tzimmes, I like butternut squash for its more delicate taste and lighter texture, especially if I'm adding matzo balls. If you want to substitute sweet potatoes, use 1 1/4 to 1 1/2 pounds of the orange-fleshed type.

Tzimmes should be moist and saucy but not soupy. Some cooks thicken it from the beginning with a roux, made by cooking flour with the sautéed onions. Because the stew gains body while simmering and standing, most people wait until it's done to decide to thicken it or not. The preferred techniques are adding a flour slurry or baking the tzimmes. (See the note at the end of the recipe.)

Matzo balls make tzimmes particularly festive. Some cooks make one large substantial chicken fat–enriched matzo ball or a flour-and-margarine dumpling, simmer it directly in the stew, and then slice it for serving. My family preferred light matzo balls enriched with a little oil, as in the recipe below, although for tzimmes they are a bit less fluffy than for serving in chicken soup. Like my mother always did, I poach them apart so they cook evenly, then add them to the finished tzimmes so they won't break up.

If you're making tzimmes ahead, it's best to heat the matzo balls separately and add them to the reheated stew. Once you've added them to the pan, you can thicken the sauce by baking, but not by stirring in a flour slurry, because the matzo balls might fall apart. Instead of putting them in the pan of tzimmes, add a few to each dish at serving time.

1 1/2 pounds boneless lean veal stew meat, trimmed of fat	2 large eggs, or 1 egg and 2 egg whites
2 tablespoons vegetable oil	1/2 cup matzo meal, plus 1 to 2 tablespoons more, if needed
1 large onion, chopped	2 pounds butternut squash
2 large carrots, cut into 1-inch chunks	2 tablespoons honey
Salt and freshly ground black pepper	1/4 teaspoon ground cinnamon
2 to 2 1/2 cups water	1 1/4 cups pitted dried plums, or prunes

Cut veal into 1- to 1 1/4-inch pieces and pat them dry. Heat 1 tablespoon oil in a heavy stew pan. Add veal cubes in two batches, browning each lightly on all sides over medium heat and removing browned meat with a slotted spoon to a plate.

Add onion to pan and sauté over medium heat, stirring often, until brown, about 10 minutes; cover and add 1 tablespoon water if pan becomes dry. Return meat to pan with any juices on plate. Add carrots, salt, pepper, and enough water to just cover. Bring to a boil, skimming occasionally. Cover and simmer over low heat, stirring occasionally, for 1 hour or until meat is tender.

For a lighter sauce, refrigerate cooked meat and its sauce separately for several hours, then skim fat from top of sauce. Return meat to sauce and reheat.

Meanwhile, prepare matzo balls. Lightly beat eggs with 1 tablespoon oil in a medium bowl. Add ½ cup matzo meal, ½ teaspoon salt, and pinch of pepper. Stir with a fork until batter is smooth. Slowly stir in 1 tablespoon broth from tzimmes. Cover batter and refrigerate for 20 minutes. Batter will thicken.

In a medium saucepan, bring about 2 quarts water to a boil with 1 teaspoon salt. Reduce heat so water barely simmers.

With wet hands, take about 1 teaspoon batter and shape it lightly in a small, roughly round dumpling by gently rolling it between your palms. Batter should be too soft to form a neat, smooth ball. If you're not sure if the matzo balls will hold together, cook one in simmering water for 10 minutes, remove it with a slotted spoon, and taste it for firmness and seasoning. If it is too soft, stir in matzo meal by tablespoons. If it is too firm, gradually stir in more broth by tablespoons.

Continue shaping matzo balls, wetting your hands before each one and slipping them carefully into simmering water. Cover and simmer over low heat for 30 minutes or until just firm. Keep them warm in their covered pan until ready to serve; or refrigerate in their cooking liquid and reheat gently in liquid.

Peel squash and cut it in half lengthwise. Discard seeds and stringy parts in cavity. Cut squash into 1-inch cubes.

Stir honey and cinnamon into sauce. Add squash and push pieces into liquid. Cover and simmer for 10 minutes. Turn squash pieces over. Add plums. Cover and simmer for 15 minutes or until squash is tender. Taste and adjust seasoning.

To serve, remove matzo balls gently from water with a slotted spoon. You can add matzo balls to sauce or put a few in each portion at serving time. If you add them to pan, spoon a little sauce over them, cover, and let stand so they absorb flavor for 10 minutes or until ready to serve. Serve stew from a casserole or deep serving dish.

NOTE: If you would like to thicken the sauce, choose one of these methods:

Baking: Bake tzimmes, uncovered, at 350°F for 20 to 30 minutes.

Using a slurry: Mix 1 tablespoon cornstarch or flour with 2 tablespoons water to a smooth paste in a medium bowl. Bring tzimmes to a gentle simmer. Gradually ladle about 1 cup tzimmes sauce into cornstarch paste, stirring until smooth. Return mixture to pan and bring to a simmer, stirring as gently as possible to avoid breaking up squash and prunes. Simmer over low heat for 5 minutes.

Makes 4 to 6 servings

Moroccan and other Sephardi cooks often stud rice with raisins. I like to embellish such classic recipes with exotic fresh fruit to grace my Rosh Hashanah table. Substitute any tender festive fruit you like. Use one kind or, even better, a colorful mixture of tart and sweet fruits.

If you'd like to use brown rice, follow the directions below, cooking the rice for 40 minutes, then adding the raisins and cooking 5 minutes more.

3 to 4 tablespoons vegetable oil
2 medium onions, halved and cut into thin slices
2 cups long-grain rice
4 cups hot chicken broth, water, or a mixture
    of the two
1 bay leaf
1½ teaspoons salt
Freshly ground black pepper

2 tablespoons raisins
½ cup pomegranate seeds
¹/₂ cup quartered pitted dates, preferably yellow
    barhi dates
½ cup fresh figs, quartered lengthwise
⅔ to 1 cup diced mango or papaya
½ cup half-slices of peeled kiwi
½ cup toasted cashews or almonds

Heat oil in a stew pan. Add onions and sauté over medium heat for 12 to 15 minutes or until tender and deep brown. Remove half of onion mixture and reserve.

Add rice to pan and sauté, stirring, for 2 minutes. Add broth, bay leaf, salt, and pepper to taste, and bring to a boil. Stir once. Add raisins. Cover and cook over low heat for 18 minutes, or until rice is just tender. Let stand off heat, covered, for 10 minutes. Discard bay leaf.

Reserve half of fruit and half of nuts. Using a fork, fluff rice lightly and gently stir in reserved onions and half of fruit and nuts. Taste and adjust seasoning. Serve rice in a shallow bowl, garnished with reserved fruit and nuts.

Makes 8 servings

LATE SUMMER FRUIT COMPOTE

Whether you eat this healthy dessert on its own or with Rosh Hashanah honey cake, the combination of lightly cooked plums, pears, peaches, and papaya is beautiful and delicious. This recipe is easy to remember—all the fruits begin with the letter P. You can also add pomegranate seeds, a Jewish New Year favorite, for a finishing touch.

Some cooks add red wine to the syrup whenever they poach plums for extra flavor. Even sweet red wine will do, as long as you reduce the amount of sugar; start with 1/3 cup and add more to taste. You can keep the fruit in its syrup for several days in a covered container in the refrigerator.

1 cup dry red wine and 2 cups water, or
    3 cups water
3/4 cup sugar
2 cinnamon sticks, or 1/2 to 1 teaspoon
    ground cinnamon
1/4 teaspoon ground cloves

A few pared strips of lemon zest
1/2 pound peaches
1/2 pound pears, ripe but firm
3/4 pound plums, ripe but firm, quartered
1 1/2 to 2 cups diced papaya or mango
1 tablespoon fresh lemon juice, or to taste

Combine wine and water mixture, sugar, cinnamon, cloves, and lemon zest in a heavy, medium saucepan. Heat over low heat, stirring gently, until sugar dissolves. Bring to a boil. Reduce heat to a simmer and add peaches. Cook 1 minute. Remove syrup from heat. Remove peaches with a slotted spoon. Peel peaches and quarter them.

Peel pears and halve them lengthwise. With point of peeler, remove flower end and core of each pear. Cut each half in 2 lengthwise quarters.

Return syrup to a boil. Add pears and plums. Cover with a lid slightly smaller than diameter of saucepan to keep fruit submerged. Reduce heat to low and cook fruit for 4 minutes. Add peaches and papaya and continue cooking for 3 to 5 more minutes or until fruit is tender when pierced with a sharp knife. Cool fruit in syrup to room temperature. Add lemon juice. Refrigerate for at least 30 minutes before serving. Remove cinnamon sticks and lemon zest strips if you like. Serve cold.

Makes 4 to 6 servings

✠ SHEHECHEYANU SALAD

This salad is the perfect way to welcome a sweet and healthy New Year. The medley of biblical fruits—pomegranates, grapes, figs, and dates—combined with a modern fruit of Israel—oranges—is beautiful and packed with great nutrition. Figs and dates are full of fiber. Pomegranate seeds and red grapes have valuable protective phytochemicals called flavonoids, a large class of plant chemicals that act as antioxidants, helping to prevent oxygen-containing molecules from damaging cells. Some flavonoids are believed to protect the body from cancer and heart disease.

The bowl of jewellike ruby pomegranate seeds, luscious fresh figs with their crimson interior, and shiny seedless grapes looks like a mixture of precious stones. If you can get yellow barhi dates, add some too. Their color and texture perfectly complement the other fruits. You can also add melon, which has a long history in the region and was longed for by the ancient Hebrews when they wandered in the desert. To vary the color, you might choose green grapes or green-skinned figs but, most important, select the best-quality fruit you can get.

Follow the method given here for removing the seeds from the pomegranate immersed in water, to minimize the mess.

1 pomegranate, or about ¾ cup pomegranate seeds
¾ cup seedless green or red grapes
⅔ cup fresh figs, quartered lengthwise
⅔ cup fresh dates, preferably yellow barhi dates,
     pitted and halved or quartered (optional)

1 cup diced ripe cantaloupe or honeydew melon
     (optional)
2 to 3 tablespoons fresh-squeezed orange juice
1 orange, peeled and diced

Cut a thin slice off top and bottom of pomegranate. With a knife, score rind from top to bottom several times, like cutting peel from an orange. Put pomegranate in a large bowl of cold water. Holding fruit under water, remove rind and break fruit in sections. With your fingers, pull seeds out of membranes. Remove membranes from water, then remove pomegranate seeds from bottom of bowl. Drain well. Transfer seeds to a glass bowl.

Add remaining ingredients and gently mix. Serve cool.

Makes 3 to 4 servings

ALMOND APPLESAUCE CAKE WITH CHOCOLATE CHIPS AND HONEY

Honey lends only a subtle accent to this cake, so it is more delicate than traditional honey cakes. Before baking, I like to soak the raisins in brandy or juice so they are plump and moist. You can substitute ½ cup whole wheat flour for ½ cup of the white flour.

Late Summer Fruit Compote with its wine syrup (page 19) is a good accompaniment. For a luscious frosting, make Spiced Chocolate Wine Glaze (page 373) and sprinkle the glazed cake with ¼ cup toasted slivered almonds.

¼ cup raisins
2 tablespoons apple brandy, rum, or apple juice
2¼ cups all-purpose flour
2¼ teaspoons baking powder
¾ teaspoon baking soda
1 teaspoon ground cinnamon
3 large eggs

1⅓ cups brown sugar
⅓ cup honey
⅔ cup canola oil or light olive oil
½ cup plus 2 tablespoons unsweetened applesauce
½ cup semisweet chocolate chips
½ cup blanched almonds, chopped

Put raisins in a jar, add brandy, cover jar, and shake to combine. Let stand at least 30 minutes or up to a few hours.

Preheat oven to 350°F. Lightly grease a 9-inch square pan, line it with parchment paper or wax paper, and grease paper. Sift flour with baking powder, baking soda, and cinnamon.

Beat eggs lightly. Add brown sugar and honey and beat until mixture is smooth and lightened in color. Gradually add oil and beat until blended. On low speed, beat in flour mixture alternately with applesauce, each in two batches. Last, beat in chocolate chips, almonds, and raisins with their liquid.

Pour batter into prepared pan. Bake for about 30 minutes or until your finger does not leave an indentation when you press lightly on top of cake, and a cake tester inserted in center of cake comes out clean. Cool in pan for about 15 minutes. Turn out onto rack and carefully peel off paper. Cover tightly when completely cool. Serve at room temperature. Cut into squares or bars.

Makes 9 to 12 servings

Yom Kippur

FASTING AND FEASTING

Yom Kippur could be called the holiday of comfort food. Well, not exactly the day of Yom Kippur, which is a 25-hour total fast, with no liquids allowed either. But the copious meal before Yom Kippur and the break-the-fast meal afterward are usually made up of food that is hearty and satisfying.

Before fasting, many of us want to pamper ourselves with the foods we have loved since childhood. That may help explain the popularity of chicken soup on Jewish tables for this important meal (in addition to the practical reason that a chicken is used for the Yom Kippur custom of *kapparot* to atone for one's sins). Chicken soup with noodles or matzo balls is soothing, and most people love it, even children. In fact, for many of us it's part of fond childhood memories.

The dinner before Yom Kippur is moderately festive and, most of all, filling. After all, the food needs to sustain you during the fast. Therefore, people eat a meal with plenty of protein, usually with a main course of chicken. The dishes should be tasty, but not too salty or spicy to avoid provoking thirst during the fast. This doesn't mean the food has to be bland, however. You can add a touch of spice as long as you don't overdo it.

Sometimes, instead of the usual chicken soup I grew up with, I like to cook a soup that's a little different. One is a soup loved by Jews from Yemen, with a hint of cumin, a bit of turmeric to give it a warm, golden hue, and the bright taste of fresh cilantro.

For the feast before the fast, it's a good idea to keep another guideline in mind. Try to take it easy. Don't put a great amount of effort into cooking the meal so that you become exhausted. That goes double for the meal following the fast. After abstaining from food and drink for a whole day, the last thing anyone wants to do is cook!

A useful solution is preparing ahead as much as possible for both meals. Yet there's no need to cook two completely different menus in advance. Let some of the dishes do double duty at your dinners.

If you're making the standard main course of chicken in the pot for the prefast meal, cook it ahead and refrigerate it. This will make it easy to skim the congealed fat from the top of the soup.

Plan on side dishes that reheat well or can easily be turned into salads. To accompany the chicken, you can make a two-way rice pilaf. First, prepare a gently spiced, colorful brown rice pilaf with raisins, carrots, squash, and herbs. Transform it into a lively salad the next day by adding cucumbers, corn, lemon juice, and a sprinkling of toasted nuts on top. This takes only a few minutes and it refreshes the dish.

A savory stew of seasonal vegetables also fits the bill perfectly. Gently cook some beau-

---

SOUP TO BREAK THE FAST

When I was growing up in Washington, D.C., my family always broke the Yom Kippur fast with a dairy meal. It was essentially brunch food. Items such as scrambled eggs with buttered toast, bagels with cream cheese and lox, noodle and cottage cheese kugel, and sour cream coffee cake were on our menu. This was the custom in the homes of my relatives and friends too. My mother explained that such a light meal is easier on your system after a day spent without food.

So when my husband and I were invited to break the fast with our neighbor Hayim Alon and his family, I was surprised to learn that some Sephardi Jews opt for a meat meal after the fast. On the table the main course was harira, a satisfying soup of lentils, chickpeas, and meat. Serving such a strength-restoring soup is the tradition in the homes of Jews of Moroccan origin. And not just among Jews. Many Moslems prepare the same soup in the evenings during the month of Ramadan, after having fasted during the day.

There's a regional rationale behind this tradition—dairy foods are not plentiful on the Maghreb menu. Besides, the soup was balanced nutritionally and turned out to be hearty but not heavy. The small dice of meat served mainly to flavor the broth, which was punctuated with chickpeas and vegetables. The lentils melded into the soup and provided body.

There is another reason why harira is ideal for the occasion—it tastes even better when made in advance. Naturally, after Yom Kippur nobody wants to start cooking.

Like many time-honored dishes, there are numerous interpretations of harira. This whole-meal soup

---

tiful eggplants, sweet peppers, and luscious tomatoes with garlic and oregano, as in Vegetable Medley with Toasted Almonds (page 309), to accompany the chicken. This is one of the best dishes to make in advance. The next day, for breaking the fast, you can serve the vegetables hot with an omelet or scrambled eggs or as a sauce for pasta. It's also delicious cold with bread. All you need to perk it up is extra seasoning, a few olives on top, and a drizzle of extra virgin olive oil.

When you bake a Rosh Hashanah honey cake or Almond Applesauce Cake with Chocolate Chips and Honey (page 21), you might like to bake two of them. Honey cakes keep well if tightly wrapped, and your cake should taste fine. At the meal before the Yom Kippur fast, you can serve the cake with some fresh figs, plums, or grapes to make it more festive and nutritious. This way you have a taste of something sweet ready for breaking the fast.

varies according to the cook's pantry and the family's tastes. Some make it hearty, chunky, and thick, while others, like my neighbor, prefer it lighter. Custom calls for lamb or chicken, but our version was made with beef. Legumes are the meat's main partners, usually chickpeas, often lentils, and sometimes fresh or dried fava beans. The soup can also be vegetarian, the way my husband's relative Dvora Cohen makes it (see the recipe on page 209).

Onions, celery, parsley, and ginger are favorite flavors, while tomatoes and spices—saffron, turmeric, or both—give the soup a golden-orange glow. A squeeze of lemon juice and a sprinkling of fresh cilantro enliven the soup with a fresh finish. Sometimes there is a thickener—either plain or toasted noodles, rice, flour, or a combination of these.

Serving couscous is not the custom with harira, but everyone in the Alon family loves it after Yom Kippur. We were all glad when a bowl of the golden pasta grains appeared on the table. It was a terrific accompaniment for the soup.

We also enjoyed several seasonal salads—marinated peppers, Israeli tomato-cucumber salad, eggplant with olives, and cooked greens with lemon and cumin, followed by apples for dessert. Compared to such a healthy selection, whether a dairy-laden dinner is lighter on your system or not is a matter of opinion.

Normally, the salads are appetizers, but for this day they were served as accompaniments. All the food, except the dessert, was put on the table from the beginning. Serving this way made perfect sense. Everyone was ravenous, and had little patience for the niceties of eating one course at a time. Besides, on this day you don't need an "appetizer" to stimulate your appetite!

❧

Apple Walnut Green Salad with a Sweet Touch

Poached Turkey with Mushrooms, Wheat Berries, and Dill

Chicken with Chickpeas and Eggplant—Easy Baraniya

Two-Way Brown Rice Pilaf with Vegetables and Raisins

The B.L.A.—Bagel with Lox and Avocado

Chocolate Walnut Ice Cream Cake

❧

❈ APPLE WALNUT GREEN SALAD
WITH A SWEET TOUCH

My friend Valerie Alon makes this delicious salad for Shabbat and holidays. She flavors the dressing with seasoned rice vinegar, which is slightly sweet and beautifully complements the apples and red onions in the salad. To this basic recipe she sometimes adds cubed fresh tomatoes, strips of sun-dried tomatoes, diced Persian cucumbers, or dried cranberries. There are always plenty of toasted nuts—usually walnuts and sometimes cashews—for a festive finishing touch.

½ red onion

1 tablespoon seasoned rice vinegar

1 to 2 tablespoons fresh lemon juice

Salt

2 to 4 tablespoons extra virgin olive oil

1 tart apple, such as Granny Smith

4 to 5 cups mixed baby lettuces, baby spinach,
     or bite-sized pieces of green-leaf lettuce

2 tablespoons dried cranberries (optional)

⅓ to ½ cup walnut halves, toasted

Halve the onion half and thinly slice each quarter. Separate slices in slivers. To make dressing, whisk vinegar with lemon juice and salt to taste in a small bowl. Whisk in oil.

A short time before serving, halve apple and cut into thin slices, leaving peel on. Combine onion, apple, greens, and cranberries (if using) in a shallow bowl, and toss. Pour dressing over salad and toss gently. Taste and adjust seasoning, adding more oil if needed. Garnish with walnuts and serve.

Makes 4 to 5 servings

❧ POACHED TURKEY WITH MUSHROOMS, WHEAT BERRIES, AND DILL

This hearty entrée is ideal sustenance before the Yom Kippur fast. The flavor of this savory stew somewhat recalls old-fashioned mushroom-barley soup, although it's made of a different grain—wheat—and is inspired by a dish from Persia.

Lamb is a popular choice in the Persian version, but turkey is a healthier option. For many Americans, this moist, savory way of preparing the popular bird will come as a discovery. As the turkey cooks, its tasty juices give the wheat a wonderful flavor. If you like, use kamut, a large-grained variety of wheat.

The classic dish consists only of wheat and meat, but I find that fresh and dried mushrooms, carrots, and fresh dill make it livelier. For a colorful, nutritious addition, add 1 to 2 cups frozen shelled edamame (green soybeans) for the last 5 minutes of cooking.

To minimize the saturated fat, refrigerate the poaching liquid after cooking the turkey and the wheat, and thoroughly skim the fat.

2½ to 3 pounds turkey drumsticks or thighs

1½ cups wheat berries, sorted and rinsed

2 large onions, coarsely chopped

5 cups water, or more if necessary

Salt and freshly ground black pepper

2 ounces dried porcini or shiitake mushrooms

2 carrots, diced

6 large garlic cloves, chopped

¼ teaspoon turmeric

6 to 8 ounces mushrooms, quartered

2 to 3 tablespoons chopped fresh dill

Cayenne pepper

In a large stew pan, combine turkey, wheat berries, and onions, and add 5 cups water, or enough to cover ingredients generously. Add a pinch of salt and bring to a boil. Cover and simmer over low heat, turning turkey pieces over from time to time, for 2 hours or until turkey is very tender when pierced in thickest part with a knife, and wheat berries are tender. Remove turkey from liquid. Cool broth and thoroughly skim fat from surface.

Meanwhile, soak dried mushrooms in a bowl of enough hot water to cover them for 30 minutes. Remove mushrooms and rinse them. If using shiitake mushrooms, remove stems; you can save them for making vegetable broth. Cut mushrooms into bite-sized pieces.

Remove turkey skin with aid of a paring knife. Discard turkey bones, cartilage, and visible fat. Pull or cut meat into wide strips.

Add carrots, dried mushrooms, garlic, and turmeric to pan. Bring to a boil. Cover and cook over medium-low heat for 5 minutes. Add fresh mushrooms and cook for 5 more minutes, or until fresh and dried mushrooms are tender. Season to taste with salt and pepper.

If casserole is too soupy, remove wheat and vegetables with a slotted spoon and boil sauce until it thickens. Return turkey meat, wheat, and vegetables to pan, and add dill. Taste for salt, and add black pepper and cayenne to taste. Serve hot.

Makes about 6 servings

CHICKEN WITH CHICKPEAS AND EGGPLANT— EASY BARANIYA

In North Africa, chickpeas are associated with Yom Kippur. They appear on Tunisian tables, together with chicken and eggplant, in an aromatic stew called baraniya that is served to break the Yom Kippur fast. This labor-intensive specialty calls for skinning soaked chickpeas and splitting each chickpea in two. The dish is rich; you deep-fry eggplant, mash it, return it to the skillet with additional oil, and fry it again until deep brown. Before flavoring the chicken with garlic, cinnamon, turmeric, and vinegar, you brown it with more oil.

To make this dish healthier as well as simpler to prepare, instead of frying the eggplant, I sauté it a little and braise it in the sauce with the chicken. In addition, I use skinless chicken; I just ask the butcher to pull the skin off.

I find that baraniya is tasty even without the chicken, and with vegetable broth instead of chicken broth, and is perfect for a meatless break-the-fast meal, accompanied by a hard-boiled egg, a little cottage cheese or yogurt, and perhaps a salad. It's faster too; cook the sauce for only 25 minutes or until the eggplant is tender.

3 pounds chicken pieces, preferably skinless
Freshly ground black pepper
1 to 2 tablespoons olive oil
1 large onion, cut into thin slices
4 large garlic cloves, chopped
One 1- or 1¼-pound eggplant, peeled if desired, diced

One 14-ounce can diced tomatoes, drained (optional)
1 to 2 cups chicken broth
Pinch of saffron, or ¼ teaspoon turmeric
¼ teaspoon hot red pepper flakes
Salt
1½ to 2 cups cooked chickpeas (garbanzo beans), or one 15-ounce can chickpeas, drained

Sprinkle chicken lightly with pepper. Heat oil in a large, deep sauté pan or stew pan. Add chicken in batches and brown lightly on all sides. Remove chicken to a plate.

Add onion to pan and cook over low heat for 7 minutes or until soft but not brown. Add garlic and cook for ½ minute. Stir in eggplant. Add tomatoes, if you like, or 1 cup chicken broth, saffron, pepper flakes, salt, and black pepper. Cook for 3 minutes, stirring often. Return chicken to pan; if you didn't add tomatoes, add remaining cup of broth. Cover and simmer over low heat for 35 minutes, or until chicken is tender. Add chickpeas and heat through. Taste sauce and adjust seasoning. Serve hot.

Makes 4 servings

TWO-WAY BROWN RICE PILAF WITH VEGETABLES AND RAISINS

Serve this colorful pilaf as a tasty accompaniment for chicken in the pre-Yom Kippur feast, or for Shabbat.

If you would like to turn the pilaf into Brown Rice and Vegetable Salad with Pistachios for the next day, to eat after the fast, set aside half the mixture and let it cool. You can also make the pilaf ahead for serving hot; simply reheat it in a covered container in the microwave.

3 tablespoons extra virgin olive oil
1 zucchini or pale green Mexican zucchini
    (also called white or Tatuma squash),
    cut into ½-inch dice
Salt and freshly ground black pepper
1 onion, chopped
1½ cups long-grain brown rice

1½ teaspoons ground coriander
1 teaspoon ground cumin
3 cups hot vegetable broth or water
1 bay leaf
1 thyme sprig, or ½ teaspoon dried thyme
1 large carrot, diced
¼ cup raisins or dried cranberries

Heat 1 tablespoon oil in a large sauté pan or stew pan. Add zucchini, salt, and pepper and sauté over medium heat, stirring, about 2 minutes. Remove with a slotted spoon.

Add 2 tablespoons oil to pan. Add onion and cook over medium heat for 4 minutes or until soft but not brown. Add rice, coriander, and cumin and sauté, stirring, about 2 minutes or until rice grains begin to change color.

Pour hot broth over rice and stir once. Add bay leaf, thyme, 1 teaspoon salt, and a pinch of pepper. Bring to a boil over high heat. Reduce heat to low, cover tightly, and simmer, without stirring, for 20 minutes. Scatter carrot over top. Cover and simmer for 20 minutes. Scatter zucchini and raisins over top. Cover and simmer for 3 minutes, or until rice is tender and liquid is absorbed. Discard bay leaf and thyme sprig.

Fluff rice gently with a large fork. Transfer very gently to a large bowl. Taste and adjust seasoning. Serve hot.

Makes 4 to 6 servings

THE B.L.A.—BAGEL WITH LOX AND AVOCADO

The idea for this sandwich came to me when my mother and I were about to have bagels and lox for brunch. I wanted a more nutritious spread than cream cheese, and I happened to have on hand a ripe avocado, which is rich in beneficial monounsaturated fat and organic minerals. Mashed with a bit of lemon juice, it turned out to be the perfect choice. Its mild, delicate flavor provides the ideal balance for the salty lox, and its smooth creamy texture resembles that of cream cheese.

Use whatever bagel you like. A whole-grain one has the best nutrition, but the sandwich will taste better if the bagel is not sweet; often whole-grain bagels also contain honey. The lox-and-avocado combination is also good in a whole wheat pita. Whether you're serving it to break the fast or for brunch, the sandwich is good accompanied by a green salad and a few high-quality olives.

1 small ripe avocado, preferably Hass (see Note)
1 teaspoon fresh lemon juice, or to taste
Salt and freshly ground black pepper
2 bagels

2 slices or 4 thin strips of lox, or smoked salmon
2 thin slices of red onion
4 thin slices of tomato
1 teaspoon capers, rinsed (optional)

A short time before serving, mash avocado and add lemon juice. Season with pepper and only a bit of salt, as there will be enough in the lox. Split bagels and spread each half with avocado. Top with lox. Put onion, tomato, and capers (if using) on bottom half, then set top half of sandwich in place. Serve at once.

NOTE: To halve an avocado, run a knife lengthwise around fruit, then twist to separate the two halves. Remove pit by hitting it with the heel of a chef's knife, using just enough force that knife sticks in pit. Then lift knife, with pit attached.

Makes 2 servings

✦ CHOCOLATE WALNUT ICE CREAM CAKE

After Yom Kippur, ice cream cake makes a sweet reward for fasting. This one is composed of meringues and chocolate ice cream. Walnuts give the dessert flavor, richness, and a healthy boost as well. They are a good source of omega-3 fatty acids, which are believed to help protect the heart. They were the first food the FDA allowed to be labeled with a health claim based on promising scientific evidence.

Choose light ice cream or frozen yogurt to keep the amount of saturated fat in the dessert low. Instead of chocolate ice cream, coffee ice cream makes a tasty partner for walnut meringues. For a pareve dessert, use soy-based ice cream, but read the nutrition label; not all soy desserts are low in calories. Perhaps this matters less after the fast, but it is good to keep in mind for other occasions.

Make this dessert a day ahead so it has time to freeze. You can bake the meringues up to 5 days ahead and keep them in an airtight container, if the weather is dry; or freeze them. Another option is to make the entire dessert 4 or 5 days ahead and keep it in the freezer. Be sure to use fresh walnuts; taste them before using them to be sure they are not rancid.

⅔ cup walnuts plus 8 extra walnut halves, toasted
⅔ cup sugar
1 tablespoon plus 1 teaspoon cornstarch
4 large egg whites, at room temperature

⅛ teaspoon cream of tartar
3 pints light chocolate or coffee ice cream
   or frozen yogurt

Position rack in center of oven and preheat to 300°F. Lightly grease and flour two nonstick medium baking sheets, tapping each to remove excess flour. Using an 8-inch springform pan rim as a guide, trace a circle onto each baking sheet, drawing it around outside of springform rim. Fit a ½-inch plain tip in a pastry bag.

Grind walnuts with ½ cup sugar in a food processor until as fine as possible, scraping mixture down often. Do not overprocess, so mixture won't become pasty. Transfer to a medium bowl. Sift cornstarch over walnut mixture. Stir lightly.

Beat egg whites with cream of tartar in a large bowl to soft peaks. With mixer at high speed, gradually beat in remaining 2⅔ tablespoons sugar; beat 15 seconds or until whites are just stiff and shiny but not dry.

Sprinkle walnut mixture over whites, using one-third of mixture at a time, and fold it in as gently and as quickly as possible, until just blended.

Immediately transfer mixture to the pastry bag, using a rubber spatula. Beginning at center of circle marked on baking sheet, pipe meringue in tight spiral until circle is covered. If there are holes, pipe small dots of meringue in each one. Pipe another spiral on second baking sheet. Pipe any remaining meringue in mounds about 1 inch in diameter and ¾ inch high, giving them rounded tops.

Bake meringues for 30 minutes. (If both baking sheets do not fit on central rack, bake them on two racks and switch their positions after 15 minutes.) Reduce oven temperature to 275°F. Continue baking for 10 to 15 minutes or until meringues are light brown, dry, and just firm but not hard; to check, touch center of each meringue very lightly—your finger should not leave an impression in mixture. Meringues burn easily if overbaked, but remain sticky if underbaked. They become firmer as they cool.

Immediately release meringues gently from baking sheets, using a large metal spatula. If they are sticky on bottom, bake 5 more minutes or until dry. Cool on a rack.

Carefully trim meringue circles, using point of a sharp paring knife, so that one just fits into an 8-inch springform pan and second is about ¼ inch smaller than the first, to leave a small space between this meringue's edge and side of pan.

Set larger meringue round in springform pan, with sides of pan closed. Soften half the ice cream briefly in refrigerator just until spreadable. Spoon it in dollops over meringue in pan. Carefully but quickly spread smooth. Set second meringue on top, centering it so that sides do not touch pan. Freeze for 10 minutes.

Soften remaining ice cream in refrigerator just until spreadable. Spoon enough ice cream around edge of top meringue to cover edge generously. Gently push vanilla ice cream between edge of meringue and edge of pan so it meets bottom ice cream layer. Spoon remaining ice cream over top of meringue. Gently smooth top. Cover and freeze for 8 hours or overnight. Garnish with toasted walnut halves.

Set cake on platter. Run a thin-bladed flexible knife around edge of cake. Release spring and remove sides of pan. Serve immediately.

Makes 8 servings

Sukkot—
The Harvest Holiday

In recent years celebrating the late summer and early fall harvest has become trendy among American food lovers. Harvest parties are given by restaurant chefs, farmers' market vendors, specialty nursery growers, home cooks, and gardeners. Honoring the season's bounty of produce is a delightful way to entertain and a joyous reason to get together. Of course this is not a new custom to Jewish cooks. Our ancestors have been doing this for millennia, to celebrate Sukkot.

Sukkot takes place in early autumn and is known as the Festival of Booths or the Festival of Tabernacles. The picniclike atmosphere of dining in a hut called a *sukkah* makes the holiday a children's favorite. Crowned with a roof of leafy branches and decorated with hanging fruit, such as pears, bananas, and clusters of grapes, the huts, or booths, are a colorful celebration of nature. The importance of respecting the natural world pervades the holiday prayers as well, which involve a ritual of holding a citron (an aromatic, large, lemonlike citrus fruit with a thick rind), called the *etrog*, along with leafy branches.

With the Sukkot theme of giving thanks for the harvest and appreciating nature, the holiday's message for healthy eating is clear—eat plenty of produce. In Jewish families, both Ashkenazi and Sephardi, it is traditional to include a wealth of vegetables on the holiday menus.

The glorious array of produce available during the Sukkot season—September or October—makes creating festive, vegetable-rich menus a snap. Stuffed vegetables, notably peppers, eggplant, and zucchini, are a holiday highlight. It's easy to understand why they are so popular on Sukkot menus. Since these vegetables are at their peak at this time of year, they are an obvious choice for celebrating nature's bounty. Stuffed vegetables are festive, easy to serve, and can be made ahead. Besides, they are portable, an important consideration for serving meals in the sukkah. You have a whole main dish—vegetable combined with grains, meat, or both—in one savory package.

To make serving in the sukkah easier, many cooks concentrate on casseroles and one-pot dishes. Elaborate or delicate dishes that demand last-minute attention are better for other occasions. I prefer to plan a relaxed, seasonal feast around soups and stews that I can cook ahead.

A vegetable soup is great for beginning the meal. At this time of year, my family and I are not ready for the hearty, long-simmered soups of autumn and winter. But a light vegetable soup is perfect: we can enjoy it hot or cold, according to our mood and the weather.

I find it convenient to serve such whole-meal dishes as Turkish Autumn Vegetable Casserole with Chicken (page 42), the perfect dish to make use of the season's profusion of veggies at the market—sweet ripe tomatoes, green beans, corn, summer squashes, and peppers of all colors, shapes, and sizes.

For casual, dairy meals for Sukkot, you might like to serve a big salad, like Mediterranean Bean Salad with Baby Greens, Feta Cheese, and Olives (page 222). For a festive meat-free sukkah party, I might serve Buckwheat Blintzes with Goat Cheese and Ratatouille (page 118).

Ripe fall fruits, especially apples, pears, grapes, dates, and persimmons, are a highlight of festive Sukkot meals. Enjoy them on their own or turn them into desserts like Double Pear Cake or Apple Cinnamon Tart. If you're feeling adventurous, make a vegetable dessert, like Carrot Compote in Cinnamon Clove Syrup (page 339).

Quick Broccoli-Vegetable Soup with Garlic and Rice

Eggplant Soup with Beans

Broiled Salmon with Rosemary, Green Beans, and New Potatoes

Turkish Autumn Vegetable Casserole with Chicken

Chicken Breasts with Red Peppers, Zucchini, and Sage

Veal and Sweet Vegetables in Ginger Sauce

Peppers with Braised Beef Stuffing

Sukkot Penne Casserole with Mediterranean Vegetables

Braised Calabaza Squash with Chiles and Ginger

Apple Apricot Whole Wheat Noodle Kugel

QUICK BROCCOLI-VEGETABLE SOUP WITH GARLIC AND RICE

With a variety of vegetables, this soup fits in nicely with the Sukkot harvest theme. For the soup base, I make use of the broccoli's cooking liquid, with the flavor reinforced by leeks, onions, carrots, and vegetable broth. Instead of rice, you can add other cooked grains, such as barley, wheat berries, bulgur, or whole wheat couscous. To turn the soup into a main course, add 1½ to 2 cups bite-sized pieces of cooked chicken or turkey or 12 ounces cubed tofu or seitan (wheat gluten) and heat through.

3 cups small broccoli florets and sliced tender stems
Salt
1 large leek (optional), white and light green parts only, quartered lengthwise
1 large onion, chopped (or 2 onions, if omitting leek)
1 large carrot, sliced

3½ cups vegetable or chicken broth
4 large garlic cloves, minced
¼ teaspoon hot red pepper flakes
½ teaspoon dried thyme
Freshly ground black pepper
1½ cups hot cooked brown or white rice

Bring 2½ cups water to a boil in a large saucepan. Add broccoli florets and stems with a small pinch of salt. Cook, uncovered, for 5 minutes, or until florets are crisp-tender. Transfer florets with a slotted spoon to a bowl, leaving stem slices in pot.

Rinse leek (if using) well to remove sand between layers. Cut into thin slices. Add leek, onion, carrot, and broth to pot. Bring to a simmer. Cover and cook over low heat for 15 minutes. Add garlic and pepper flakes. Cover and cook over low heat for 2 minutes or until vegetables are tender. Return broccoli florets to pan. Stir in thyme, black pepper, and salt if needed. Ladle into bowls and top each with a few spoonfuls of rice.

Makes 4 servings

❧ EGGPLANT SOUP WITH BEANS

Making soup is not a common way to utilize eggplant. But I make eggplant soup often, as I'm always looking for easy, healthy ways to use this satisfying vegetable, which is at the peak of its season during Sukkot.

Usually I start my soup like a typical Mediterranean eggplant stew, with the vegetable's usual partners—sautéed onions, garlic, tomatoes, and herbs. Sometimes I add zucchini, peppers, or green beans. I simply pour in a little more liquid than usual and my stew becomes soup. When I want the soup to play the role of a vegetarian main course, I add chickpeas, tofu, or both. Occasionally I add chunks of a meatless soy sausage; you can use a sliced chicken or turkey sausage or low-fat beef frank the same way. If I want the soup to be even more satisfying, I add diced potatoes or serve the soup with rice or bulgur pilaf.

For an even easier vegetable soup, I skip the sautéing and simmer the eggplant along with the other soup vegetables. With eggplant soup, unlike many other eggplant dishes, you can use little or no oil, and it will still be tasty. And eggplant soup doesn't need much attention. If it cooks for a long time and the eggplant cubes disintegrate, that's fine; they simply thicken the soup.

Actually, eggplant soup appears wherever people cook lots of this vegetable. You can find variations of it in India, where eggplant is said to have originated, and in Persia; in both countries the eggplant is combined with legumes, as I like to do. For a Tunisian eggplant soup, cooks add fava beans, chiles, and tomatoes. An innovative Israeli chef makes soup from roasted eggplants, sautéed onions, chicken stock, and fresh basil.

Depending on how fond your family is of tomatoes, use either a small or a large can. I like to serve this soup with crusty, country-style bread.

One 1- to 1¼-pound eggplant
1 to 3 tablespoons extra virgin olive oil
1 large onion, chopped
Salt and freshly ground black pepper
¾ pound pale green Mexican zucchini
    (also called white or Tatuma squash) or
    zucchini, cut into ¾-inch dice
4 garlic cloves, chopped
One 14- or 28-ounce can tomatoes, drained
    (juice reserved), coarsely chopped
1 small yellow or green bell pepper, diced (optional)

1 to 2 cups chicken or vegetable broth
1 cup frozen green beans
One 15-ounce can white beans or chickpeas,
    not drained
1½ teaspoons dried thyme, crumbled
¼ teaspoon hot red pepper flakes
12 to 16 ounces regular or firm tofu, cut into cubes,
    or 6 to 12 ounces meatless or beef frankfurters,
    sliced
2 tablespoons chopped green onion or parsley

If skin is not tough, you can leave eggplant unpeeled. Cut eggplant into small dice of about ¾ inch.

Heat 1 to 2 tablespoons oil in a sauté pan. Add onion and sauté over medium heat for 7 minutes or until beginning to turn golden; if using a small amount of oil, cover pan and add 1 tablespoon water if necessary to prevent burning. Add eggplant, salt, and pepper. Cover and cook over low heat for 5 minutes, stirring occasionally. Add squash, cover, and cook for 3 minutes.

Add garlic, tomatoes, diced bell pepper (if using), and 1 cup broth. Bring to a boil. Cover and cook over low heat for 25 minutes or until eggplant is tender. Add green beans, white beans with their liquid, thyme, pepper flakes, and juice from canned tomatoes. Add more broth if soup is too thick. Return to a boil. Add tofu. Simmer for 5 minutes or until green beans are tender. Taste and adjust seasoning. If you like, add 1 tablespoon oil to enrich the soup. Serve hot, sprinkled with green onion.

Makes 3 to 4 main-course servings

BROILED SALMON WITH ROSEMARY, GREEN BEANS, AND NEW POTATOES

When I prepare this French-inspired entrée and savor the rich fish, the sweet, crisp-tender beans, and the delicate poached potatoes, I am reminded of the beauty of simple ingredients prepared with minimum fuss. At the table we like to follow a Mediterranean tradition popular in Israeli restaurants—we drizzle our salmon, potatoes, and beans lightly with excellent, very fruity olive oil. The warm fish and vegetables bring out the flavor of the oil so we really notice its luscious character; yet the oil complements the fish without overpowering it. With a full-bodied extra virgin olive oil, a little goes a long way.

Instead of green beans, you can serve the fish with fresh spinach or, in springtime, with asparagus. Instead of the rosemary, flavor the fish with 1 1/2 teaspoons fresh thyme or 1/2 teaspoon dried thyme.

8 to 12 small whole potatoes
Salt and freshly ground black pepper
1 1/4 pounds salmon fillet, preferably tail section,
    about 1 inch thick
1 tablespoon fresh lemon juice
2 tablespoons extra virgin olive oil, plus extra
    for drizzling

1 to 1 1/2 teaspoons minced fresh rosemary,
    plus a few sprigs for garnish
1 pound slim green beans, preferably French–style
    haricots verts, ends removed
Lemon wedges (for serving)

To poach potatoes, cover them with water in a saucepan, add a generous pinch of salt, and bring to a boil. Cover and cook over low heat for 25 to 30 minutes or until tender. Drain well. Peel if you want. Cover and keep warm.

Sprinkle salmon with lemon juice and 1 tablespoon oil and rub them over fish. Sprinkle fish evenly with minced rosemary and salt and pepper to taste.

Preheat broiler. Line broiler rack with foil if you like, or brush it lightly with oil. Set salmon on broiler rack and broil 4 minutes. Turn salmon over and broil 4 minutes more. To check whether fish is done, make a small cut with a sharp knife in thickest part; color of flesh should have changed all the way through.

Meanwhile, boil green beans, uncovered, in a large saucepan of enough boiling salted water to cover them generously, over high heat for 5 to 7 minutes or until crisp-tender. Drain well.

To serve, toss green beans with salt, pepper, and 1 tablespoon oil. Serve fish, potatoes, and beans on plates or a platter, garnished with lemon wedges and rosemary sprigs. Set out a cruet of olive oil for drizzling.

Makes 4 servings

TURKISH AUTUMN VEGETABLE CASSEROLE WITH CHICKEN

For Sukkot many Sephardi Jews take advantage of the plentiful late summer vegetables. Families are fond of sitting down to dinners of grand casseroles of vegetables flavored with olive oil and herbs. Components vary from one table to another and usually include the Mediterranean standards familiar from Provençal ratatouille—onions, peppers, eggplant, zucchini, and tomatoes. But traditional cooks of Balkan origin don't stop there, including green beans, okra, peas, and potatoes in their stew.

Most Israelis call this dish *guvec* (pronounced "givech"), Turkish for an earthenware casserole, but some Sephardi Jews call it *turlu*, which means mixture. It makes sense that the dish takes its name from Turkish, since most of the Balkan region, where Sephardi Jews have a long history, was part of the Ottoman Empire for centuries.

Seasonings tend to be subtle—either salt and pepper alone, or perhaps a touch of garlic, paprika, or fresh herbs, especially parsley and dill. Still, some like it hot and throw in plenty of red pepper flakes, while others prefer a blend of sweet spices, such as cinnamon, allspice, and nutmeg.

In old-fashioned recipes, the vegetables are first deep-fried, and the casserole then cooks for hours. To-day many opt for shorter cooking times, resulting in vegetables that retain more of their individual character. Once the casserole has been assembled, it simmers pretty much on its own.

To update it, I skip frying the vegetables; they absorb plenty of flavor from the sauce. This not only makes more nutritional sense, but also makes the preparation faster and easier. A popular custom is to turn the gu-vec into a main course by adding meat; I follow the custom of some cooks who use chicken, turkey, or even fish for a lighter dish. I keep the simmering time to a minimum by using fast-cooking boneless chicken and stewing the vegetables briefly, just until they are tender. The vegetables acquire a delicious richness from the savory chicken juices, especially if you use dark meat. Best of all, their taste intensifies when you make the casserole in advance, ready to be served hot or warm.

2 tablespoons extra virgin olive oil

2 large onions, halved and sliced

8 ounces fresh green beans, cut into 3 pieces, or frozen cut green beans

1 to 1¼ pounds boneless chicken, preferably thigh meat, cut into 1-inch cubes

2 large garlic cloves, coarsely chopped

2 bell peppers, green or red, or one of each, cut into large dice

One 1-pound eggplant, unpeeled, cut into ¾-inch dice

1 pound small zucchini, cut into 1-inch dice

1½ cups chicken broth, or more if needed

Salt and freshly ground black pepper

1½ teaspoons chopped fresh thyme or dill, or ½ teaspoon dried thyme or dill

¼ teaspoon hot red pepper flakes, or to taste (optional)

2 tablespoons tomato paste

2 large tomatoes, peeled and sliced thin

Choose a shallow stew pan, preferably one that's ovenproof; in that case, preheat oven to 375°F. Heat oil in stew pan. Add onions and sauté over medium heat, stirring occasionally, for 7 minutes or until they begin to turn golden. If using fresh green beans, cook them in a saucepan of boiling salted water for 4 minutes, or until nearly tender. Rinse and drain well.

Add chicken to onions and brown it lightly. Add garlic, bell peppers, eggplant, zucchini, 1 cup broth, salt, pepper, thyme, and pepper flakes (if using). Bring to a boil. Cover and simmer over medium-low heat for 20 minutes or until chicken and vegetables are nearly tender. Add green beans. Mix tomato paste with remaining ½ cup broth and stir into sauce. Taste sauce and adjust seasoning. Top stew with tomato slices and sprinkle with salt and pepper.

At this point finish casserole in oven or, if pan is not ovenproof, continue cooking it on stovetop. If using oven, bake casserole, uncovered, for 10 to 15 minutes or until vegetables are tender, checking sauce once or twice and adding a few tablespoons hot broth or water if necessary to prevent burning. Sauce should be concentrated and should just coat components but should not be soupy.

To finish casserole on stovetop, cook it, covered, over low heat for 10 minutes, or until vegetables are tender, adding a little more broth as necessary to prevent burning. Serve hot or warm.

Makes 4 to 6 servings

CHICKEN BREASTS WITH RED PEPPERS, ZUCCHINI, AND SAGE

Chicken breasts won't be boring when you enhance them with sweet peppers and fresh herbs following this recipe, which is my lightened twist on the traditional Roman pollo alla romana, made of chicken with roasted peppers. You can sauté the peppers as in the recipe, or char and peel them (see page 376); or, to save time, use roasted red peppers from a jar. This entrée is practical because your supper vegetables are part of the quick-cooking chicken dish. With all in one pan, it's portable, and thus perfect for Sukkot.

If you'd like pasta as a partner for the chicken, choose a small kind, such as orzo or short spirals. For a lighter accompaniment, serve the chicken with colorful mixed salad greens. There's no need to make a separate sauce; just use part of the chicken's juices to moisten the pasta or the greens. Wine vinegar is an especially good addition to the sauce if you're serving greens.

3 to 4 tablespoons extra virgin olive oil
2 to 3 red, orange, or yellow bell peppers,
*   or 2 roasted red peppers from a jar, cut into*
*   strips*
¾ to 1 pound zucchini or pale green Mexican
*   zucchini (also called white or Tatuma squash),*
*   cut into 2-inch sticks*
Salt and freshly ground black pepper
3 or 4 boneless, skinless chicken breasts
*   (1 to 1½ pounds), patted dry*

1 large onion, chopped
¼ cup dry white wine
2 large garlic cloves, chopped (optional)
½ cup chicken broth
1½ tablespoons chopped fresh sage
1 tablespoon chopped fresh rosemary (optional)
1 to 2 tablespoons white wine vinegar (optional)

Heat 1 to 2 tablespoons oil in a large skillet. Add bell peppers and sauté over medium heat for 5 minutes. Add squash sticks, salt, and pepper, and sauté until both vegetables are crisp-tender, about 3 minutes. Remove from skillet.

Add remaining oil to skillet and heat over medium heat. Add chicken and sauté, pressing on pieces occasionally with a spatula to flatten them, for 5 minutes on each side or until no longer pink inside when you cut into thickest part. Remove with a slotted spatula.

Add onion to pan and sauté for 5 minutes or until softened; if pan becomes dry, add 1 or 2 tablespoons wine and cover pan. Stir in garlic (if using), followed by remaining wine and broth, and bring to a boil. Simmer over low heat for 2 minutes. Return chicken to sauce, cover, and heat gently for 3 minutes, turning once. Stir in sautéed vegetables, sage, rosemary, and vinegar (if using). Taste sauce and adjust seasoning. Serve hot.

Makes 4 to 6 servings

❈ VEAL AND SWEET VEGETABLES IN GINGER SAUCE

Homey casseroles and stews have returned into vogue and can be found even at elegant restaurants. In this stew the flavors of the broth and soy sauce balance the red wine's acidity, and the ginger, vegetables, and raisins contribute sweetness. To keep the stew fairly light, I use a substantial amount of vegetables, equal to the weight of the meat, so the meat is stretched over more portions. I skip the usual step of browning the meat, so that I can use less oil. If you like, you can substitute boneless chicken thighs for the meat; cook them for a total of 45 minutes, along with the vegetables.

This dish can be prepared ahead and makes a tasty entrée for a Sukkot, Rosh Hashanah, or Shabbat dinner.

1 tablespoon vegetable oil

2 medium onions, chopped

3 tablespoons minced peeled ginger

1 tablespoon all-purpose flour

2 pounds boneless lean veal, cut into 1-inch pieces, trimmed of fat and patted dry

¾ cup dry red wine

1¼ cups beef or chicken broth

2 tablespoons soy sauce

Salt (optional) and freshly ground black pepper

1¼ pounds orange-fleshed sweet potatoes (often labeled yams)

½ pound parsnips, peeled and cut into ½-inch chunks

½ pound slim carrots, cut into ½-inch chunks

2 tablespoons raisins

Cayenne pepper

Heat oil in a large, heavy stew pan. Add onions and sauté over medium-low heat for 7 minutes or until light brown. Add ginger and sauté ½ minute. Sprinkle mixture with flour. Cook over low heat, stirring often, for 3 minutes.

Add meat to pan. Stir in wine, broth, soy sauce, and black pepper. Bring to a boil, stirring often. Cover and cook over low heat for 1 hour, stirring occasionally.

Peel sweet potatoes and cut into large dice (about 1 inch). Add parsnips, carrots, and sweet potatoes to pan. Mix well to moisten with sauce. Cover and cook for 45 minutes or until meat is very tender; check with point of a knife. Add raisins and cayenne to taste, and cook for 2 minutes to plump the raisins. Taste and add salt and pepper if needed. Serve hot.

Makes 6 to 8 servings

Meat-stuffed peppers may be one of the most popular staples of the Sukkot menu. For this dish I use a different kind of beef filling, based on Mexican beef machaca. The beef is poached, shredded, and cooked in a savory sauce accented with chiles, onions, tomatoes, oregano, and cumin. Garlic figures prominently and sometimes is added in several stages for extra punch. These flavorings also happen to be popular in the Sephardi Jewish kitchen. That's not surprising—both groups have a Spanish connection.

This filling is different from standard ground-beef stuffing because its texture tends to be more tender. Ground beef, especially if it's fairly low in fat, can become tough during cooking. But stewed shredded beef can be moist even if you choose a lean cut. With the addition of corn kernels and peppers, the stuffing makes a pleasant change from the commonplace ground meat and rice mixture. Besides, adding vegetables to the stuffing means it contains less meat.

Instead of being stuffed into peppers, the savory beef can be served as an entrée with beans and rice or with tortillas. Mexicans also like it scrambled with eggs for breakfast. And it's a good filling for meat blintzes.

This recipe gives you a bonus—a tasty broth from poaching the beef. You can use the broth to make a satisfying soup to serve in the sukkah another day; simply simmer seasonal vegetables in the broth and embellish it with cooked noodles, rice, or kneidelach (matzo balls).

If you use fresh corn, grill it so the kernels acquire a sweet caramelized flavor. Instead of beef you can use boneless veal, which often has a fat content similar to the leanest beef cuts. It will take about 1 hour to cook. Boneless chicken thigh meat will need even less time—30 to 40 minutes.

1½ pounds lean stewing beef, trimmed of fat, cut into 1-inch pieces
2 onions, 1 sliced and 1 chopped
6 garlic cloves, peeled, 3 whole and 3 chopped
1 bay leaf
Salt and freshly ground black pepper
About 3 tablespoons vegetable oil
2 small jalapeño peppers, chopped
1 teaspoon ground cumin
1 teaspoon dried oregano

One 14-ounce can diced tomatoes, drained and chopped
3 tablespoons tomato paste
1 cup grilled (see Note) or cooked frozen corn kernels, or drained canned corn
2 red bell peppers, diced, plus 6 fairly small whole red or green peppers (for stuffing)
2 poblano chiles (called pasilla in California), grilled and peeled (page 376) and cut into strips
Cayenne pepper (optional)

Put beef in a saucepan with sliced onion, whole garlic cloves, bay leaf, and salt. Add 3 cups water or enough to just cover beef. Bring to a boil, skimming foam from surface. Cover and cook over low heat for 2 hours or until meat is very tender. Cool meat in broth for 30 minutes. Drain broth and reserve it; skim fat thoroughly. Shred meat into long, thin strips with your fingers, discarding any fat or gristle.

Heat 2 tablespoons oil in a stew pan. Add chopped onion and cook over medium-low heat for 7 minutes or until softened. Add chopped garlic and chopped jalapeño peppers, and sauté a few seconds, stirring. Add shredded beef, cumin, oregano, tomatoes, 1 tablespoon tomato paste, and ¼ cup reserved beef broth, and bring to a simmer. Simmer uncovered, stirring often, for 20 minutes or until mixture is thick but still moist. Add corn, diced red bell peppers, and grilled poblano chile strips, and cook for 3 minutes. Add a few tablespoons broth if filling is dry. Season to taste with salt, pepper, and cayenne (if using).

Preheat oven to 375°F. Halve whole peppers for stuffing lengthwise, discarding cores and seeds. Cook pepper halves in a saucepan of boiling water for 3 minutes; or steam them, covered, in a steamer basket above boiling water. Drain well. Lightly oil a shallow baking dish large enough to hold peppers in a single layer. Set peppers, cut side up, in dish.

Spoon stuffing into pepper halves, filling them generously. Mix remaining 2 tablespoons tomato paste with ½ cup beef broth and pour into baking dish around peppers. Drizzle them with remaining oil. Cover and bake for 30 minutes or until peppers are very tender. Serve peppers hot or warm, with a little sauce spooned over them.

NOTE: To make grilled corn kernels, husk the corn and grill it briefly on the barbecue or in the broiler, turning it often, until it is lightly charred and barely tender; it will cook more inside the peppers.

Makes 6 servings

SUKKOT PENNE CASSEROLE WITH MEDITERRANEAN VEGETABLES

It might seem that the Mediterranean trio of eggplant, tomatoes, and peppers has been part of traditional Sukkot meals from time immemorial, but this is not the case. Eggplant would have been the first to appear on the menu, as it arrived in the Mediterranean from Persia in the ninth or tenth century, according to my friend Clifford A. Wright, the author of *Mediterranean Vegetables*. Peppers and tomatoes came later, from the New World.

These vegetables are great in this healthy casserole flavored with garlic, thyme, hot pepper flakes, and a little Parmesan. For the best nutrition, use whole wheat or other whole-grain pasta, or one made with part soy flour. For a pareve version, substitute 1/4 cup bread crumbs for the cheese, or use soy cheese.

3 to 4 tablespoons extra virgin olive oil

2 green or red bell peppers, or 1 green and 1 red pepper, seeds and ribs discarded, cut into strips

1 large eggplant (about 1 1/4 pounds), cut into 1/2-inch dice

Salt and freshly ground black pepper

6 garlic cloves, minced

3/4 to 1 pound ripe tomatoes, peeled and diced, or one 14-ounce can tomatoes, drained and diced

1 bay leaf

1/4 teaspoon hot red pepper flakes, or more if desired

1 tablespoon chopped fresh thyme, or 1 teaspoon dried thyme

2 teaspoons chopped tarragon (optional)

8 ounces penne (diagonal macaroni), preferably whole wheat (2 1/3 to 2 1/2 cups)

3 to 5 tablespoons grated Parmesan

Heat 2 tablespoons oil in a large skillet. Add bell peppers and sauté over medium-high heat for 5 minutes. Add eggplant, sprinkle with salt and pepper to taste, and sauté, stirring, for 5 minutes. Cover and cook over medium heat, stirring once or twice, for 7 to 10 minutes or until eggplant and peppers are tender, adding water by tablespoons as necessary to prevent sticking. Remove from skillet.

Preheat oven to 375°F. Add 1 teaspoon oil to skillet and heat briefly. Add garlic and sauté for 1/2 minute. Add tomatoes, bay leaf, pepper flakes, salt, and pepper, and cook over medium-high heat, stirring often, for 10 minutes or until sauce is thick. Discard bay leaf. Add thyme and tarragon (if using).

Cook penne in a large pot of boiling salted water for 8 minutes or until just tender (al dente). Drain, rinse, and drain well. Transfer to a large bowl. Add tomato sauce, eggplant, and peppers to pasta and toss. Add 2 tablespoons Parmesan and toss again. Taste and adjust seasoning.

Oil a 2-quart casserole. Spoon pasta mixture inside. Sprinkle with remaining oil, then with remaining Parmesan. Cover and bake for 10 minutes. Uncover and bake for 10 more minutes or until dotted with brown. Serve hot.

Makes 4 servings

BRAISED CALABAZA SQUASH WITH CHILES AND GINGER

The slight spiciness of ginger and mild chiles complements the sweetness of hard-shelled orange squash. I use a vegetable braising technique, popular among Sephardi and Indian cooks, of cooking the vegetable with very little water so the taste remains concentrated.

Meaty calabaza squash, which can be purchased by the piece in Latin American markets, is a good choice, and so are butternut squash and Japanese kabocha squash. I like to use heart-shaped poblano chiles, which are labeled pasilla chiles in California. They are sometimes mild and sometimes hot, and give the dish a pleasing aroma.

One 2-pound piece calabaza squash
1 tablespoon canola oil or other vegetable oil
2 onions, chopped
1½ tablespoons chopped peeled ginger

1 or 2 poblano chiles (called pasilla in California), seeds discarded, cut into strips
Salt and freshly ground black pepper
1 teaspoon ground coriander

Cut squash into pieces and cut off peel with a heavy, sharp knife. Remove any seeds or stringy flesh. Cut flesh into about 1-inch cubes.

Heat oil in a stew pan. Add onions, cover, and sauté over medium-low heat, stirring often, for 5 minutes. Add ginger and chile strips and sauté for 5 more minutes. Add squash pieces and a little salt and pepper. Cover and cook over low heat for 10 minutes. Add 3 tablespoons water, cover, and cook for 15 more minutes or until tender, stirring from time to time and adding water by tablespoons if necessary. Stir in coriander. Taste and adjust seasoning. Serve hot or warm.

Makes 3 to 4 servings

Dried apricots, pecans, maple syrup, and sweet spices add good flavor to this apple-noodle kugel, made more wholesome with whole wheat noodles. Be sure to slice the apples thin so they will become tender as the kugel bakes. If you're making this for a dairy meal, you might like to substitute butter for half the oil.

1 pound whole wheat noodles
Pinch of salt
3 to 4 tablespoons vegetable oil
⅓ cup pecans, chopped
½ cup diced dried apricots
2 or 3 tender apples, such as Golden Delicious
    or Braeburn (total about 1½ pounds)
2 tablespoons maple syrup, brown rice syrup,
    or agave nectar

1 teaspoon ground ginger
Pinch of cloves
1 teaspoon ground cinnamon
4 large eggs, separated, or 2 eggs, separated, and
    3 egg whites
3 to 4 tablespoons sugar

Preheat oven to 350°F. Grease a 13×9×2-inch baking dish. Cook noodles in a large pot of boiling salted water, uncovered, over high heat until barely tender, about 5 minutes. Drain, rinse with cold water, and drain well. Transfer to a large bowl. Mix with 2 to 3 tablespoons oil, pecans, and apricots.

Peel apples, halve, core, and slice thin. Transfer to a bowl. Add maple syrup and sprinkle with ginger, cloves, and ½ teaspoon cinnamon. Mix well. Add to noodle mixture and mix well.

Whip egg whites to soft peaks. Beat in 3 to 4 tablespoons sugar and whip at high speed until whites are stiff but not dry. Stir egg yolks into noodles. Stir in one-fourth of whipped whites. Fold in remaining whites.

Transfer noodle mixture to greased baking dish. Sprinkle with ½ teaspoon cinnamon, then with remaining tablespoon oil. Cover dish and bake for 30 minutes. Uncover and bake for 15 to 20 minutes or until set. Serve hot.

Makes 8 servings

Hanukkah

The eight-day holiday of Hanukkah commemorates a miracle. It occurred after the Temple of Jerusalem was liberated, as a result of the Maccabees' victory over a foreign army, earning religious freedom for the Jews. A minute quantity of ritually pure oil needed for kindling the Eternal Light of the Temple, normally enough for one day, miraculously lasted for eight days.

American Jews celebrate this event by eating potato latkes. Yet potatoes had nothing to do with the Hanukkah miracle. They were unknown in the land of Israel at the time of the Maccabees. Potatoes, native to the New World, became familiar to Europeans long after Columbus's historic voyage. Latkes, or potato pancakes, most likely developed in Eastern Europe or Russia. Ashkenazi Jews adopted them and made them Hanukkah favorites.

It is the oil used to fry the latkes that represents the miracle. Here lies Hanukkah's healthy message. In ancient Israel the oil used for lighting lamps, as well as for cooking, was olive oil. Nutritionists recommend using olive oil more than other fats because of its beneficial qualities.

But nobody said you have to use the oil for deep-frying. After all, deep-fried foods absorb substantial amounts of fat. There are plenty of delicious, healthy dishes that contain oil and thus fit in beautifully with the spirit of Hanukkah, but are not fried. Oil can be used to flavor salads and vegetables, for example, or to lightly moisten roasted potatoes. In theory, you eat one of these dishes, and you have memorialized the Hanukkah miracle.

Still, even someone motivated to eat healthy foods would be disappointed if there were no latkes for Hanukkah. My mother, who was always nutrition conscious, found a solution to make latkes healthier. She turned latke mixtures into kugels by baking them in casserole dishes. I bake individual potato kugels in muffin pans and moisten each one with just a little oil. Baked latkes are not as crisp as fried ones, but when it comes to preparing healthy food, compromise is a good thing. Another solution is to pan-fry latkes in a heavy skillet rather than using a bath of oil as deli cooks often do.

Latkes don't have to be made of potatoes. All sorts of other latkes are prepared in Jewish kitchens. Depending on the cook's origin, they might be made from leeks, greens, carrots, apples, cottage cheese, or buckwheat. I like to use cauliflower, mushrooms, and New World ingredients—corn, pumpkin, and sweet potatoes.

In addition to latkes, other traditional dishes are made for Hanukkah. Israelis love sufganiyot, or jelly doughnuts. Italian Jews might prepare fish turnovers, fried chicken, eggplant fried with parsley, and as a sweet, fried pastry nuggets in honey. Still, all are fried.

There are plenty of nutritious possibilities when it comes to accompaniments for the latkes. Applesauce, the most popular partner, is nutritious and can be delicious if home-

LATKES FROM SPICY LANDS

*T*he first time I ate aloo tikki, spicy potato patties, at an Indian restaurant, I immediately thought of latkes. They reminded me of the type of potato pancakes I've eaten at Jewish delis—crisp on the outside and with a smooth interior, like latkes made with mashed rather than grated potatoes. These Indian "latkes" have become one of my favorite Indian dishes. Every time I eat them, no matter what the time of year, I think of Hanukkah.

In fact, Indian cooks have developed potato-pancake making to a fine art and serve them often. On festive occasions, these exotic potato patties might be stuffed, and then they somewhat resemble the fried kubeh familiar from Sephardi eateries. Usually the stuffings are meatless, but there are notable exceptions. The Jews of Cochin, for example, stuff their holiday potato cakes with chicken, according to Dina Levy and Miriam Dekel, the editors of a Hebrew book on this group's food, Not Just Rice and Curry. *Ran Shinar, the author of* Hari Curry Indian Cuisine *(also in Hebrew), fills his potato cakes with ground-meat curry and notes that you can use any leftover curry.*

Seasonings for these crusty potato appetizers vary from a gentle pinch of ground ginger, nutmeg,

made. (See Out-of-This-World Applesauce, page 70.) The other traditional associate for latkes, sour cream, is best spooned on in a small dollop or replaced by yogurt or low-fat sour cream.

Since latkes go well with savory as well as sweet tastes, pancake toppers can range from crumbled goat cheese, lox strips, and caviar to roasted peppers and marinated mushrooms. Some people like spicy toppings like Yemenite zehug (page 363) or Mexican-style salsa. Sometimes I prepare a topping of tomatoes and garlic, accented with a little basil and olive oil (Fresh Tomato Basil Dip, page 163). Even a fruity-spicy chutney, such as one of pineapple and mango mixed with sweet and hot peppers, is an inviting topping for those with adventurous palates. Those with a sweet tooth will welcome such offerings as cinnamon-and-sugar, strawberry jam, or vanilla-accented pear compote.

One smart strategy for healthy Hanukkah eating is to avoid making a meal out of latkes. They are best served as an accompaniment. Prepare a big, festive salad or a hearty bowl of bean soup, and follow it with an aromatic baked fish such as Sesame Salmon with Spinach (page 122). Serve the latkes as an appetizer or side dish rather than the main dish

or cumin to a liberal dose of hot chiles—fresh, dried, or a mixture of both. Some chefs accent their patties with the lively flavors of fresh onions, garlic, fresh ginger, cilantro leaves, or lemon juice. For a little extra richness, many cooks enhance their potato cakes with coconut, peanuts, almonds, or cheese.

Latkes made of cooked mashed potatoes need not be fried. You can bake them instead. (See the note following the recipe for Spicy Potato Latkes, page 66.)

Like latkes, which usually come with applesauce or sour cream, Indian potato cakes are often served with fruity or dairy dips. Or, instead of applesauce, there might be mango chutney. For a creamy partner for the pancakes, often yogurt is served. Those who prefer spicy sauces top their potato cakes with a spoonful of chile-spiked cilantro-mint chutney.

Neela Paniz, who serves tasty Indian snacks at her Bombay Café in Los Angeles, noted in her book, The Bombay Café, that potato pancakes "are a favorite street food all over India" and are served with bowls of chopped onion, green chiles, and tamarind chutney. With her lemony potato pancakes, she offers a choice of accompaniments: sweet-and-sour tamarind-date chutney, spicy green chile chutney or, bowing to the American custom, sour cream.

of the meal or party. You will end up eating fewer of them, and the menu will be more balanced.

At Hanukkah parties, even if you prepare fried latkes, include plenty of other foods. Add a selection of colorful vegetable salads, such as jicama salad with oranges, carrot salad, and Israeli salad. A festive way to serve latkes is to provide an array of healthy toppings. Each person can add these toppings to his or her plate as they please.

With latkes and other fried treats, the best way to keep the calories down is to savor them in moderation. If you're watching your weight, decide ahead of time to eat only one or two latkes, and enjoy every bite.

THE LATKE LOVERS' OLYMPICS

*L*atkes, or levivot *as they are called in Israel, are among the best-loved Jewish specialties.*

One Hanukkah I enjoyed the ultimate latke experience. I was invited to be a judge at the annual latke contest at the James Beard House in New York, where latke mavens compete with each other to see who can make the most tempting one.

Contestants entered their latkes in two separate categories, one for professional chefs and one for anyone who likes to make latkes. There was excitement in the air as the cooks scrambled to get their latkes ready in the kitchen of the townhouse. The atmosphere was friendly and everyone was in good spirits, freely sharing their secrets. We sat, sipped wine, and sampled one latke after another.

Sampling a multitude of latkes was a fascinating exercise. Some were exceptionally moist, others crisp and crunchy. Sour cream made one latke tender and tasty, but too soft. One contestant put lox in his latke batter—a good idea except that the flavor didn't come through; personally, I prefer lox as a topping. A third added a generous amount of smoked meat that proved overwhelming—too much of a good thing doesn't work either.

A young chef created the latke that took the first place. Jill Conklin, who at the time was the chef of Walter Potenza's Restaurant of Historical Cuisine in Providence, Rhode Island, made a tasty vegetable latke topped with raita, an Indian sauce, and accompanied by a sweet-and-savory green tomato marmalade. It turned out hers was the best from a nutritional standpoint too, combining potatoes with carrots, red peppers, zucchini, and onions, then topping the latkes with a sauce of sour cream (which you could prepare with yogurt), minced cucumbers, onion, lemon juice, and fresh mint.

Festive Winter Spinach Salad with Papaya

Country Chard Soup

Lior's Lentil Soup

Sesame Chicken Satays

Rosemary Chicken Drumsticks with Sweet and Hot Peppers

Baked Chicken with Spiced Red Wine and Fig Sauce

Beans with Diced Meat in Cumin Tomato Sauce

Baked Tofu with Sweet-and-Sour Ginger Sauce

Spicy Potato Latkes

Baked Potato and Apple Latkes with Walnuts

Honey Cinnamon Hanukkah Pastry Balls

Out-of-This-World Applesauce

This colorful deep green salad, studded with orange cubes of tender Maradol papaya and white dice of jicama, is easy to make and most welcome on the Hanukkah table. Even sworn latke lovers will enjoy the relief of something fresh and green in between bites of their holiday treat. Another good occasion for serving this salad is for Shabbat lunch, before the cholent.

Instead of spinach, you can make this salad with romaine leaves. The sweetness of the jicama and the papaya beautifully complements the taste of the greens. In many markets Maradol papaya is labeled "Mexican papaya." In my house we use it as our winter substitute for tomatoes in cold-season salads. Because it lacks the acidity of tomatoes, we use more lime or lemon juice than in our usual Israeli salad.

¾ pound fresh spinach (1 medium bunch), or
    one 10-ounce bag of cleaned spinach
One 8- to 12-ounce piece of jicama
½ to 1 cup finely shredded green or red cabbage
    (optional)
2 to 4 thin slices of red onion, halved and
    separated into half moons

2 cups peeled diced Maradol (Mexican) papaya
1 to 3 tablespoons extra virgin olive oil
1 to 2 tablespoons strained fresh lime juice
Salt and freshly ground black pepper

If using a bunch of spinach, remove stems and any wilted leaves and wash remaining leaves in several changes of water, lifting leaves out of liquid so sand falls to bottom of bowl. Dry spinach well in a salad spinner or towel. Tear any large leaves in 2 or 3 pieces.

Cut jicama in half and cut off peel with a sturdy knife, removing fibrous layer below skin as well. Cut jicama in thin slices, then into dice.

In a large bowl, combine spinach, cabbage (if using), and red onion. Toss to mix. Add two-thirds of the jicama and half the papaya and toss lightly. Add oil, lime juice, and salt and pepper and toss. Taste and adjust seasoning. Spoon salad onto a platter or shallow serving dish. Scatter remaining jicama and papaya over salad.

Makes 4 servings

❧ COUNTRY CHARD SOUP

For a healthy beginning to a Hanukkah meal, choose this easy-to-make French soup based on nutritious chard. You can also make it with spinach or other greens. Unlike many classic soups, it doesn't require a roux of butter and flour. All you do is thicken the soup with a little rice. There's no need to push the soup through a strainer either. The soup's rustic texture contributes to its satisfying quality.

Instead of the common French choice of butter, the soup is enriched with olive oil to commemorate Hanukkah's miracle as well as to promote good health; for a buttery flavor, use half butter and half oil. To further lighten the soup, I omit the old-fashioned enrichment of egg yolks and cream. The milk—or soy milk for a nondairy version—gives it a pleasing creaminess, heightened by the aroma of freshly grated nutmeg, the usual French partner for creamy greens.

If you'd like a thicker soup, puree it in the blender. If it's too thick, gradually add several tablespoons milk or water to the hot soup to bring it to the desired consistency.

1 pound green or red chard, rinsed well, stems
   peeled if ribs are thick
1 to 2 tablespoons extra virgin olive oil, or
   1 tablespoon oil and 1 tablespoon butter
½ onion, finely chopped

1½ cups vegetable broth or water
3 tablespoons uncooked long-grain white rice
Salt and freshly ground black pepper
1⅓ to 1½ cups milk or soy milk
Freshly grated nutmeg

Cut chard stems in thin strips. Chop leaves; keep them separate from stems.

Heat 1 tablespoon oil in a medium saucepan over low heat. Add onion and cook, stirring often, for 5 minutes. Add chard stems and stir briefly over heat until coated with onion mixture. Add broth, rice, and salt and pepper and bring to a boil. Cover and simmer over low heat for 15 minutes or until rice is tender. Add chard leaves and bring to a simmer. Cook for 5 minutes or until chard is tender. Stir in milk, add nutmeg, and simmer, uncovered, for 5 minutes or until soup thickens to your taste. Remove from heat. If you like, stir in remaining oil or butter. Taste and adjust seasoning. Serve hot.

Makes 4 servings

Lentils have everything going for them. They are wonderfully healthy, containing valuable vegetable protein and plenty of fiber, and they make tasty, satisfying soups.

This soup is based on a recipe from my old friend Lior Moore, who lives in Givatayim, Israel, and publishes an Internet newsletter, "Lior's Kitchen Talk," devoted mostly to Middle Eastern and Jewish cooking. Lior's lentil soup technique is interesting because she uses both red and brown lentils. I asked her if she decided to use both kinds to benefit from two different lentil textures—the red ones to give her a smooth, thick soup, since they fall apart as they cook, and the brown ones to contribute distinct whole lentils to the soup. Lior laughed and said the way her soup came about was much simpler and less calculated. Once she was cooking the soup, and had finished her bag of red lentils, so she added some brown ones. The soup came out better and she continued making it that way.

Lior prepares her soup for festive meals and flavors it with onions fried in butter, garlic, tomato, cumin, and soup powder. Instead of using butter, I cook the onions in a small amount of olive oil. I add more vegetables for extra flavor and nutrients and to give the soup greater volume so that it makes a good main course.

1 cup red lentils	2 celery ribs, sliced
1 cup brown lentils	1 or 2 carrots, diced (optional)
1½ to 2 tablespoons extra virgin olive oil	4 ounces green beans, cut into 1-inch pieces
2 onions, chopped	(optional)
3 cups vegetable or chicken broth	2 zucchini or pale green Middle Eastern squash, diced
3 cups water	2 teaspoons ground cumin
4 large garlic cloves, chopped	Salt and freshly ground black pepper
1 tomato, fresh or canned, chopped	Lemon wedges (for serving)

Spread red and brown lentils on a plate in batches. Pick through them carefully, discarding any stones; rinse and drain lentils.

Heat 1½ tablespoons oil in a large, heavy saucepan. Add half of chopped onions and cook over medium-low heat, stirring often, for 10 minutes or until soft and deep brown; if pan looks dry, add 1 tablespoon water. Transfer onion mixture to a bowl.

Add broth and water to saucepan and bring to a boil. Add both kinds of lentils, remaining onion, garlic, tomato, celery, and carrot if you like. Return to a boil. Partially cover and simmer soup over low heat for 30 minutes, adding more water if soup becomes too thick. Add green beans (if using), zucchini, cumin, and salt and pepper and simmer for 10 minutes or until lentils are very tender. Taste and adjust seasoning; add remaining oil if you like. At serving time stir in sautéed onions. Serve with lemon wedges.

Makes 6 servings

❧ SESAME CHICKEN SATAYS

Satays, or mini-kebabs, said to have originated in Indonesia, have become popular around the world. They even appear on bar mitzvah menus. Most people love them because they have layers of flavor—the meat is soaked in a spiced soy marinade, next it is basted with the marinade as it grills, and finally served with a peppery, sweet-sour sauce.

Part of the charm of satays lies in the dipping sauce. Frequently it's a thick peanut sauce made with coconut milk. But recipes vary greatly, and satays might come with soy-based, curry, or hoisin sauces. I've even seen them served with pesto.

Some people who avoid peanuts make the sauce with an Israeli favorite—tahini, or sesame paste. You can combine tahini with peanut butter for a creamy sauce without coconut milk, which is high in saturated fat.

Serve satays as appetizers at Hanukkah parties, or make them into entrées by setting them on hot steamed rice, with fresh sliced vegetables alongside; favorites are cucumbers, sweet peppers, onions, and tomatoes.

If you want a coconut flavor, substitute light or regular coconut milk for half the chicken broth. If you have Indonesian sweet soy sauce (kecap manis), you can substitute it for the soy sauce and sugar. You can also make these satays with fresh tuna instead of chicken, or vegetarian ones with firm tofu, eggplant chunks, zucchini slices, and mushrooms.

1¼ pounds boneless chicken breasts,
skin removed

MARINADE

2 teaspoons vegetable oil
2 teaspoons tamarind paste, mixed with
1 teaspoon water, or 1 tablespoon strained
fresh lemon juice
1 shallot, minced
1 teaspoon minced peeled ginger
1 large garlic clove, minced
1 tablespoon soy sauce
1 teaspoon brown sugar
1 teaspoon ground coriander
½ teaspoon ground cumin
¼ teaspoon Asian hot chili paste or chili sauce

PEANUT-SESAME SAUCE

2 teaspoons vegetable oil
½ cup minced onion
2 large garlic cloves, minced
¾ cup chicken broth or water
½ teaspoon Asian hot chili paste, chili sauce, or
hot red pepper flakes, or more to taste
¼ cup peanut butter
2 tablespoons tahini (sesame paste) or additional
peanut butter
1 to 2 teaspoons Asian (toasted) sesame oil
1 to 2 tablespoons soy sauce
1 teaspoon brown sugar, or more to taste
1 teaspoon tamarind paste or lemon juice, or
more to taste
2 teaspoons grated peeled ginger

1 to 2 tablespoons toasted sesame seeds (page 380)

Cut chicken into thin strips, about ¾ to 1 inch wide and about 2 inches long. Put in a bowl. Add marinade ingredients and mix well. Cover and marinate for 1 to 2 hours in refrigerator. If using bamboo skewers, soak them in cold water for 30 minutes so they won't burn.

For peanut-sesame sauce, heat vegetable oil in a saucepan. Add onion and sauté over medium-low heat for 7 minutes or until softened; cover if pan becomes dry. Add garlic and sauté for ½ minute. Add broth and chili paste and bring to a boil. Remove pan from heat. Add peanut butter in 2 portions, whisking after each addition. Whisk in tahini. Bring to a simmer. If sauce is too thin, simmer 2 to 3 minutes or until thickened; if it is too thick, stir in 1 to 2 tablespoons water. Stir in sesame oil, soy sauce, sugar, tamarind paste, and ginger. Taste and adjust seasoning, adding more sugar or tamarind if needed.

Thread chicken on skewers. Brush with marinade. If using bamboo skewers, put foil on ends to prevent burning.

Reheat sauce over low heat, cover, and keep warm. Preheat broiler or prepare grill. Put skewered chicken on lightly oiled broiler rack set about 4 inches from flame or on lightly oiled grill above glowing coals. Grill or broil about 6 minutes, turning often. To check, cut into a large piece—chicken should be white inside, not pink.

At serving time, brush satays with sauce and sprinkle them with sesame seeds. Serve with small bowls of sauce for dipping.

Makes 6 to 7 appetizer or 4 to 5 main-course servings

ROSEMARY CHICKEN DRUMSTICKS
WITH SWEET AND HOT PEPPERS

This simple chicken dish is one of the easiest entrées to cook and to serve. I love it with potato latkes, or with Rice Pilaf with Caramelized Onions and Mushrooms (page 322), as both go so well with the chicken's rosemary-scented juices. Use green, red, or yellow peppers, or a mixture for the most colorful result. To vary the flavor, I occasionally use mild or medium-hot chiles instead of green peppers. If you like, add 1 or 2 chopped jalapeño peppers for a bit of heat. You can substitute cilantro sprigs for the rosemary.

To reduce the amount of fat, have the butcher remove the chicken skin. Baking the skinned pieces in a covered pan will keep the chicken moist.

2 ½ pounds chicken drumsticks or thighs,
    skin removed
Salt (optional) and freshly ground black pepper
½ teaspoon paprika
2 large onions, halved and sliced
8 rosemary sprigs

1 red bell pepper, cored, quartered lengthwise
1 green bell pepper or Anaheim or poblano chile
    (pasilla in California), cored, cut into
    thin strips
2 jalapeño peppers, chopped (optional)

Preheat oven to 400°F. Lightly oil a baking dish. Add chicken pieces and season on both sides with salt and pepper to taste and paprika. Top with sliced onions and add 4 rosemary sprigs to dish. Cover and bake for 30 minutes.

Reduce oven temperature to 350°F. Add a few tablespoons water to dish if pan is dry. Put red and green bell pepper pieces in dish and turn chicken pieces over; if using jalapeño peppers, stir them into juices. Cover and bake chicken for 30 minutes, checking to make sure dish doesn't become dry. Uncover and bake for 15 to 20 more minutes, or until chicken is tender and light brown; juices should no longer be pink when thickest part of chicken is pierced. Discard cooked rosemary sprigs. Serve chicken topped with onions and peppers. Garnish with fresh rosemary sprigs.

Makes 4 servings

✺ BAKED CHICKEN WITH SPICED RED WINE AND FIG SAUCE

When I attended a Medieval Feast cooked by Los Angeles chefs, it was clear from our menu that cuisine in the Middle Ages had more in common with Middle Eastern cooking than with that of contemporary Europe. This food had plenty of spice. Cinnamon, nutmeg, saffron, ginger, and cloves seasoned the meat and fish entrées, which often had almond-thickened sauces. Figs and raisins were used liberally in savory dishes. So was verjuice, the sour juice of unripe grapes, still loved in Persian cooking.

Michael Cimarusti, then chef of the Water Grill, told me it took two days to simmer the red wine sauce that he served with a grilled striped bass. He flavored the sauce with port, chicken stock, dried figs, currants, star anise, and coriander and fennel seeds, then finished it with rosewater. The wonderful sauce was strikingly different from today's sauces.

The sauce for this chicken dish is inspired by his version, but is easy to make. Instead of spending two days simmering it, you need only a few minutes. The fruit and port give the sauce a sweet note, which is balanced by the dry wine and the spices. Although you can serve it with grilled robust-flavored fish such as tuna, mackerel, or salmon, you may enjoy it more with baked chicken, as in this recipe, or with turkey or beef. You can find star anise at Chinese grocery stores, but if you don't have it, omit it or add 1 to 2 teaspoons of Pernod or other anise liqueur to the finished sauce.

1 cup dry red wine
1 green onion, minced
1 fresh thyme sprig or ½ teaspoon dried thyme
1 bay leaf
2 or 3 whole star anise (optional)
½ teaspoon fennel seeds
1½ cups chicken broth
¼ cup port
⅓ cup dried figs, diced
3 tablespoons dried currants
2½ teaspoons potato starch or cornstarch, dissolved in 3 tablespoons cold water

1 teaspoon ground coriander
Salt and freshly ground black pepper
2 to 3 teaspoons tomato paste (optional)
Pinch of sugar or squeeze of lemon juice (optional)
1 large onion, sliced
2½ pounds chicken breasts, with skin and bones
2 to 3 teaspoons vegetable oil
½ teaspoon paprika
1 teaspoon rosewater or pure vanilla extract (optional)

In a medium saucepan, combine red wine with green onion, thyme, bay leaf, star anise (if using), and fennel seeds. Bring to a boil, cover, and simmer for 5 minutes. Uncover and cook over medium-high heat until wine is reduced to about ½ cup.

Add broth, port, figs, and currants and bring to a boil. Cover and simmer for 7 minutes or until figs are just tender, then cook, uncovered, for 2 to 3 more minutes to reduce the liquid slightly. With a slotted spoon, remove fruit, thyme sprig, bay leaf, and star anise pieces. Set fruit aside; discard herbs and star anise.

Whisk potato starch mixture and gradually pour into simmering sauce, whisking. Bring to a boil, whisking constantly. Add coriander, salt, and pepper. If you'd like a reddish color, whisk in tomato paste. Simmer sauce for 1 or 2 minutes until thickened. Remove from heat. Return figs and currants to sauce. Taste and adjust seasoning. If sauce is too tart, add a pinch of sugar; if it's too sweet, add a little lemon juice. You can make the sauce up to 2 days ahead and refrigerate it in a covered container.

Preheat oven to 375°F. Lightly oil a roasting pan or spray it with oil spray. Put sliced onion in roasting pan. Lightly rub chicken with oil and sprinkle it with paprika and freshly ground pepper. Set chicken pieces on onion slices in one layer. Bake chicken, uncovered, for 20 minutes.

Reduce oven temperature to 350°F. Remove skin from chicken. If necessary, reheat sauce over low heat.

Spoon about ¼ cup sauce over chicken. Cover and bake for 15 minutes. Turn chicken pieces over and coat them with another ¼ cup sauce. Bake for 15 minutes longer or until meat is no longer pink in thickest part; cut into chicken to check.

Stir rosewater, if you like, into remaining sauce. Serve chicken hot with remaining sauce.

Makes 4 to 6 servings

BEANS WITH DICED MEAT
IN CUMIN TOMATO SAUCE

This traditional Sephardic stew is a good choice during Hanukkah. With its healthy proportion of beans to a rel-atively small amount of meat, it is sometimes referred to as beans with meat rather than beef stew with beans. These stews were undoubtedly developed due to the need to be frugal, but they are very nutritional. The meat flavors the sauce, while the beans increase the protein content of the dish without adding fat, and con-tribute good fiber as well. Beef is the favorite meat, but some cooks use lamb or veal. If possible, cook the beef in the sauce ahead, then refrigerate and skim off the fat. Substitute chicken or turkey for the meat if you like, or make the bean stew without meat and cook the tomato sauce for only 20 minutes. Garlic, cumin, and pepper give this stew a typical Israeli flavor, with plenty of well-browned onions contributing sweetness. You can make it with great Northern beans, pinto beans, chickpeas, lima beans, or black-eyed peas.

1 pound dried pinto beans or white beans
    (about 2½ cups), sorted and rinsed, or
    three or four 15-ounce cans beans, drained
Salt and freshly ground black pepper
½ to 1 pound lean beef or lamb, fat trimmed
1½ tablespoons olive oil or vegetable oil
2 large onions, chopped
3 large garlic cloves, chopped

2 teaspoons ground cumin
1½ pounds ripe tomatoes, peeled, seeded, and
    chopped, or one 28-ounce can tomatoes,
    drained and chopped
2 teaspoons paprika (optional)
¼ to ½ teaspoon hot red pepper flakes or
    cayenne pepper (optional)

Combine dried beans with 6 cups water in a medium saucepan. Bring to a boil. Cover and cook over low heat for 1 hour. Add a pinch of salt and cook for 15 to 30 more minutes or until beans are just tender.

Cut meat into ³/₄-inch cubes. Heat oil in a heavy stew pan. Add meat in batches and brown cubes on all sides over medium-high heat. Remove from pan. If necessary, pour off excess fat from pan, leaving only 1¹/₂ to 2 tablespoons. Add onions and sauté over medium heat for 10 minutes or until golden brown; cover if pan becomes dry. Add garlic and cumin, and sauté for ¹/₂ minute. Stir in tomatoes and cook for 2 minutes. Return meat to pan. Add salt, pepper, paprika, and pepper flakes (if using), and 1 cup water. Stir and bring to a boil. Cover and simmer until meat is tender. Lamb takes about 45 minutes and beef 1¹/₂ to 2 hours.

Skim as much fat as possible from sauce. Drain beans, reserving their cooking liquid. Add cooked or canned beans to stew. Simmer over very low heat for 5 to 10 minutes to flavor the beans, cooking it uncovered if stew is too soupy, or adding a few tablespoons bean cooking liquid or water if stew is too thick. Taste and adjust seasoning. Serve hot.

Makes 4 to 5 servings

❊ BAKED TOFU WITH
SWEET-AND-SOUR GINGER SAUCE

Sweet-and-sour sauce is a good match for tofu. The resulting dish is much lighter than the familiar sweet-and-sour chicken, which is often coated in a thick batter and deep-fried. Baking the tofu gives it a slightly chewy, meatier texture. If you like tofu's natural texture, you can skip the baking step and simply heat it through in the sauce.

To serve the tofu as an appetizer, cut it into 1-inch cubes and serve it on toothpicks. For an entrée, cut tofu in slices. Include the sautéed diced peppers if you're serving the tofu as a main course, and accompany it with brown rice. On Hanukkah, this dish is a tasty accompaniment for potato latkes.

12 to 16 ounces firm or extra-firm tofu
Freshly ground black pepper
2 tablespoons soy sauce
1 red or yellow bell pepper, cut into large dice
    (optional)
1 green bell pepper, cut into large dice (optional)
1 tablespoon peanut oil or canola oil (optional)
2 tablespoons rice vinegar
¼ cup ketchup

1 to 2 tablespoons honey or brown sugar
2 to 3 teaspoons minced peeled ginger
1 large garlic clove, minced
1 green onion, chopped
¼ cup orange juice
⅓ cup vegetable broth or water
1½ teaspoons cornstarch
½ teaspoon Chinese chili garlic paste, a few drops
    hot pepper sauce, or cayenne pepper

Preheat oven to 400°F. Lightly oil a baking dish. Remove tofu from liquid in its container and pat dry. Either cut tofu into 1-inch cubes, or halve tofu horizontally to make 2 thin slices and cut each slice into 4 pieces. Set them in the dish, side by side. Sprinkle with pepper to taste and 1 tablespoon soy sauce. Bake for 10 to 15 minutes or until slightly dried.

If using bell peppers, heat oil in a skillet, add peppers, and sauté over medium heat for 5 to 7 minutes or until softened.

Combine vinegar, remaining soy sauce, ketchup, honey, ginger, garlic, green onion, orange juice, broth, and cornstarch in a small saucepan and mix well. Cook over medium-high heat, stirring constantly, until sauce thickens and comes to a simmer. Stir in sautéed peppers. Add chili garlic paste to taste.

Brush tofu lightly with sauce. Bake for 5 minutes. Turn tofu pieces over and brush with more sauce. Bake 5 to 10 minutes more, or until glazed and browned. Serve hot. Serve remaining sauce separately.

Makes 6 appetizer or 4 main-course servings

If you like falafel, the seasonings of these Indian-inspired latkes will have an appealing familiarity and will add variety to your Hanukkah menus. Serve them with mango chutney. For a dairy meal you might like to serve them with plain yogurt as well.

There's no need to stand in the kitchen and keep frying latkes as people eat them. Contrary to a widespread notion, latkes can be reheated. This makes them convenient for entertaining at the holidays. To make them ahead, fry them and put them on a cookie sheet, then refrigerate or freeze them. Once they are frozen, you can transfer them to a freezer bag. If your latkes are frozen, partially thaw them before reheating. Bake them on an ungreased cookie sheet in a preheated 450°F oven for 5 to 7 minutes or until they are hot.

Instead of frying the latkes, you can bake them on a greased baking sheet. The crust is not as delicate, but baking yields pleasing results and is more practical than frying if you're making a large amount. Besides, you'll use less oil (see Note).

1 pound potatoes, preferably large baking potatoes
Salt and freshly ground black pepper
1 small onion, finely chopped (optional)
1 jalapeño pepper, finely chopped, or
     cayenne pepper to taste
1 teaspoon ground coriander

½ teaspoon ground cumin
¼ teaspoon turmeric
3 large eggs
2 to 3 tablespoons bread crumbs or flour, if needed
3 to 5 tablespoons vegetable oil, or more, if needed
     (for baking instructions, see Note)

Put potatoes in a saucepan, cover with water, and add salt. Bring to a boil, cover, and simmer for 25 minutes or until tender. Drain, peel, and mash potatoes. Add onion, jalapeño pepper, coriander, cumin, turmeric, and salt and pepper to taste. Beat eggs and mix with potatoes. Add bread crumbs, if necessary, so mixture is thick enough to be formed into patties. Mix well.

Preheat oven to 300°F to keep latkes warm. Heat 3 tablespoons oil in a heavy, large skillet over medium heat. Using a large tablespoon, add a spoonful of batter to oil, pushing it off with another spoon. Flatten slightly to make a small pancake of 2- to 2½-inch diameter. Mixture should spread, but pancake does not need to be very thin. If mixture is too thick to spread at all, add a little water to batter. If pancakes do not hold together, add 1 tablespoon more bread crumbs to batter.

Make more pancakes of the same size and fry for 5 minutes or until they are golden brown on both sides; turn them carefully with two pancake turners. Transfer to paper towels spread on an ovenproof tray. Keep warm in oven while frying rest of pancakes. Stir batter occasionally; add more oil to skillet if needed.

The pancakes can be kept warm for 30 minutes. You can also make them 1 day ahead and refrigerate them; heat in 1 layer on a baking sheet in a 300°F oven.

NOTE: To bake pancakes, preheat oven to 350°F, oil two nonstick baking sheets generously, and heat them in oven. Shape pancakes, spooning batter onto hot baking sheets. Bake for 10 minutes. Turn pancakes over carefully and bake for 10 more minutes or until light brown. If you'd like them browner, broil briefly.

Makes about 4 servings

BAKED POTATO AND APPLE LATKES WITH WALNUTS

Grated apples add a subtle sweet accent to these latkes. They are baked in muffin tins instead of being fried, which makes them substantially lower in fat.

If you prefer, top the latkes with applesauce instead of honey; or use applesauce sweetened with a little honey. For a meatless meal, you might like to garnish each with a small dollop of low-fat sour cream or plain yogurt, before drizzling with honey and sprinkling with walnuts and cinnamon.

About 2½ tablespoons canola oil, grapeseed oil, or other vegetable oil
1 medium onion, chopped
1¾ pounds baking potatoes
1 large apple, tart or sweet
2 large eggs
2 tablespoons finely chopped walnuts, plus more for sprinkling

1 teaspoon salt
¼ teaspoon freshly ground black pepper (optional)
¼ teaspoon ground cinnamon, or to taste, plus more for sprinkling
Honey (for drizzling)

Preheat oven to 400°F. Heat 1½ tablespoons oil in a heavy nonstick skillet. Add onion and sauté over medium-low heat until softened, about 7 minutes; during sautéing, if pan becomes dry, cover it to create steam. Let onion cool.

Peel potatoes and apple. Coarsely grate them, using large grater disk of a food processor or with hand grater. Put grated potatoes and apple in a large strainer and squeeze out excess liquid. Transfer mixture to a bowl. Add sautéed onion, eggs, 2 tablespoons walnuts, salt, pepper (if using), and ¼ teaspoon cinnamon. Mix well.

Oil 12 nonstick muffin pans, making sure to oil edges of bases. Using a ⅓-cup measure, add scant ⅓ cup batter to each muffin pan. Smooth tops lightly. Spoon ¼ teaspoon oil over each one. Bake about 45 minutes or until brown at edges and firm.

Remove from oven and run a small sturdy rubber spatula around edges of muffins to release them. You can then leave them in pan for 15 to 30 minutes to keep hot. Serve hot, drizzled lightly with honey and sprinkled with cinnamon and walnuts.

Makes 12 muffins, 4 to 6 servings

HONEY CINNAMON HANUKKAH PASTRY BALLS

Israelis usually fill their sufganiyot, or Hanukkah doughnuts, with jam and sprinkle them with powdered sugar. These Hanukkah pastries, inspired by Greek loukoumades, are sweetened with honey instead, a little inside the dough and more drizzled on the finished pastries. As a Turkish variation, you can drizzle them with lemon syrup (see page 374). You can also finish the sweet with chopped walnuts.

There's another difference too. Instead of being fried in oil, these pastry balls are brushed with oil and baked. Baking them is not only more healthy, it's much easier. You can use light olive oil for its mild flavor, or vegetable oil.

FOR DOUGH

¼ cup plus 1 tablespoon all-purpose flour

¼ cup whole wheat flour or additional white flour

½ cup water

1 tablespoon honey

¼ teaspoon salt

3 to 4 tablespoons mild olive oil or vegetable oil

3 large eggs, or 2 eggs plus 1 to 2 egg whites

Grated zest of 1 lemon

1 to 2 tablespoons mild olive oil or vegetable oil

4 to 6 tablespoons honey (for drizzling)

Cinnamon (for sprinkling)

2 to 3 teaspoons chopped walnuts (optional)

Position rack in lower third of oven and preheat to 400°F. Oil two baking sheets.

Mix both kinds of flour. Combine water, 1 tablespoon honey, and salt in a small, heavy saucepan. Add 3 or 4 tablespoons oil. Bring to a boil and remove from heat. Add flour mixture immediately and stir quickly with a wooden spoon until dough is smooth. Set pan over low heat and cook mixture, stirring, for about 30 seconds. Let cool for a few minutes.

Add 1 egg and beat it thoroughly into mixture. Beat in second egg until mixture is smooth. In a small bowl, beat third egg or egg white with a fork. Gradually beat enough of this egg into the dough until dough becomes very shiny and is soft enough so that when some is lifted, it just falls from the spoon. Stir in lemon zest.

Using 2 teaspoons, or a pastry bag and ½-inch plain tip, shape mounds of dough of about 1 inch diameter, spacing them about 2 inches apart on baking sheets. Pour 1 to 2 tablespoons oil into a small dish. Brush mounds with oil, gently giving them a round shape.

Bake for 30 minutes or until dough is puffed and browned; cracks that form during baking should also be brown. Serve hot or warm.

To serve, put puffs on a platter or divide among plates. Serve drizzled with honey and sprinkled with cinnamon and walnuts, if you like.

Makes about 6 servings

Most people don't give much thought to applesauce. They simply open a jar when they need a partner for potato pancakes. But when I lunched at Milky Way, a popular kosher restaurant in Los Angeles, the applesauce caught my attention. It was simply scrumptious.

You wouldn't really call it sauce. There were fairly firm apple cubes in a small amount of syrup. A liberal dose of cinnamon gave the applesauce plenty of punch and a dark brown hue, almost as if it had been caramelized. It was sweeter than standard applesauce but it had a lemony tang. Leah Adler, the owner of the restaurant (and also known as Steven Spielberg's mother), assured me they use only three ingredients—Granny Smith apples, cinnamon, and sugar. The tart apples gave it a hint of lemonlike flavor.

Like French apple compote, it was chunky, but its flavor was fresher and brighter than most versions of this classic. The texture of the apple cubes was distinct. The secret? This applesauce was cooked briefly, and thus is an ideal dessert for cooks in a hurry. Also, unlike French compote, it doesn't use any butter.

My cousin Mildred Greenberg sometimes adds apple juice instead of water and, for a lower-calorie version, sprinkles in a little calorie-free sweetener instead of sugar. For variations, sweeten it with brown rice syrup, found at natural food stores, maple syrup, honey, or brown sugar, or add raisins.

Some chefs like applesauce made from a mix of apples, as each contributes different qualities. The soft ones break down and thicken the applesauce, and the firm, greenish ones give it texture.

This applesauce is easier to make than old-fashioned smooth applesauce because you don't have to mash or puree the apples or strain them through a food mill. As soon as the apples are cooked, it's done.

You can leave the peels on to save time and to benefit from their nutrients; they soften enough during the cooking. But first taste the raw fruit; if their skin is bitter or very green and tough, peel them.

The applesauce thickens as it cools, so don't worry if it appears too thin when you finish cooking it. You can eat the applesauce right away, but it will taste even better if you refrigerate it overnight—the flavors mellow and come together. Serve it with latkes, blintzes, or crepes. It also makes a tasty dessert on its own or topped with plain or vanilla yogurt and nuts or granola.

2 pounds apples—tart, sweet, or a mixture
1 cup water
½ cup sugar, or more to taste

2 teaspoons ground cinnamon
Lemon juice to taste (optional)

Peel apples if you like. Cut them into small dice, ½ inch or smaller. Cook water, sugar, and cinnamon in a medium saucepan over medium heat, stirring, until mixture comes to a boil. Add apples. Cover and cook over medium-low heat for 10 minutes, then over low heat for 5 minutes or until they are just tender. Stir only if apples appear to be sticking. Taste, and add more sugar or lemon juice if needed. Serve warm or cold.

Makes about 4 servings

Purim

A CELEBRATION WITH SEEDS AND BEANS

Purim could be called the "eat, drink and be merry" holiday. Of all the Jewish festivals, Purim is surely the most fun. Drinking wine and spirits is a mitzvah. Exchanging gifts of sweet treats is a custom loved by everyone. Children are supposed to make noise, and not just anywhere—in the synagogue! The holiday dress code calls for costumes, the funnier the better. At the synagogue people see not only the children masquerading in colorful costumes, but sometimes the rabbi too.

With all this, it may seem surprising that healthy eating is an integral part of Purim's customs. Purim commemorates the heroism of Esther, whose story is related in the Book of Esther, or the Megillah of Esther, which is read on Purim. You could say the Purim Megillah's dramatic story sounds like a movie script—Esther wins the "Miss Persia" contest, and the prize is that she gets to marry the king! Later the heroic Jewish queen saves her people from the evil designs of Haman.

The Purim *seudah* (festive dinner) celebrates this story. It's the custom to serve a lavish spread with plenty of wine, to commemorate the victory of the Jews and to recall the palace banquets. Yet Queen Esther didn't do much feasting. She had a problem when she moved into the king's palace—the meat served there wasn't kosher. Legend relates that she became a vegetarian and subsisted only on seeds and legumes. For this reason Jews traditionally include such foods in their Purim menus—hence, the popularity of the poppy seed filling for hamantaschen.

In most households the holiday feast is not vegetarian. However, many families honor Esther by adding some kind of legume to their menu. A common custom is starting the Purim dinner with plain cooked chickpeas, which are delicious if you cook dried ones instead of opening a can. Black-eyed pea patties are prepared in Russian Jewish homes, and chickpeas with rice and honey appear on Romanian tables.

Among Israelis the favorite Purim entrée is turkey, because of a play on words of the Hebrew term for turkey and a reference in the Book of Esther. Turkey is a great choice, as it is widely considered the healthiest of meats.

For Purim, the saying goes, drink until you don't know the difference between "cursed is Haman" and "blessed is Mordecai" (Esther's cousin, a hero in the story). This rabbinical recommendation to imbibe is avidly followed by some. Of course, there's no nutritional merit to overdoing it, but a modest amount of wine or spirits is recommended by some. For example, Walter Willett, head of the Department of Nutrition at

HEALTHIER HAMANTASCHEN

*T*here are more ways to make delicious hamantaschen than references to the evil Haman in the Megillah. After all, hamantaschen are the most popular Purim treat, and creative bakers have come up with numerous versions. Some use yeast dough, others use sweet pie dough, and still others use cream cheese dough. Fillings range from orange marmalade, dried fruit, and preserves to chocolate and even peanut butter.

Yet the old-fashioned standard—poppy seed hamantaschen in crisp cookie dough—remains the favorite. I love the classic recipe, but decided to make a healthier version too. "Why bother?" some friends asked. "Purim comes only once a year, and is a time to celebrate."

One reason is to help nutrition-conscious eaters partake in the enjoyment. With all the feasting, some people feel so guilty about eating rich foods that they avoid hamantaschen completely, but regret missing the treasured treat. Besides, even if Purim lasts only one day, hamantaschen often are around for longer. Either you baked a batch or you received some for mishloah manot—the traditional exchange of treats. Making hamantaschen somewhat healthier means feeling better about eating a few.

The emphasis is on "somewhat." I'm not suggesting that such hamantaschen make a substitute for your breakfast oatmeal; nor am I encouraging anyone to overindulge.

When it comes to holiday treats, I'm in favor of slight adjustments to classic recipes, not drastic changes. I have tasted fat-free hamantaschen made with applesauce, but I don't make mine that way. People look forward to their Purim hamantaschen, and I wouldn't want mine to disappoint.

the Harvard School of Public Health, and co-author (with Mollie Katzen) of *Eat, Drink & Weigh Less*, feels that for most adults, a glass of wine or other alcohol a day is beneficial for health.

I mastered imbibing for Purim not at the synagogue but at cooking schools in France, where appreciating alcohol is a yearlong passion. When I studied at the Parisian École de Cuisine La Varenne and at École Le Nôtre, a professional pastry school located, how appropriately, in a town called Plaisir (meaning pleasure), our chefs always instructed us to "Bien imbiber vos gâteaux"—"Imbibe your cakes well." What they meant was to moisten our baked cakes with a simple syrup punched up with spirits.

Rum, kirsch (clear cherry brandy), and Grand Marnier are frequent choices. Cooks often select a liqueur that complements the filling—orange liqueur with orange cake,

Instead, I keep modifying the hamantaschen in subtle ways. My customary recipe had a very rich, sweet pastry, with lots of butter and egg yolks—the kind of dough used for French fruit tarts. One year, when I was baking hamantaschen with my mother, we used margarine to make them pareve. Always practical, my mother suggested we use whole eggs instead of just yolks, and thus we would need fewer. Naturally, I agreed. My mother was a good hamantaschen baker. Besides, she had taught me how to make them when I was a girl.

She also suggested adding baking powder. My French dough had none. The Parisian chefs with whom I had studied regarded baking powder with suspicion. Even the word for it, levure chimique, *or chemical leavening, was not appealing. The baking powder proved a good addition and gave our dough a pleasing lightness; it also made the hamantaschen look a bit bigger.*

With scientific research showing that it's best to avoid the trans fats found in most margarines, I replaced it with canola oil. Since dietary guidelines now encourage us to eat more whole grains, I made another small change. I substituted whole wheat flour for part of the white flour in the dough.

Personally, I liked poppy seed filling only when I learned to cook the seeds with milk, honey, and butter when I lived in Israel. Today, for my pareve poppy seed filling, I cook them in soy milk, which, like the milk and butter, gives the filling a luscious flavor. I slip in a little bit of oats, which adds to the creamy texture. Chopped figs contribute natural sweetness, and healthy fiber too.

There is no need to make a big fuss over the nutritious boost in these hamantaschen. After all, Purim is a holiday celebrating intrigue, and the fact that these hamantaschen are healthier can remain the baker's secret.

coffee liqueur with chocolate cake, or pear brandy with pear-filled cake. After splitting a cake into layers, you dab them with the syrup, using a pastry brush. This method is almost always used for layer cakes made from light batters, like sponge cakes and the French standard, génoise, a whole-egg sponge cake enriched with a little butter.

For some desserts, such as Light Peach Trifle (page 343), there's no need to make a syrup; you simply brush the cake—in this case, ladyfingers—lightly with liqueur.

Imbibing does wonders for a light cake's texture and taste. The lively syrup flavors the cake and helps it to keep longer. Without this treatment, the cake would quickly become dry.

These spirited syrups play a nutritional role too. They enable you to enjoy cakes that contain less saturated fat than pound cakes or other butter cakes by keeping them moist.

POPPY SEEDS

*P*oppy seeds have a pleasing nutty flavor. Although we tend to associate them with Central and Eastern European specialties like poppy seed breads, cakes, strudels, and buttered noodles, poppies have long been grown in the Middle East and are used to flavor Indian vegetable dishes.

Raw poppy seeds are quite perishable because of their high oil content. They should be stored in a cool place. If they have been ground, it's safest to keep them in the refrigerator and to use them promptly. I know this from experience. The first time I bought them to make my own filling for hamantaschen was when I lived in Israel over thirty-five years ago. I didn't know this rule then, and after leaving the poppy seeds three days at the warm room temperature, I had to throw them out.

It's easiest to buy poppy seeds ground, but if they are whole, you can grind them in a coffee grinder. You can also crush them in a mortar with a pestle or roll them with a rolling pin, but you'll need to soak them first in a little warm water to soften them.

Roasting or cooking raw poppy seeds brings out their flavor. Of course, they become toasted when baked on breads. For hamantaschen, some filling recipes simply call for mixing the seeds with sugar and dried fruit. I find the flavor is far superior when the poppy seeds are cooked with the other filling ingredients.

✦

Carrot and Beet Salad with Sunflower Seeds

Early Springtime Salad with Raw Asparagus

Black Bean Soup with Curry and Tofu

Spicy White Bean Soup with Kale

Purim Pizza with Onions, Olives, and Capers

Purim Turkey with Chile Almond Chocolate Sauce

Baked Turkey Schnitzel with Sweet-Sour Onion Compote

Three Sisters Chili

Purim Pasta Primavera with Pecans

Pareve Poppy Seed Hamantaschen

✦

CARROT AND BEET SALAD WITH SUNFLOWER SEEDS

Queen Esther, the heroine of the holiday, is said to have subsisted on seeds and for that reason many people include them in their Purim menus. Poppy seeds are the common choice, but other seeds make good additions to menus too. In this recipe the toasted sunflower seeds enliven the salad of winter vegetables and contribute vitamin E. You can use raw carrots, but I cook them lightly to bring out their sweetness.

You can vary the seeds and the oil in the dressing to your taste. If you like, substitute Mexican pumpkin seeds (pepitas) or use toasted walnuts or pecans, and make the dressing with pumpkin seed, walnut, or pecan oil.

2 large beets

2 large carrots, cut into thin strips

4 cups red-leaf or green-leaf lettuce, cut into wide strips

2 medium cucumbers, cut into thin strips

1 to 2 tablespoons white or red wine vinegar

2 to 3 tablespoons sunflower oil or canola oil

Salt and freshly ground black pepper

2 tablespoons toasted sunflower seeds

Rinse beets, taking care not to pierce their skins. Put in a pan, cover with water, and bring to a boil. Cover and simmer over low heat for 40 to 50 minutes or until tender. Let cool. Run beets under cold water and slip off skins. Halve beets, place cut side down, and slice them.

Meanwhile, put carrot strips in a saucepan of boiling water to cover and cook over medium heat for 3 minutes or until barely tender but still crisp. Remove with a slotted spoon and let cool.

Combine lettuce strips, cucumbers, and carrots in a bowl. Toss to mix. Add vinegar, oil, salt, and pepper and mix well. Serve topped with sliced beets and toasted seeds.

Makes 4 servings

Not many people think of eating asparagus raw but when it is very tender, it makes a delicious, beautiful addition to salads. I love its "green" flavor in the salads I make in late winter and early spring, when the asparagus has just come to the market and when the jicama, which is at its best during the cool months, is still fresh and moist. The jicama's sweetness is the perfect foil for the subtle bitterness of the asparagus and that of my garden's arugula shoots, which I add to this seasonal salad. Italian parsley and green onions are other standard elements in my mix, as well as a few baby radishes, making this salad a healthy, colorful prelude to the Purim feast.

10 pencil-thin asparagus spears
½ long (hothouse or Japanese) cucumber,
*   4 Middle Eastern or pickling cucumbers, or*
*   1 medium cucumber*
2 medium tomatoes, or 4 plum tomatoes
6 small red radishes
1 to 1½ cups diced jicama (see Note)

¼ cup chopped flat-leaf parsley
2 green onions, white and green parts, chopped
1 to 2 cups mixed baby lettuces, baby spinach, or
*   coarsely chopped arugula*
2 tablespoons extra virgin olive oil
1 to 2 tablespoons strained fresh lemon juice
Salt and freshly ground black pepper

Discard bottom quarter of asparagus spears (or save for flavoring vegetable broth). Cut rest of each spear into 1-inch pieces.

Peel cucumbers if they have been waxed, cut into ½-inch dice, and put in a glass serving bowl. Cut tomatoes in similar dice and add to bowl. Halve radishes, cut in ¼-inch slices, and add to bowl. Add jicama, parsley, and green onions and mix to combine. Add lettuces and half the asparagus pieces and toss mixture. Add oil, lemon juice, and salt and pepper and toss again. Taste and adjust seasoning. Serve cool or cold, topped with remaining asparagus.

NOTE: To prepare jicama, cut off the peel with a sharp knife. Cut into thin slices, then into dice.

Makes 4 servings

❧ BLACK BEAN SOUP WITH CURRY AND TOFU

Black bean soup is loved in Latin America, but I find it benefits enormously from Asian additions. White cubes of tofu add a refreshing light taste and contrasting color and texture to the dark, earthy soup. A last-minute accent of fresh garlic and curry paste gives depth of flavor to the soup.

Full of wholesome ingredients—the high fiber of beans, the nutritious plant protein of tofu, and the vitamins from the vegetables—this rich-tasting, satisfying soup has no additional fat besides the natural fat in the tofu and a trace of fat in the beans. I cook the vegetables briefly so they keep their color. With canned black beans, the soup is ready in a short time. We like it as a vegetarian Purim entrée, preceded by Early Springtime Salad with Raw Asparagus (page 77), or as a one-pot main course for lunch or supper.

1 large onion, chopped	1 zucchini, quartered and diced
1 medium boiling potato, diced	One 14- or 15-ounce can black beans, or 1 1/2 cups
4 to 6 cups vegetable broth or water	cooked, drained black beans (see Note)
Salt and freshly ground black pepper	3 large garlic cloves, chopped
2 carrots, sliced	1 teaspoon curry paste or curry powder
1 to 1 1/2 cups chopped cabbage	4 to 8 ounces firm tofu, cut into cubes

Cook onion and potato in 4 cups broth with salt and pepper for 15 minutes. Add carrots and return to a boil. Cover and cook for 3 minutes. Add cabbage, zucchini, and beans and cook for 3 minutes or until vegetables are just tender, adding more broth if soup becomes too thick. Just before serving, add garlic, curry paste, and tofu and heat for 1 minute. Taste and adjust seasoning. Serve hot.

NOTE: You can use 3/4 cup dried black beans. Rinse, drain, and cook them in water to cover generously for 1 1/4 to 1 1/2 hours or until tender.

Makes 4 servings

❈ SPICY WHITE BEAN SOUP WITH KALE

This recipe evolved from the pasta e fagioli (pasta with beans) I tasted in Verona, Italy, where it was made with whole wheat spaghetti. Like minestrone, the composition of this Italian favorite varies from one season to another. Cold-weather versions like this one are more likely to include hearty greens than tomatoes. Classic versions of the soup are often flavored with smoked meat. In kosher kitchens the meat is usually omitted and the soup is pareve, although some cooks simmer meatballs in the soup to turn it into a meaty main course. You can substitute chopped frozen spinach or other greens for the kale.

Persian cuisine also features hearty bean soups like this, known as *aash*. If Queen Esther had ordered this soup, it probably would have included Persian toasted vermicelli, which resembles whole wheat spaghetti.

1½ cups small dried white beans (about 10 ounces),
*   sorted, or three 15-ounce cans white beans,*
*   undrained*
2 cups vegetable broth
About 6 cups water
2 tablespoons extra virgin olive oil
1 medium onion, chopped
2 celery ribs, diced
½ cup diced carrot

½ pound kale, mustard greens, or chard, cleaned,
*   trimmed, and chopped*
2 large garlic cloves, minced
1 cup whole wheat spaghetti, broken in
*   2-inch pieces*
2 teaspoons chopped fresh rosemary, or
*   1 teaspoon chopped dried rosemary*
½ teaspoon hot red pepper flakes, or to taste
3 tablespoons chopped fresh parsley leaves

Pick over beans, discarding any pebbles and any broken or discolored beans. Rinse beans, drain, and place in a large saucepan. Add broth and 1 quart water, and bring to a boil. Cook, uncovered, over medium-low heat, adding hot water occasionally so beans remain covered, for 1¼ hours, or until beans are tender. Drain beans, reserving cooking liquid. Measure bean cooking liquid; add enough water to make 6 cups; if using canned beans, mix broth with bean liquid and enough water to make 6 cups.

Puree about one-third of the cooked or canned beans with 1 cup water.

Heat 1½ tablespoons oil in saucepan. Add onion, celery, and carrot and cook over medium-low heat, stirring often, for 10 minutes or until onion is soft but not brown. Add measured liquid and bring to a boil. Add kale. Cook, uncovered, over medium heat for 15 minutes or until vegetables are tender.

Bring soup to a boil. Add garlic and spaghetti and cook, uncovered, over medium-high heat, stirring occasionally, for 5 to 8 minutes or until pasta is tender but firm to the bite. Add bean puree and whole beans; if soup is too thick, add more water. Stir in rosemary, pepper flakes, and parsley. Taste and adjust seasoning. Serve drizzled with a little more oil.

Makes 4 to 5 servings

PURIM PIZZA WITH ONIONS, OLIVES, AND CAPERS

Around Purim my mother often emphasized the importance of trying to use up your flour before Passover. A pizza is a great way to do this and is perfect for a Purim party. This one is vegetarian, in honor of Queen Esther's diet, and contains no cheese. With its topping of sweet, tender, slowly sautéed onions, it's inspired by the Provençal pissaladière, but I omit the usual anchovies and flavor the topping instead with a sprinkling of capers and black olives, as is sometimes done in southern Italy. You can add a few sliced tomatoes too.

When it comes to pizza, this one is a wholesome choice. The dough, made with part whole wheat flour, is easy to make by hand; or see the Note following the recipe for using a processor or mixer. Use a fruity extra virgin olive oil and serve the pizza warm from the oven.

¾ cup whole wheat flour
¾ cup all-purpose flour
1 envelope (¼ ounce) dry yeast, or
    1 cake fresh yeast
½ cup lukewarm water, or more if needed
4 to 5 tablespoons extra virgin olive oil
¾ teaspoon salt
5 medium onions, halved and cut into thin slices

Freshly ground black pepper
1 tablespoon chopped fresh basil (optional)
3 ripe tomatoes, sliced (optional)
1½ teaspoons chopped fresh thyme leaves, or
    ½ teaspoon dried thyme, crumbled
3 to 5 teaspoons capers, drained
⅓ cup pitted black olives

Sift whole wheat flour and all-purpose flour into a bowl and make a well in center. Sprinkle dry yeast or crumble fresh yeast into well. Pour ¼ cup lukewarm water over yeast and let stand for 10 minutes or until foamy. Stir until smooth. Add remaining water, 1 tablespoon oil, and ¾ teaspoon salt, and mix with ingredients in middle of well. Stir in flour mixture and mix well, to obtain a fairly soft dough. If dough is dry, add more water by tablespoons. Knead dough lightly, slapping it on working surface, until it is smooth and elastic. If dough is very sticky, flour it occasionally while kneading.

Lightly oil a medium bowl. Add dough, turning to coat entire surface. Cover with plastic wrap or with lightly dampened towel. Let dough rise in a warm draft-free area for 1 hour or until nearly doubled in volume.

Heat 3 tablespoons olive oil in a large skillet over low heat. Add onions, salt, and pepper. Cook over medium-low heat, stirring occasionally, for 5 minutes. Cover and cook for 10 more minutes or until very tender. Stir in basil (if using).

Oil a 10- or 11-inch tart pan; or oil a baking sheet. With oiled hands, pat dough to a round in tart pan or to a 10- or 11-inch round on baking sheet; make edges higher than center.

Fill dough with onion mixture. If you like, top with tomato slices. Sprinkle with thyme and capers. Garnish with olives. If you like, drizzle with a little more oil. Let rise in a warm place for 15 minutes. Preheat oven to 400°F.

Bake for 20 minutes or until dough is golden brown and firm but not hard. Serve warm.

NOTES: If you prefer, make dough instead by blending ingredients in a food processor, then process 1 minute to knead, or in a mixer with dough hook. (See Apple Cinnamon Tart, page 346.)

If you have a pizza stone, you can bake pizza on preheated stone at 425°F to 450°F for 12 to 15 minutes for a crunchier crust.

Makes 4 to 6 servings

PURIM TURKEY WITH CHILE ALMOND CHOCOLATE SAUCE

This Mexican-inspired recipe is a perfect way to enjoy the customary Purim turkey. In honor of Queen Esther's diet, the sauce has plenty of nuts and seeds. The sauce is a lighter, kosher version of mole poblano that I make with a small amount of vegetable oil rather than animal fat. I have simplified the recipe, which can be exceedingly complicated when made the traditional way, by using one type of dried chile instead of three and skipping the steps of browning the turkey and straining the sauce several times.

Try to cook the turkey a day ahead so you can thoroughly skim the fat from the broth.

3 pounds turkey thighs or drumsticks

1 quart water

Salt and freshly ground black pepper

5 dried ancho chiles

One 15-ounce can tomatoes, drained

6 tablespoons almonds, toasted (page 379)

1½ tablespoons sesame seeds, toasted (page 380)

1 dry corn tortilla, torn into pieces

½ medium onion, cut into chunks

1 large garlic clove, peeled

3 tablespoons raisins

¼ teaspoon ground cinnamon

¼ teaspoon ground coriander

¼ teaspoon anise seed

Pinch of ground cloves

1 tablespoon vegetable oil

1 ounce unsweetened chocolate

Combine turkey and water in a stew pan with salt and pepper. Bring to a boil. Cover and simmer for 1½ hours or until tender. Remove turkey from broth.

Pour broth into a bowl; let cool and skim off fat.

Rinse chiles, remove stems and seeds, and tear chiles in pieces. Cover with hot water and soak for 1 hour or until softened. Drain chiles, discarding liquid.

Put chiles in blender or food processor. Add tomatoes, toasted almonds, 1 tablespoon toasted sesame seeds, tortilla, onion, garlic, raisins, cinnamon, coriander, anise seed, cloves, and ½ cup turkey broth. Process to a coarse puree.

In pan used to cook turkey, heat oil over medium-high heat. Add chile puree and cook over medium-low heat, stirring, for 5 minutes or until thickened. Add 2 cups turkey broth and chocolate, stirring often over low heat for 15 minutes or until sauce is thick. Season to taste with salt and pepper. Skim excess fat from sauce.

Discard turkey skin and cut meat from bones in large strips. Put in a shallow baking dish. Pour sauce over turkey.

Preheat oven to 350°F. Bake turkey, covered, for 30 minutes or until hot. If sauce is too thick, thin it with a few tablespoons turkey broth. Sprinkle turkey with remaining toasted sesame seeds and serve.

Makes 6 to 8 servings

BAKED TURKEY SCHNITZEL WITH SWEET-SOUR ONION COMPOTE

Among Jews from Israel to Alsace, turkey is a Purim favorite. For a delicious option that's much faster to prepare than a roast turkey, turn the breasts into savory schnitzels and set them on a bed of a meltingly tender stewed onion. From a nutritional standpoint, the lean turkey breasts are a good choice, and so are the onions, which contain good amounts of vitamin C, folate, and fiber, as well as disease-fighting phytonutrients. Instead of frying the schnitzel the usual way, I bake it in its light bread-crumb coating with a drizzle of extra virgin olive oil. A green salad, such as festive Apple Walnut Green Salad with a Sweet Touch (page 27), is a great accompaniment.

You can easily make the delicately sweet-and-sour onion compote ahead and reheat it before serving the turkey. The compote also makes a delicious bed for grilled chicken or fish.

3 tablespoons extra virgin olive oil or
   vegetable oil
1½ pounds white or yellow onions, halved and
   thinly sliced
Salt and freshly ground black pepper
1 to 2 teaspoons white wine vinegar
¼ to ½ teaspoon sugar
⅓ cup whole wheat or all–purpose flour

¾ cup unseasoned dried bread crumbs, preferably
   whole wheat
1 teaspoon paprika
1 pound turkey breast slices, about ¼ inch thick
1 teaspoon dried thyme, crumbled
2 egg whites
1 tablespoon chopped parsley
1 lemon, cut into wedges

In a heavy stew pan heat 2 tablespoons oil. Add onions, salt, and pepper. Cover and cook over low heat, stirring often, for 20 minutes. Uncover and cook, stirring very often, for 15 minutes longer or until onions are golden and tender enough to crush easily with a wooden spoon. Stir in vinegar and sugar and heat until absorbed.

Preheat oven to 475°F. Spread flour on one plate, the bread crumbs with paprika on another. Arrange turkey in one layer on a third plate and sprinkle pieces with thyme, salt, and pepper on both sides. Lightly oil a baking sheet with olive oil or oil spray.

Beat egg whites in a shallow bowl. Lightly coat a turkey slice with flour on both sides. Tap and shake to remove excess flour. Dip slice in egg whites. Last, dip both sides in bread crumbs so turkey is completely coated; pat and press lightly so crumbs adhere. Repeat with remaining slices. Set pieces side by side on oiled baking sheet.

Drizzle turkey with 1 tablespoon oil. Bake turkey, uncovered, for 5 minutes per side or until golden brown and cooked through. Meanwhile, reheat compote. To serve, spoon onion compote onto plates, set turkey schnitzels on top, and sprinkle with chopped parsley. Serve with lemon wedges.

Makes 4 to 5 servings

This hearty casserole features the healthy, Native American "three sisters" combination—beans, corn, and squash—developed by resourceful farmers. The three elements are known as the "three sisters" because, when planted together, they help each other to grow. Whether you make this colorful, tasty dish meaty or serve it as a meatless Purim entrée, it's easy to prepare. Serve it with hot sauce if you like it extra spicy.

½ pound fresh green beans, ends removed, broken
    in two, or 1½ cups frozen green beans
1½ to 2 cups frozen lima beans or cooked dried
    lima beans, or one 15-ounce can lima beans
½ pound extra-lean ground beef, chicken, or turkey
    (optional)
1 to 2 tablespoons olive oil or vegetable oil
1 large onion, chopped
2 or 3 zucchini, or pale green Middle Eastern or
    Mexican squash
2 garlic cloves, chopped

2 jalapeño or serrano peppers, chopped, or
    ¼ teaspoon hot red pepper flakes, or
    more to taste
2 teaspoons paprika
1 teaspoon ground cumin
One 28-ounce can tomatoes, drained and diced
1 teaspoon dried oregano
Salt and freshly ground black pepper
½ cup water
1½ cups frozen corn kernels
Cayenne pepper

Cook fresh green beans in a pan of boiling salted water to cover for 6 minutes or until crisp-tender; drain. Cook frozen green beans and lima beans according to package instructions until barely tender; drain.

If using meat or chicken, heat 1 tablespoon oil in a large sauté pan or stew pan, add meat and sauté over medium heat, stirring to separate, for 5 minutes or until color of meat changes. Remove from pan. Add remaining tablespoon oil to pan and heat it. Add onion and sauté over medium heat for 5 minutes, adding water by tablespoons if pan becomes dry. Add zucchini, garlic, and jalapeño peppers. Cover and cook for 2 minutes. Stir in paprika and cumin, followed by tomatoes, oregano, salt, pepper, and water.

Return meat to pan. Stir and cook over medium heat for 5 minutes or until sauce has thickened. Add corn and cook for 5 minutes or until meat, corn, and squash are tender. Add all of beans, salt, pepper, and cayenne to taste. Cover and heat through. Taste and adjust seasoning.

Makes 4 to 5 servings

Nuts are often on the Purim menu, in honor of Queen Esther's vegetarian diet, and they are terrific in pasta dishes. This one is based on the classic pasta primavera, which means springtime pasta in Italian. The dish appears on so many menus that it gives the impression that it is an age-old Italian standard. In fact it was invented fairly recently, in the 1970s, and not in Italy but by a chef in New York City. The original recipe calls for sautéing the vegetables in olive oil with garlic and adding a tomato-basil sauce and a cream sauce with butter and Parmesan cheese. I prefer not to overpower the vegetables by heavy sauces. Instead I prepare this lighter, healthier pasta dish flavored with olive oil and garlic.

Broccoli, asparagus, and peas are perfect for Purim, but you can treat this colorful dish as a basic recipe and vary the vegetables according to the seasons. To save time, buy sliced mushrooms. If you like, buy packaged shredded carrots and add them at the same time as the frozen peas. You can serve the dish with fresh grated Parmesan cheese. Or, for a heartier main course, add lean protein, like roasted turkey breast, cooked salmon or sea bass, a touch of lox, or edamame (green soybeans).

8 ounces small broccoli florets
8 ounces thin asparagus, ends trimmed,
*   spears cut into 3 or 4 pieces*
Salt and freshly ground black pepper
8 ounces spaghetti, vermicelli, or linguine,
*   preferably whole wheat*
1 cup fresh shelled or frozen peas, or fresh
*   sugar snap peas*

3 to 4 tablespoons extra virgin olive oil
6 ounces sliced mushrooms
4 large garlic cloves, minced
2 or 3 plum tomatoes, diced
2 tablespoons thin strips fresh basil or
*   chopped flat-leaf parsley*
⅓ cup pecan halves, toasted (page 380)

Add broccoli and asparagus to a large saucepan of boiling salted water and cook, uncovered, over high heat for 2 minutes or until crisp-tender. Remove with a slotted spoon, rinse, and drain.

Return water to a boil, adding enough to cover pasta generously. Add pasta and boil, uncovered, over high heat, separating strands occasionally with a fork, for 7 minutes. Add peas and continue cooking for 2 or 3 minutes or until pasta is tender but firm to the bite. Drain, reserving ¼ cup cooking liquid.

Meanwhile, heat 3 tablespoons oil in a very large skillet. Add mushrooms, garlic, and salt and pepper and sauté over medium heat for 2 minutes. Add broccoli and asparagus and sauté for 2 more minutes. Add pasta and peas to skillet and toss for 1 minute over low heat, adding 2 or 3 tablespoons pasta cooking liquid if mixture is too thick. Add tomatoes and basil and toss mixture well. Season to taste with salt and pepper. Add remaining oil, if desired. Serve immediately, topped with toasted pecans.

Makes 4 servings

PAREVE POPPY SEED HAMANTASCHEN

These hamantaschen contain a luscious filling of poppy seeds simmered with honey, dried fruit, and soy milk, enclosed in a dough containing some whole wheat flour and canola oil instead of all-white flour and butter or margarine. The dough is easy to make in a food processor. Use freshly ground poppy seeds for the filling, if possible, and keep them in the refrigerator until ready to use. You can find them in Jewish, Middle Eastern, or Eastern European grocery stores. Either leave them whole or, for a finer, smoother filling, grind them in a spice grinder. If you like, serve the hamantaschen sprinkled with powdered sugar.

¾ cup whole wheat flour
1¼ cups all-purpose flour
¾ teaspoon baking powder
Pinch of salt
½ cup sugar (for dough), plus 3 tablespoons
    (for filling)
1 large egg
6 tablespoons canola oil

1 teaspoon grated orange zest
2 to 3 tablespoons orange juice
½ cup poppy seeds (about 2½ ounces), preferably
    freshly ground
½ cup soy milk
3 tablespoons honey
¼ cup dried dark figs, chopped, or raisins
2 tablespoons fine oats

Combine whole wheat and all-purpose flours, baking powder, salt, and ½ cup sugar in a food processor. Process to blend. Beat egg with oil and add to processor. Add orange zest. Pulse until dough is the texture of meal.

Add juice 1 tablespoon at a time, pulsing after each addition, until dough becomes sticky crumbs; if dough is too dry, sprinkle with a little more juice or water and process again. Transfer to a bowl and press together. Wrap in plastic wrap and refrigerate 4 hours or overnight.

In small saucepan combine poppy seeds, soy milk, honey, figs, oats, and 3 tablespoons sugar, and bring to a simmer. Cook over low heat, stirring often, about 10 minutes or until thick. Remove from heat and let cool. Refrigerate for at least 1 hour before using.

Grease a baking sheet. Cut dough into 4 pieces. Roll out 1 piece on a lightly floured surface until about ⅛ inch thick. Using a 3-inch cookie cutter, cut into circles. Brush edges lightly with water. Put 1 teaspoon poppyseed filling in center of each circle. Pull up edges of circle in 3 arcs that meet in center above filling. Close them firmly. Pinch edges to seal. Put on greased baking sheet and refrigerate. Wrap and refrigerate scraps at least 30 minutes.

Roll and shape more hamantaschen from remaining dough and from scraps. Refrigerate 1 hour or up to overnight to firm dough.

Position rack in center of oven and preheat to 375°F. Bake hamantaschen for 12 to 14 minutes or until they are light golden at edges and golden brown on bottom. Cool on a rack.

Makes about 2 dozen hamantaschen (including scraps)

Passover

I have always loved the eight-day holiday of Passover. Eating matzo and dishes made from it was a different, fun way to eat. For my mother, like other Jewish mothers, it was a challenge to make Passover food that tasted better than the food of the rest of the year, in spite of the extra "kosher-for-Passover" restrictions.

Passover, which is also called Pesach or Pessah, is as important on the Jewish holiday calendar as Thanksgiving is on the American one. Passover's main event is the Seder, the ceremonial dinner on the first night of the holiday. In the homes of observant Jews who live outside Israel, there's a Seder on the second night as well. For many families, getting together for the Seder is a must, even if relatives live far from each other. Because Passover is celebrated in a big way, Passover meals stand out in people's memories as wonderful feasts.

Known as the "Festival of Spring" and the "Time of Liberation," the Passover message promotes healthy eating. Even the Seder ceremony calls for eating a celery stick or parsley sprig to remind us that this is the springtime holiday, a time to eat more vegetables. Liberation refers to freedom from slavery, but it could be a metaphor for freedom from bad habits, like an unhealthy living style.

Long before the holiday, anticipation builds. There is plenty to do to get ready, like thorough cleaning of the kitchen, shopping for new clothes and, of course, purchasing the special kosher-for-Passover ingredients to use during the eight-day holiday.

WHAT MAKES FOODS KOSHER FOR PASSOVER?

Matzo is the best-known Passover food. During the eight days of Passover, this unleavened bread is the only bread that is eaten, as a reminder of the flatbread the ancient

Hebrews ate as they rushed to escape from Egypt. Wheat flour is prohibited, because it can "leaven" or ferment naturally upon contact with liquid, as it does when you make a sourdough starter. Although matzo itself is made of wheat flour, speedy mixing and baking techniques prevent it from leavening. For Passover, Ashkenazi Jews also avoid corn, rice, other grains, and legumes, but many Sephardi Jews do eat them; it's simply a difference in customs.

Instead of flour, baked goods are prepared using matzo meal, made from ground matzo, and potato starch. Matzos, matzo meal, and finely ground matzo cake meal are the basis for dumplings, casseroles, stuffings, cakes, and boxed breakfast cereals.

When I was growing up, we made a large percentage of our Passover dishes from plain matzo and matzo meal. Today an impressive array of holiday ingredients is available at the market, making it easy to create a variety of holiday meals. Now there is Passover breakfast cereal, stuffing mix, pancake mix, and cake mix, and there are even Passover noodles and Passover couscous. Matzo comes in flavors from garlic to grape juice, and is also available as whole wheat and spelt matzo.

Some people complain that because matzo isn't as satisfying as bread, in order to feel

SEDER PLATE FOODS

*T*he Passover table is set for the predinner Seder ceremony, which features wine as well as foods to recall the Hebrews' slavery and flight to freedom. On one plate there are three matzos. Other symbolic foods are displayed on a beautiful Seder plate, with Hebrew words indicating their positions. Fresh horseradish or bitter greens represent the bitterness of servitude. A small piece of roasted lamb or poultry commemorates the sacrifices in the Temple in Jerusalem, as does a roasted hard-boiled egg.

Haroset is a star of the Seder. This reddish-brown mixture of chopped nuts and fruit stands for the mortar the slaves were forced to make. Although contemplating such labor is not a cheery thought, guests quickly put it out of mind when the sweet, tasty spread arrives. In addition to the spoonful of haroset for the Seder plate and a bowlful for sampling during the ritual, some families prepare extra to have on hand for snacks during the holiday.

A celery rib or parsley sprig on the Seder plate reminds us that Passover is the holiday of spring.

A SEDER IN THE MEDITERRANEAN MODE

*W*hen it comes to planning our Seders, it's natural that many of us should "think Mediterranean." After all, the Jewish homeland is at the heart of the region, and a wonderful profusion of Mediterranean ingredients thrives there. Making good use of these foods results in menus that are perfectly suited to Israel's environment. Although it is the Sephardi Jews whose direct culinary heritage is Mediterranean, all Jews claim this origin. The Mediterranean land of Israel is the birthplace of Jewish culture, kashrut, and, of course, Jewish cuisine. Even matzo resembles some of the flatbreads that are common throughout the area.

History, geography, and culture aren't the only reasons for "going Mediterranean." By now many of us have heard the nutritionists' message about the beneficial effects of the Mediterranean diet.

But the best reason for cooking a Seder menu in the Mediterranean spirit is that this cuisine is delicious. With its exuberant use of herbs, spices, aromatic vegetables, citrus fruits, and olive oil to enliven food, the variety of tasty meals is endless. Cooks are always delighted to discover that the Mediterranean manner of cooking is convenient too, as this relaxed style is full of easy dishes. The ingredients speak for themselves, without the need for complex sauces or intricate techniques.

There are plenty of choices to help simplify Seder preparation. For a festive starter, cooking artichokes and fava beans in white wine accented with thyme and olive oil (see recipe on page 286) is a perfect balance for the vegetables' distinctive flavors. Fresh garlic and a sprinkling of cumin do wonders for all sorts of meat main courses, like the chicken stew with zucchini and peppers. Chopped dates added to haroset give this Passover tradition a new dimension of flavor. For dessert, serve fruit with luxurious meringues embellished with pistachios.

full they end up eating too much matzo and thus consume too many calories. But there's no reason for this to be the case. In a meal with meat, chicken, fish, or dairy foods, plenty of cooked and raw vegetables, a moderate amount of potatoes, and fruit, diners should be satisfied and should not feel the need to gorge on matzo.

In planning the Seder dinner, timing is the tricky part. You don't always know when you'll be putting dinner on the table. The meal follows the recital of the Haggadah—the book of songs and narration of the Passover story, and it's hard to predict how long this reading will take.

To make cooking and serving simpler, I compose my menu of dishes that can be made in advance and kept hot. Doing this helps prevent the fatigue that can set in if you embark on an exhausting marathon of cooking just before the holiday. I choose some dishes that keep warm or reheat easily and others that taste good at room temperature.

Since the biblical era, Jewish cooks have had plenty of time to perfect their Passover preparation strategies, and quite a few holiday specialties are convenient for cooking in advance. This is not the night for soufflés, sautés, or grilled meats. It's much better to opt for soups, braised dishes, and salads.

Be sure to include some cold dishes on the Seder menu. The traditional Ashkenazi

THE VEGETARIAN PASSOVER PUZZLE

*D*esigning meatless meals for Passover can be difficult, but vegetarians worldwide have come up with interesting solutions. These days, even people who plan their holiday meals around meat try to incorporate more vegetable dishes into their menus.

Cooks of diverse origins have created Passover casseroles based on vegetable purees, potatoes, or matzo. Sephardi cooks prepare lasagnelike mina, composed of matzo layered with fillings of spinach, potatoes or eggplant, or, for dairy meals, with cheese. I've often had Moroccan mashed potato pashtidah (a casserole), flavored with onions, garlic, and turmeric as an appetizer, but it makes a good meatless main course too; it also goes well with chicken (see the recipe on page 100). My mother, who was born in Warsaw, often baked mushroom and matzo kugel with sautéed onions, which made a savory vegetarian entrée or pareve side dish, or could be enriched with cottage cheese for a milchig meal.

Passover meals present a greater challenge for vegans, who do not eat eggs or dairy products and base their meals mainly on grains and legumes. Bean and vegetable stew served over rice, a common vegan entrée, works for many Sephardi Jews but is problematic for observant Ashkenazim, who do not eat grains or legumes, which are called kitniyot in Hebrew (and on labels of kosher-for-Passover items).

But even with these restrictions, you can prepare substantial meals. In my household, our menus are often vegan. We discovered that certain vegetables can be very satisfying, even without grains and legumes. Obviously, tubers and roots like potatoes, sweet potatoes, carrots, and turnips can fill you up and, when spiced well, are delicious.

Ashkenazi Jews created many delectable dishes from mushrooms, taking advantage of their unique, meaty texture. If you chop them into fine bits and sauté them with shallots or onions, they become a French dish called duxelles, a tasty topping for matzo or filling for peppers, tomatoes, or zucchini.

gefilte fish is a great choice—it's not difficult to cook and is simple to serve. Although it has a reputation for being complicated, my gefilte fish is easy to make. No more scaling whole fish, picking out bones, and chopping the fish in a wooden chopping bowl. I buy fillets and grind them in my food processor. If you don't want to make gefilte fish, you can buy it frozen and ready to cook in your homemade vegetable broth, or even ready-made in a jar. You might like to try it in a healthy new presentation—in Springtime Green Salad with Gefilte Fish Balls, Sugar Snap Peas, and Asparagus (page 97).

To truly celebrate Passover as the springtime festival, it's a good idea to include plenty

---

Eggplant, the king of Middle Eastern vegetables, is also meaty and satisfying. Normally I serve Mediterranean stews of eggplant with tomatoes, peppers, and zucchini over rice, but they taste fine with baked or steamed potatoes or with whole wheat matzo.

Even leafy greens can become filling when cooked at length. Braised cabbage with onions and carrots is served as a side dish in France, but I occasionally eat it as an entrée with creamy mashed potatoes. Cooks from India simmer spinach with sautéed onions, chiles, and spices to create a thick, concentrated puree. It's great with boiled potatoes, spread on matzo, or just eaten with a spoon. Naturally, these dishes also make good accompaniments for chicken or meat.

A delectable, filling way to enjoy light vegetables such as asparagus, broccoli, and cauliflower is to combine them with plenty of onions sautéed in extra virgin olive oil.

Olive oil is a year-round favorite of many Sephardi Jews, but on Passover it gains prominence on the menus of observant Ashkenazim also. This is due to the kitniyot issue. According to How to Keep Kosher *by Lise Stern, many of the foods used to make vegetable oils—corn, sunflower seeds, sesame seeds, and soy beans—are included in lists of kitniyot. Canola oil, made from a plant in the mustard family, is considered kitniyot-derived too. Rabbi Shraga Simmons of aish.com, the Web site of Aish HaTorah, notes that those who are strict about kitniyot-based oils use only olive or walnut oil. Since walnut oil is expensive and not always easy to find, olive oil is the choice of many cooks.*

A fine, fruity olive oil enhances most vegetables, raw or cooked. Passover is a good time to try some of the fine kosher-for-Passover olive oils now being produced in Israel. A luscious, aromatic extra virgin olive oil makes vegetable dishes sing.

Let's not forget nuts, another useful, and healthy, Passover ingredient. For a finishing touch, I like to sprinkle my vegetable dishes with pecans or toasted almonds. They make the dish festive, a perfect celebration of spring.

of fresh produce every chance you get. Add extra carrots, celery, and squash to your chicken soup and slip vegetables into your savory matzo kugels.

Follow a custom of the French, who enjoy the season with dishes *à la printanière*, "in the springtime style," meaning surrounded by a selection of spring vegetables. If you're preparing roast turkey breast (see page 263), serve it not just with roasted potatoes, but also with asparagus tips, new carrots, small turnips, and spring onions heated together. You can also include fresh green peas, if it's your family's custom to eat them during Passover (some people who avoid legumes do not eat peas).

Many of the old-fashioned Passover specialties are still suitable for today, even with our faster-paced lifestyles. These perennially popular dishes tend to be convenient to serve. I give time-honored favorites a lively, healthy twist by including generous amounts of vegetables and herbs. I have developed some quicker, lighter versions of these favorites that keep their character intact but use only modest amounts of fat.

I make sure to include the quintessential Passover dish, matzo balls, in my Seder menu. As Whole Wheat Matzo Balls (page 201) they might embellish chicken soup with asparagus; or they might act as a partner for a colorful chicken stew—Chicken with Matzo Balls, Peppers, and Zucchini. Instead of the usual plain potato kugel, my version is a delicious, creamy casserole of cauliflower and potato punctuated with browned mushrooms and onions. Potato kugel is also good with plenty of onions and a few carrots added; or try a grated apple for a different effect.

Remember to prepare a big bowl of Israeli salad of diced tomatoes, cucumbers, onions, and chopped parsley. With its color and crunch, it can be the easiest way to get children to eat vegetables.

At dessert time, don't concentrate only on cake and cookies. Before you get to the sweets, set out a beautiful bowl of fruit salad. Slice some fresh, bright red strawberries and add orange wedges, banana slices, and diced apples and pears, moisten them with a little orange liqueur or orange juice, and, for a real treat, add chopped toasted hazelnuts or pecans. The family will greet this beautiful dessert with enthusiasm and enjoy its fresh taste. Then follow it with small portions of a sweet finale: either Macadamia Orange Cake with Red Berry Sauce or Passover Chocolate Cinnamon Brownies with Almonds (pages 108 and 107).

Persian Haroset with Pistachios and Pomegranate Juice

Springtime Green Salad with Gefilte Fish Balls,
Sugar Snap Peas, and Asparagus

Passover Salmon Cakes

Moroccan Potato and Diced Chicken Casserole

Chicken Stew with Matzo Balls, Peppers, and Zucchini

Passover Matzo Balls

Veal in Tomato Wine Sauce with Rosemary Gremolata

Roasted Asparagus with Citrus Dressing

Strawberry Soup with Yogurt

Passover Chocolate Cinnamon Brownies with Almonds

Macadamia Orange Cake with Red Berry Sauce

Hazelnut Macaroons

Passover Cinnamon Mandelbrot

PERSIAN HAROSET WITH PISTACHIOS AND POMEGRANATE JUICE

Pistachios and pomegranate juice make Persian haroset unique, and unlike most other kinds of haroset, it contains bananas too. This haroset is based on a recipe from Nilu Saadian, whom I often met at Chabad of Woodland Hills. She buys a special haroset spice blend at Persian kosher stores, but I add each spice separately. Nilu feels that pomegranate juice, a traditional element of the haroset, is very healthy, and this is borne out by modern research.

Nilu says the proportions of fruits and nuts are to taste, but she advises using a high proportion of nuts so the haroset will keep during the whole week of Passover, to be spread on matzo as a tasty, nutritious snack.

⅓ to ½ cup unsalted shelled pistachios, plus a few
    extra for garnish
⅓ to ½ cup walnuts
⅓ to ½ cup almonds
¾ to 1 cup dates, halved and pitted
¼ cup pomegranate juice, or to taste
2 to 4 tablespoons grape juice, or to taste
¾ teaspoon ground cinnamon

Pinch of ground cloves
½ teaspoon ground ginger
¼ teaspoon ground nutmeg
¼ teaspoon ground cardamom (optional)
1 small apple, peeled, cored, and halved
1 small pear, peeled, cored, and halved
1 small banana, diced fine
Matzos (for serving)

In a food processor, grind pistachios, walnuts, and almonds by pulsing them until fairly fine, leaving a few small chunks. Transfer to a bowl. Put dates in processor with pomegranate juice, 2 tablespoons grape juice, and spices, and grind to a paste. Add to nut mixture.

Coarsely grate apple and pear. Add to nut-and-date mixture. Stir in banana dice and mix well. Taste, and add more juice if needed—either pomegranate or grape juice, so the haroset can spread easily. If you prefer a finer paste, return mixture to food processor and process briefly.

Coarsely chop a few pistachios for garnish. Serve haroset at room temperature or cold, garnished with pistachios and accompanied by matzos.

Makes 10 to 12 servings

SPRINGTIME GREEN SALAD WITH GEFILTE FISH BALLS, SUGAR SNAP PEAS, AND ASPARAGUS

The first time we tasted kamaboko, the Japanese fish cakes shaped like a half-cylinder, we called it "Japanese gefilte fish" because of its delicate flavor. In Hawaii it's popular in pasta salads. We've also seen it in Japanese soups and as a garnish for Filipino rice noodles.

For this recipe, inspired by the Hawaiian salads, I use homemade gefilte fish matched with baby greens and spring vegetables instead of pasta. Making the gefilte fish from salmon gives the salad a lovely color contrast and the healthy benefits of the salmon's omega-3 content. (See "Safe Fish," page 237.) You can shape the gefilte fish in small balls for the salad as in the recipe below, and it will cook faster. When the weather is warm and I want a quick lunch, I sometimes use slices of prepared gefilte fish to garnish a bowl of green salad. Use any gefilte fish you prefer.

I like an Asian dressing for the salad, but I also serve red horseradish (horseradish with beets) on the side for anyone who wants a dab of this traditional accompaniment on the gefilte fish.

SALMON GEFILTE FISH BALLS

1 pound salmon fillet, free of skin and any small bones, cut into pieces

1 large egg

1 medium onion, finely chopped

¾ teaspoon salt

¼ teaspoon ground black pepper

2 tablespoons chopped fresh dill

1½ tablespoons matzo meal

3 cups Quick Fish Stock (page 371) or vegetable broth

GREENS, COOKED VEGETABLES, AND DRESSING

6 to 8 ounces thin asparagus, ends trimmed, spears cut into 2 pieces

4 to 6 ounces sugar snap peas

1 to 2 tablespoons rice vinegar, or more to taste

1 to 2 teaspoons low-sodium soy sauce (optional)

Salt and freshly ground black pepper

1 tablespoon vegetable oil

1 tablespoon Asian (toasted) sesame oil or additional vegetable oil, or more to taste

4 to 6 cups mixed baby greens, rinsed and dried

1 green onion, chopped

For salmon gefilte fish balls: Grind salmon in a food processor until very fine. Add egg, chopped onion, and measured salt and pepper, and process to blend. Transfer to a bowl. Stir in dill and matzo meal.

Combine fish stock and 1 cup water in a medium saucepan and bring to a simmer. Taste broth and add salt if needed. With moistened hands, shape fish mixture in balls, using about 2 tablespoons mixture for each. Carefully drop fish balls into simmering stock. If necessary add enough hot water to barely cover them, pouring it carefully near edge of pan, not over fish balls. Return to a simmer, cover, and simmer over low heat for 30 minutes. Let fish balls cool in their broth.

To cook vegetables for salad: Add asparagus to a saucepan of boiling salted water and cook, uncovered, over high heat for 3 minutes or until crisp-tender. Remove with a slotted spoon, rinse, and drain. Return liquid to a boil. Add sugar snap peas and boil, uncovered, for 2 minutes or until crisp-tender. Remove with a slotted spoon, rinse, and drain. Pat peas and asparagus dry.

For the dressing: Whisk rice vinegar with soy sauce (if using) and pepper in a small bowl. Whisk in vegetable oil and sesame oil.

A short time before serving, cut each gefilte fish ball in half. Put greens in a shallow serving bowl. Add green onion, half the asparagus, and half the sugar snap peas. Add dressing and toss lightly. Taste, adjust seasoning, and add more oil or vinegar if needed. Top with remaining asparagus, sugar snap peas, and gefilte fish.

Makes 4 to 6 servings

❈ PASSOVER SALMON CAKES

At a Passover party given by Women's American ORT, I met eighty-five-year-old Faye Waldman, who made delicious salmon cakes and gave me the recipe. The secret to their refined flavor was the fresh salmon that Ms. Waldman poached in white wine. Ms. Waldman enriched the cakes with real mayonnaise and sautéed them in butter. I have adapted the recipe to make them lower in saturated fat.

3 tablespoons olive oil or vegetable oil
1 large onion, chopped
½ cup dry white wine
2 pounds skinless salmon fillet, cut into cubes
Salt and freshly ground black pepper
Pinch of lemon pepper, or ½ teaspoon grated
   lemon zest

2 eggs
2 tablespoons low-fat mayonnaise
2 to 3 teaspoons snipped dill or chopped parsley
½ to ¾ cup matzo meal, plus ½ cup more for
   dipping

Heat 1 tablespoon oil in a deep skillet, add onion, and cook over medium-low heat until soft but not brown. Add wine and bring to a simmer. Add fish, salt, and pepper. Cover and cook for 1 to 2 minutes. Let stand off heat, covered, for 5 minutes or until salmon is cooked through. Drain any liquid remaining in pan. Adjust seasoning, adding lemon pepper to taste. Let cool.

Preheat oven to 400°F. Lightly beat eggs in a bowl and add salmon. Add mayonnaise, dill, and ½ cup matzo meal, or enough for mixture to hold together. Let mixture stand for 15 minutes to absorb the matzo meal.

Oil a baking sheet. Put ½ cup matzo meal on a plate and season it with salt and pepper. Form fish mixture in small cakes, using 3 to 4 tablespoons mixture for each.

Dip cakes in seasoned matzo meal and set them on baking sheet. Drizzle them with remaining 2 tablespoons oil. Bake for 15 to 20 minutes or until lightly browned. Serve hot or warm.

Makes about 8 appetizer servings

MOROCCAN POTATO AND DICED CHICKEN CASSEROLE

My husband's Moroccan cousin, Dvora Cohen, taught me how to make this favorite dish from her native land. Served year-round, it's especially popular for Passover and makes a festive lunchtime main course. Using the base of golden potato puree enriched with eggs and accented with turmeric, cooks add whatever meats and vegetables they have on hand, or omit the meat for a pareve version. Old-fashioned recipes call for large amounts of oil and eggs, but I have reduced the quantities for this healthy version.

If your family avoids peas and green beans on Passover, substitute 1 cup diced zucchini. As in Cauliflower and Potato Kugel with Mushrooms (page 148), you can substitute cauliflower for half the potato for extra nutrients.

2 pounds boiling potatoes, scrubbed, halved if large
1 medium carrot (about 4 ounces), halved crosswise
½ cup green beans, cut into 1-inch pieces
½ cup fresh shelled or frozen peas
3 to 4 tablespoons vegetable oil
2 large onions (1 pound total), chopped
2 large eggs

2 egg whites
¼ teaspoon turmeric
1 teaspoon salt
½ teaspoon freshly ground black pepper
1 to 1½ cups diced cooked chicken
⅓ cup chopped cilantro, flat-leaf parsley, or a
    mixture of both

Preheat oven to 350°F. Put potatoes in saucepan, cover with water, and add a pinch of salt. Bring to a boil and cook for 30 minutes or until tender. Remove with a slotted spoon to a colander. Add carrot and green beans to saucepan and cook for 5 minutes or until tender; remove with a slotted spoon. Add peas and cook fresh ones 2 to 5 minutes or until tender, or frozen ones for 1 minute. Drain well.

Heat 2 to 3 tablespoons oil in a large skillet. Add onions and sauté over medium heat for 10 to 15 minutes or until they begin to brown.

Peel potatoes and finely mash with potato masher. Add eggs one by one, beat well after each addition, then beat in egg whites. Stir in turmeric, salt, and pepper. Fold in chicken, carrots, green beans, peas, and cilantro. Taste and adjust seasoning.

Heat 1 tablespoon oil in a 2-quart casserole in oven for 2 minutes or until hot. Remove with pot holders and swirl casserole carefully so oil coats sides. Carefully add potato mixture without stirring in oil from sides of pan. Bake for 50 minutes or until a knife inserted in center comes out dry. Serve hot or warm.

Makes 4 to 6 servings

CHICKEN STEW WITH MATZO BALLS, PEPPERS, AND ZUCCHINI

This colorful entrée is perfect for the Seder, as it can be made in advance and reheated. If you like, substitute asparagus or green beans for the zucchini, or use pale green skinned Mexican zucchini (also called white or Tatuma squash). Cumin adds a good flavor, but if your family doesn't eat seeds on Passover, omit it; the chicken will still have plenty of flavor.

One 3½-pound chicken, cut into 8 serving pieces, skin removed
Salt and freshly ground black pepper
½ teaspoon turmeric
1½ teaspoons ground cumin
2 tablespoons extra virgin olive oil
1 large onion, thinly sliced
2 bell peppers, any color, cut into strips

3 large garlic cloves, minced
½ cup drained, chopped canned tomatoes
1½ cups chicken broth, or more if needed
1½ pounds zucchini, ends removed, cut into 2-inch sticks
3 tablespoons chopped cilantro, parsley, or dill (optional)
Passover Matzo Balls (page 102)

Sprinkle chicken on both sides with salt, pepper, turmeric, and 1 teaspoon cumin. Rub seasonings into chicken. Heat oil in a shallow stew pan. Add leg and thigh pieces and brown them lightly on all sides over medium-low heat. Remove them and brown remaining chicken pieces for only 1 or 2 minutes, so delicate breast meat won't be dry; remove.

Add onion to pan and cook over low heat for 5 minutes or until soft but not browned. Stir in bell peppers and garlic and cook, stirring often, about 5 minutes. Add tomatoes and remaining cumin. Set chicken on top, putting in leg and thigh pieces first to be sure they are close to base of pan. Add broth and bring to a boil. Cover and cook over low heat for 40 minutes or until chicken is tender.

Cook zucchini in a saucepan of boiling salted water for 2 minutes or until crisp-tender. Drain, rinse with cold water, and drain well.

Add zucchini to sauce and heat through. Add more stock if sauce is too thick. Stir in cilantro (if using), and salt and pepper if needed. Serve in shallow bowls or deep plates, with matzo balls.

Makes 4 servings

❖ PASSOVER MATZO BALLS

For Passover, matzo balls are made without baking powder. If you are careful to keep the batter soft, they will still be light. If you're substituting egg whites for two of the eggs, adding a little oil helps to compensate by contributing a pleasant richness to the matzo balls.

3 large eggs, or 1 egg plus 3 egg whites
¾ cup plus 2 tablespoons matzo meal
¼ teaspoon salt, or to taste
Pinch of black pepper

2 teaspoons olive oil or vegetable oil (optional)
2 to 3 tablespoons chicken broth or water
2 quarts salted water, or 1 quart water and
   1 quart chicken broth (for simmering)

In a small bowl, lightly beat eggs. Add matzo meal, salt, and pepper and stir with a fork until smooth. Stir in oil if you like. Add chicken broth by spoonfuls, adding enough so mixture is just firm enough to hold together in rough-shaped balls.

Bring salted water to a bare simmer. With wet hands, take about 2 teaspoons of dough and roll it between your palms into a ball; mixture will be soft. Gently drop matzo ball into simmering water. Continue making balls, wetting hands before shaping each one. Cover and simmer over low heat for 30 minutes. Keep them warm and covered until ready to serve; or refrigerate them in their cooking liquid, then reheat them gently in the liquid. (For an alternative method, see Note.) When serving, remove them carefully with a slotted spoon, add them to bowls, and spoon soup or sauce over them.

NOTE: Microwaving is an efficient way to reheat small amounts of matzo balls and enables you to refrigerate them without their liquid.

Transfer cooked matzo balls with a slotted spoon to a glass dish and cover them.

At this point you can refrigerate them. Reheat them in their covered dish in microwave.

Makes 4 servings

VEAL IN TOMATO WINE SAUCE WITH ROSEMARY GREMOLATA

A generous amount of vegetables complements the veal in this colorful Passover entrée. I use rosemary sprigs to flavor the wine sauce, and chopped fresh rosemary as part of the gremolata garnish, a classic Italian blend of parsley, lemon zest, and garlic. Sprinkled on the stew at the last moment, it does wonders to brighten its flavor. If you like, substitute 1 1/2 cups shelled fresh or frozen peas for the green beans, or use a mixture of both. If your family doesn't eat beans or peas during Passover, substitute 2-inch pieces of asparagus or strips of zucchini. Steamed new potatoes or rice pilaf are good accompaniments.

2 pounds boneless veal shoulder, cut into
    1- to 1 1/4-inch pieces, patted dry
2 tablespoons extra virgin olive oil
Salt and freshly ground black pepper
1 onion, chopped
1 carrot, chopped
2 parsley sprigs
3 rosemary sprigs
3 fresh thyme sprigs, or 3/4 teaspoon dried
    thyme, crumbled
1 bay leaf
1/2 cup dry white wine

One 14-ounce can tomatoes, drained and chopped
1 1/2 cups chicken broth
3 large garlic cloves, minced
1 1/2 pounds green beans, broken in 2 or 3 pieces
1 tablespoon tomato paste (optional)

ROSEMARY GREMOLATA
1 teaspoon finely grated or finely chopped lemon zest
1 medium garlic clove, very finely minced
    (1/2 teaspoon)
2 teaspoons finely minced fresh rosemary
1/4 cup minced flat-leaf parsley

Preheat oven to 350°F. Trim any fat from meat. In a heavy stew pan, heat oil over medium heat. Add half of veal, sprinkle lightly with salt and pepper to taste, and brown very lightly on all sides. Transfer veal pieces as they brown to a plate. Repeat with remaining veal.

Add onion and carrot to pan and scrape in juices from browning veal. Cook over low heat, stirring, until vegetables soften, about 7 minutes. Tie parsley, rosemary and thyme sprigs, and bay leaf in a piece of cheesecloth to make an herb bag and add to pan. Add wine and bring to a boil over high heat, stirring. Boil, stirring, until wine evaporates and pan is nearly dry.

Return veal to pan with any juices on plate. Add tomatoes, broth, and garlic and bring to a boil, stirring. Push down herb bag to immerse it in liquid. Cover and braise veal in oven for 1 1/4 hours or until veal is tender when pierced with point of a knife.

Boil green beans in a pan of boiling salted water for 6 minutes or until crisp-tender. Drain, rinse with cold water, and drain well.

Transfer veal to a plate with a slotted spoon. Discard herb bag. Stir tomato paste (if using) into sauce. Boil, stirring often, until sauce is thick enough to lightly coat a spoon. Return veal to pan of sauce and add green beans. Bring to a simmer. Taste and adjust seasoning.

To make gremolata, combine lemon zest, garlic, rosemary, and parsley in a small bowl. Mix thoroughly with a fork. At serving time, sprinkle gremolata evenly over hot veal. Cover and cook over low heat for 1 minute. Serve hot.

Makes 4 to 6 servings

❧ ROASTED ASPARAGUS WITH CITRUS DRESSING

Serving asparagus with orange sauce is a classic European custom. Olive oil and lemon juice give this asparagus salad a Mediterranean accent. It's perfect for Passover, Shavuot, or any festive springtime meal.

Low in calories but rich in nutrients, asparagus is an excellent source of vitamin A, vitamin C, vitamin K, and folate. It's a very good source of fiber and several B vitamins and a good source of calcium.

1 tablespoon plus 2 teaspoons extra virgin olive oil
2 teaspoons fresh orange juice
1 teaspoon fresh lemon juice

Salt and freshly ground black pepper
Cayenne pepper
1 pound medium-width asparagus

Combine 2 teaspoons olive oil, orange juice, lemon juice, salt, pepper, and cayenne in a small bowl. Whisk to combine. Taste and adjust seasoning.

Preheat oven to 450°F. Rinse asparagus and cut off tough bases, 1 to 1½ inches. Put asparagus in a roasting pan or large shallow baking dish so it makes one or two layers. Sprinkle evenly with 1 tablespoon oil and with salt, pepper, and cayenne to taste; toss to distribute seasonings. Roast uncovered, shaking pan once or twice to turn spears, about 12 minutes. When done, asparagus should be crisp-tender.

Put asparagus in a shallow serving dish and toss with dressing. Taste and adjust seasoning. Serve warm or at room temperature.

Makes 4 servings

❧ STRAWBERRY SOUP WITH YOGURT

This refreshing dessert soup is a fitting salute to spring during Passover week. I always reserve a few deep red strawberry slices for a lovely, natural garnish for the pink soup. You can enrich the soup with plain, vanilla, or strawberry-flavored yogurt, but pay attention to the calories—they vary widely. For the lowest-calorie version, choose a yogurt labeled "light," which is usually fat free and often uses a calorie-free sweetener. Instead of yogurt, you can enrich the soup with low-fat sour cream or leben, a mild form of yogurt available at Israeli markets.

For a pareve version, omit the dairy products or use soy yogurt (but not on Passover if your family avoids legumes).

When poaching the berries, you can substitute 1 cup dry white or rosé wine for half the water.

6½ cups strawberries, rinsed, then hulled

2 tablespoons honey

2 cups water, or 1 cup apple or white grape juice
    and 1 cup water

2 to 6 tablespoons sugar, or to taste, or
    2 tablespoons sugar and, if needed, calorie-free
    sweetener to equal 2 to 4 tablespoons sugar

1 tablespoon potato starch, dissolved in
    2 tablespoons cold water

1½ to 2 cups yogurt

2 teaspoons fresh lemon juice, or to taste

6 mint leaves

Reserve 6 strawberry slices for garnish. Make fresh strawberry puree: In a food processor or blender, puree 4 cups strawberries with honey until smooth. (There's no need to rinse food processor.)

In a saucepan bring remaining berries to a simmer with 2 cups water. Cover and simmer for 8 minutes or until berries are soft and liquid is red. Remove berries with a slotted spoon and puree them in food processor or blender until smooth. Mix with fresh strawberry puree.

To strawberry cooking liquid in pan, add 2 tablespoons sugar (but not sweetener) and dissolved potato starch, and bring to a simmer, stirring. Remove from heat.

Whisk 1¼ cups yogurt until smooth in a bowl, then gradually whisk cooking liquid from strawberries into it. Stir in strawberry puree mixture. Add lemon juice to taste, and more sugar or sweetener if desired. If soup is too thick, stir in a little more water, by tablespoons. Chill thoroughly.

Ladle into bowls. Garnish each serving with a dollop of yogurt topped with a strawberry slice and a mint leaf.

Makes 6 servings

PASSOVER CHOCOLATE CINNAMON BROWNIES WITH ALMONDS

These dark, chocolaty brownies are moist and tasty, so that even a small one satisfies as a sweet treat after dinner. They gain their richness from bittersweet chocolate and oil, combined either with a little butter (for dairy meals) or margarine (for meat meals). You can use light olive oil, which has a neutral flavor, or vegetable oil. If using margarine, choose one that is free of trans fats; soft tub margarines tend to be the best choice from a nutrition standpoint. For a special treat, frost the brownies with Spiced Chocolate Wine Glaze (page 373) and sprinkle them with 1/4 cup toasted slivered almonds.

5 ounces bittersweet or semisweet chocolate,
    chopped
3 tablespoons (1 1/2 ounces) unsalted butter or
    margarine, cut into pieces
1/2 cup brown sugar
1/2 cup granulated sugar
3 large eggs

5 tablespoons light olive oil or vegetable oil
1/2 teaspoon ground cinnamon
1/8 teaspoon salt
3/4 cup matzo meal
3 tablespoons unsweetened cocoa
2/3 cup chopped almonds

Preheat oven to 350°F. Grease a 9-inch square cake pan. Melt chocolate in a medium heatproof bowl over hot water. Stir until smooth. Remove from water; cool 5 minutes.

Soften butter. In mixer beat butter with brown and granulated sugars and eggs until very light and fluffy. Add oil, cinnamon, salt, matzo meal, cocoa, and melted chocolate. Beat slowly to combine. Stir in almonds.

Spoon batter into pan. Bake for 25 minutes or until color has changed evenly on top and a cake tester or toothpick inserted 2 inches from center comes out dry. Do not overbake. Cool in pan. Cut into squares. Serve at room temperature.

Makes 20 to 24 brownies

MACADAMIA ORANGE CAKE WITH RED BERRY SAUCE

Inspired by a French almond cake, this delicate dessert is good for Passover or any time of year. Although macadamia nuts are rich, much of their fat is monounsaturated.

Both the cake and the raspberry-strawberry sauce are flavored with a hint of citrus. Instead of serving the cake with the sauce, you can coat it with Spiced Chocolate Wine Glaze (page 373) and sprinkle it with chopped toasted macadamia nuts.

2 tablespoons unsalted butter or trans fat–free
    margarine
2 tablespoons vegetable oil
¾ cup macadamia nuts
½ cup plus 1 tablespoon sugar

3 large eggs
2 tablespoons orange juice
1 teaspoon grated orange zest
¼ cup potato starch, sifted
Red Berry Sauce (page 372)

Grease an 8-inch round cake pan, about 2 inches deep. Line base with a round of wax paper or foil; grease paper or foil. Preheat oven to 375°F.

Melt butter in a small saucepan over low heat; let cool, then stir in oil. Grind macadamia nuts with sugar in a food processor to a fine powder.

Beat 1 egg with macadamia mixture at low speed of mixer until blended, then at high speed for 2 minutes or until mixture is thick and smooth. Add remaining eggs one by one and beat at high speed about 3 minutes after each addition. Beat in orange juice and grated zest. Sprinkle potato starch over macadamia mixture and fold in gently. Gently fold in butter mixture in a fine stream.

Transfer immediately to cake pan. Bake for 28 to 30 minutes or until cake comes away from pan and a cake tester inserted into center of cake comes out clean. Carefully turn cake out onto a rack. Gently remove paper. Turn cake over again so smooth side is down. Let cool. Serve cake in slices, with sauce spooned around them.

Makes 8 servings

HAZELNUT MACAROONS

At Passover time, canned macaroons are ubiquitous at the supermarket and in kosher groceries, but these delicate cookies taste so much better homemade and they are easy to bake at home. The dough is made by simply blending the ingredients in the food processor.

Besides, the commercial ones are usually coconut based, and yours can be much healthier. Macaroons don't need any oil or egg yolks; the only fat they contain comes from nuts. Hazelnuts and almonds contain beneficial monounsaturated fat and are good to include in a heart-healthy diet.

Almonds keep the macaroons' color light and complement the taste of hazelnuts. Toast and peel the hazelnuts for the best flavor; in some markets you can purchase them already peeled.

1 cup hazelnuts
½ cup blanched almonds
1 cup sugar

2 large egg whites
1 teaspoon fresh lemon juice
1½ teaspoons grated orange zest

Position rack in upper third of oven and preheat to 350°F. Toast hazelnuts in a shallow baking pan in oven for 8 minutes or until skins begin to split. Transfer to a strainer. Rub hot hazelnuts energetically with a towel against strainer to remove some of skins. Cool nuts completely. Leave oven on.

Line a rimmed baking sheet with parchment paper or wax paper; grease paper lightly.

Grind hazelnuts and almonds with ¼ cup sugar in a food processor continuously until mixture forms fine, even crumbs. Add egg whites, lemon juice, and orange zest and process until smooth, about 20 seconds. Add remaining sugar in two additions and process for 10 seconds after each or until smooth.

With moistened hands, roll about 1 tablespoon mixture between your palms into a smooth ball. Put on prepared baking sheet. Continue with remaining mixture, spacing cookies about 1 inch apart.

Gently press to flatten each macaroon slightly so it is about ½ inch high. Brush entire surface of each with water. Bake for 18 to 20 minutes or until very lightly but evenly browned; centers should still be soft.

Remove from oven. Do not let cool. Lift one end of paper and pour about 2 tablespoons water under paper, onto baking sheet; water will boil on contact with hot baking sheet. Lift other end of paper and pour about 2 tablespoons water under it. When water stops boiling, remove macaroons carefully from paper. Cool them on a rack.

Makes about 20 macaroons

✿ PASSOVER CINNAMON MANDELBROT

These biscottilike cookies are based on a recipe I got from my friend Norma Laine after I sampled them at a Passover potluck party. To lower the fat content, I have replaced part of the oil with applesauce and added an alternative of egg whites instead of whole eggs. Almonds are the classic nut used in these crunchy cookies, but they taste good with all kinds of nuts. Sometimes I also add ½ cup chopped bittersweet chocolate. To enjoy them the traditional way, serve them with tea, for sipping and for dipping the mandelbrot.

1¼ cups matzo cake meal

2 tablespoons potato starch

¼ teaspoon salt

1 teaspoon ground cinnamon

3 eggs, or 1 egg plus 3 egg whites

¾ cup sugar

½ cup vegetable oil or light (neutral-flavored) olive oil

¼ cup applesauce

¾ cup chopped walnuts, pecans, or almonds

Sift together matzo cake meal, potato starch, salt, and cinnamon. In a large bowl, thoroughly beat eggs and sugar. Beat in oil and applesauce. Mix dry ingredients and nuts into egg mixture. Refrigerate at least 1 hour or up to 24 hours.

Preheat oven to 350°F. Lightly oil a cookie sheet. Lightly oil your hands and shape dough on sheet into logs of about 3×1 inch. Bake for 30 minutes or until lightly browned. Cool slightly. Transfer carefully to a board and let stand until cool enough to handle.

With a sharp knife, carefully cut into diagonal slices about ½ to ¾ inch thick; dough will be slightly soft inside. Return slices to cleaned baking sheets in one layer; you will need two or three baking sheets.

Reduce oven temperature to 200°F. Return cookies to oven and bake for 5 minutes on each side or until lightly browned. Don't let them brown throughout or they will be too dry. They'll become crisper as they cool. Cool on a rack. Keep in airtight containers.

Makes 20 to 24 cookies

Shavuot

THE FESTIVAL OF FIRST FRUITS AND DAIRY DELIGHTS

You'd think a holiday to celebrate cheese would be a French idea. Yet it is Shavuot, the Jewish festival that takes place in May or June, that highlights dairy foods. The official purpose of the two-day holiday is to commemorate the receiving of the Scriptures by Moses on Mount Sinai. Its unofficial raison d'être is that on this day you're supposed to indulge in creamy delights—noodle kugels with sour cream, cheese phyllo pastries, cheese blintzes, and most important of all, cheesecakes.

Yet Shavuot has a healthy message that's sometimes lost in the clamor for cheesecake. Dairy foods are not the only time-honored ingredients for Shavuot. Like other biblical holidays, Shavuot combines religious and agricultural themes. It's known as the holiday of the giving of the Torah, the festival of first fruits (*hag ha-bikurim*), and the feast of the harvest (*hag ha-katzir*).

In the Bible, grains and produce are more prominent than cheese for Shavuot. The story of Ruth, which is read on the holiday, takes place in the grain fields. Shavuot marks the end of the Omer period, referring to the days that were counted after the Omer offering—a measure of barley brought to the Temple on the second day of Passover. For Shavuot, the Temple offering also involved grains, baked as two loaves of bread.

The holiday's produce element appears as *bikurim*, the "first fruits" of the land. People arranged them in a basket and brought them ceremoniously to Jerusalem, as an expression of thanks. I can easily understand how this thanksgiving tradition came about; I am always thrilled to see the first fruits of my own garden—peaches and nectarines—at this time of year.

For Shavuot meal planning, this emphasis on produce is a good thing. Even to cheese aficionados, fresh vegetables and fruits provide a welcome balance.

Making a menu out of the grains and produce available in the region at that time, together with a modest amount of dairy foods, is a fitting way to bring Shavuot's biblical background to life. Besides, doing so can add up to a healthy holiday celebration. After all, the biblical diet was the original Mediterranean diet, so heartily recommended these days by nutritionists.

First, consider what foods were available. For someone who grew up in Israel, this is pretty easy. My husband readily recites the list of the "Seven Species" of the land of Israel, which he learned as a child—wheat, barley, grapes, figs, pomegranate, olives, and honey, which is interpreted as referring to the region's dates.

WHY WE CELEBRATE SHAVUOT WITH CHEESE

*M*any experts explain the practice of celebrating Shavuot with cheese in religious terms. On the day before the solemn event of receiving the Torah, the Hebrews abstained from eating meat for reasons of purity. In the Jewish way of thinking, if a meal is not fleishig or bsari—if it doesn't include meat—it's milchig or halavi (dairy) or pareve (neither).

According to the author of The Jewish Holidays, Rabbi Michael Strassfeld, "when the Israelites received the laws of kashrut (keeping kosher) at Sinai, they realized that all their pots were not kosher and so ate uncooked dairy dishes." Kashrut requires separating meat and dairy foods in menus and using different pans to cook them. Naturally, at this historic moment, the Hebrews did not want to incur divine displeasure due to improper pots. Desert nomads couldn't go down to their local cookware store to purchase two sets of pots and pans! So, for this unique occasion they feasted on fresh cheese.

The custom of eating dairy delicacies on Shavuot also is rooted in nature. In biblical times, early summer was the season when goats, sheep, and cows were giving an abundance of milk, and so there was a bounty of dairy foods to enjoy.

Today, I'm sure that many families observe this custom simply because they love it. When I lived in Israel, my neighbors began discussing their favorite cheesecake recipes for weeks before Shavuot. As a child, I preferred the meals of Shavuot above all others because I adored brunch-type dishes made with cheese, sour cream, butter, and eggs. I was sorry the holiday didn't last as long as Passover or Hanukkah because I wanted to enjoy these rich treats for a whole week. It's probably lucky for me that it didn't. At the time I didn't understand the importance of moderation!

Of course, the Seven Species were not the only produce items available for cooks to vary their meals. The Middle East is where agriculture began, and our ancestors enjoyed an assortment of crops. Cucumbers, eggplants, onions, melons, almonds, and pistachios were on the menu in ancient Israel's households. (But not tomatoes, peppers, or potatoes; they came from the New World.)

Dairy foods were often made from goat's and sheep's milk and undoubtedly resembled traditional Middle Eastern cheeses still popular today—strained yogurt (labneh), fresh white cheeses, and brined cheeses like feta.

These elements go together well in a menu. For example, you could make a vegetable soup with barley, a tabbouleh-type salad of bulgur wheat flavored with olive oil, and a raisin-studded cheesecake with a sauce of sliced dried figs warmed in honey. Another way to honor Shavuot is to create a single dish from most of the Seven Species, and to serve it for the holiday dinner along with your family favorites. Since the weather is warm on Shavuot, a salad is a good choice. (See Shavuot Seven Species Salad, page 115.)

Usually my Shavuot meals turn out to be eclectic. I like to prepare some classic Ashkenazi dishes that I grew up with, such as a savory noodle kugel or an easy-to-fix vegetable spread known as mock chopped liver that's made in Jewish homes in dozens of versions (page 155). One or two Sephardi specialties that I came to know and love in Israel, such as spinach cheese phyllo dough burekas (page 168), also appear on my menu, or eggplant matched with savory cheese, which I put in blintzes.

Since I spent years studying cooking in Paris, it's natural that this French culinary influence creeps into my Jewish holiday dishes too. A lox pâté is a favorite appetizer on my Shavuot table. In my kitchen, even my mother's cheesecake recipe has a subtle French twist.

For dessert, making a pudding of biblical grains cooked in milk is a wholesome way to enjoy the two Shavuot traditions. You can use barley or whole wheat berries, but a much faster-cooking choice is semolina. Semolina is simply durum wheat that is more coarsely ground than flour. Its tiny grains give puddings a more interesting texture than fine flour would. (See French Orange-Scented Semolina Pudding with Nectarines, page 130.)

❦

Shavuot Seven Species Salad

Linguine Salad with Spicy Tomato Dressing and Feta Cheese

Buckwheat Blintzes with Goat Cheese and Ratatouille

Grilled Fish with Olive-Vegetable Medley

Sesame Salmon with Spinach

Whole Wheat Blueberry Blintzes with Citrus Ricotta Filling

Lemony Blueberry Sauce

Light and Luscious Vanilla Cheesecake with Almonds

Creamy Peach Pistachio Noodle Kugel

Milk N' Honey First Fruits Salad

French Orange-Scented Semolina Pudding with Nectarines

❦

Combining the three Shavuot themes—grains and produce of ancient Israel along with dairy products—results in a nutritious, tasty salad. Start with cooked barley, bulgur wheat, or a mixture of both; each contributes a different flavor and texture. Then add raisins, dried figs, and dates, if you like. Pomegranates, one of the biblical Seven Species, are not in season on Shavuot, but you can flavor the dressing with the sweet-tart flavor of pomegranate paste, juice, or syrup. Enrich the salad with olive oil and a few olives. The ancient Israelis probably didn't have lemons, but they could season their salads with wine vinegar. (For more on the biblical Seven Species and foods available in ancient Israel, see page 112.)

Cucumbers add a refreshing quality and onions enliven the grains' flavor. For more of a sweet touch, you could add melon cubes too. If you'd like to boost the salad's nutrition with vegetarian protein, choose lentils or chickpeas from your biblical pantry. Toasted almonds or pistachios provide a festive finish.

To include the holiday's dairy theme and enhance the salad's flavor as well, add goat or feta cheese, or top each serving with a small dollop of tangy labneh (strained yogurt). Of course, if your menu features cheesecake, you may prefer to omit these rich milk products. After all, one advantage we have over the ancient Hebrews is refrigeration—so we can relax and not feel compelled to finish our dairy foods as quickly as they did!

This colorful bulgur and barley salad makes a festive meatless main course or appetizer. Serve it with a green salad, or as a buffet salad with dips and marinated vegetables.

In early autumn, when pomegranates become available, a few spoonfuls of pomegranate seeds are a lovely, tasty addition. Then it makes a delightful, strength-restoring salad for breaking the Yom Kippur fast or as a midweek Sukkot entrée.

4 tablespoons extra virgin olive oil, or more
    if needed
1 large onion, chopped
¾ cup pearl barley
2 cups vegetable broth
Salt and freshly ground black pepper
2 teaspoons fresh thyme or 1 teaspoon dried thyme
¾ cup medium bulgur wheat
⅓ cup dried figs or pitted dates, sliced, or some
    of each
¼ cup raisins

2 teaspoons pomegranate paste (optional)
2 tablespoons wine vinegar
2 teaspoons honey (optional)
¼ cup chopped green onion
¼ cup chopped flat-leaf parsley
2 or 3 small cucumbers, diced
⅓ cup pitted black olives, halved (optional)
½ to ¾ cup crumbled feta or Bulgarian cheese, or
    diced goat cheese (optional)
¼ cup sliced almonds, toasted

Heat 2 tablespoons oil in a large, heavy saucepan. Add onion and sauté over medium-low heat, stirring often, for 5 minutes or until softened but not browned. Remove half of onion and set aside. Add barley to pan and sauté, stirring, for 1 minute. Add 1¾ cups broth, salt, pepper, and thyme, and bring to a boil. Cover and cook over low heat for 40 minutes or until barley is tender, adding more broth if liquid evaporates before barley is cooked.

Spoon reserved onion into another saucepan and heat it. Add bulgur wheat and sauté, stirring, for 2 minutes. Add 1½ cups water, salt, and pepper and bring to a boil. Cover and cook over low heat for 10 minutes. Add figs and raisins, cover, and cook for 5 more minutes or until water is absorbed and bulgur and fruit are tender.

Fluff barley with a fork. Lightly fold in bulgur wheat mixture. Cool to room temperature.

For dressing, whisk pomegranate paste (if using) with vinegar, honey, salt, and pepper. Add remaining oil. Fold into barley mixture. Add green onion, parsley, cucumbers, and half the olives (if using). Taste and adjust seasoning. Serve topped with remaining olives, cheese, and almonds.

Makes 6 to 8 servings

LINGUINE SALAD WITH SPICY TOMATO DRESSING AND FETA CHEESE

Add feta and an uncooked vegetable dressing to pasta, and you have a quick dish bursting with flavor. Robust whole-grain pasta is a good match for the cheese and the spicy dressing. If you'd like a less salty cheese, use goat cheese or fresh mozzarella instead of feta. Another good choice is reduced-fat feta. For a pareve salad, you can omit the cheese or use strips of soy cheese or other nondairy cheeses. If you want the dressing to be less pungent, remove the seeds and membranes of the jalapeño peppers.

1 pound ripe tomatoes, finely diced
2 large garlic cloves, minced
1 or 2 jalapeño peppers, minced
Salt
2 or 3 green onions, sliced thin
2 teaspoons dried oregano
2 to 4 tablespoons extra virgin olive oil
8 ounces green beans, broken in 2 or 3 pieces
1 zucchini, cut into thin strips

8 ounces whole wheat, soy-enriched, or other whole-grain linguine
½ to 1 cup feta, crumbled (2 to 4 ounces)
1 poblano chile (called pasilla in California) or green or red bell pepper, roasted (page 376) and cut into strips
2 tablespoons chopped cilantro or flat-leaf parsley
⅓ to ½ cup pitted black olives, such as Kalamata (optional)

Combine tomatoes, garlic, jalapeño peppers, salt to taste, half the green onions, oregano, and 1 tablespoon oil in a small bowl. Stir to combine.

Cook green beans, uncovered, in a saucepan of boiling salted water over high heat for 4 minutes. Add zucchini and cook 1 to 2 minutes or until vegetables are crisp-tender. Drain well; if cooking vegetables in advance, rinse them with cold water to keep their color bright, and drain.

Cook pasta, uncovered, in a large pot of boiling salted water over high heat, stirring occasionally, for 5 to 8 minutes or until tender but firm to the bite.

Drain pasta well and transfer to a large heated serving bowl. Toss with 1 tablespoon oil, then with dressing. Reserve 2 to 3 tablespoons feta for garnish. Add bean mixture, roasted chile strips, cilantro, remaining green onions, and remaining cheese to pasta and toss. Taste and adjust seasoning. Top with reserved feta and with olives, if you like. Serve hot, warm, or at room temperature.

Makes 4 servings

❧ BUCKWHEAT BLINTZES WITH GOAT CHEESE
AND RATATOUILLE

In the land of Israel in biblical times, there were more goats than cows, and much of the cheese was undoubtedly goat cheese. This tasty cheese is a wonderful food to include in the Shavuot feast. With its tangy flavor, it is generally more suited to savory dishes than to desserts. I find the creamy, slightly crumbly kind that often comes in a log shape is perfect paired with ratatouille vegetables—eggplant and its Mediterranean friends—and baked inside a blintz. So is feta cheese, which can be made with milk from goats, sheep, or cows.

Blintzes resemble crepes except that blintzes are cooked on only one side before being filled. Buckwheat flour is a nutritious choice for making them. Russian cooks use it to make blinis. French creperies routinely use buckwheat crepes, or galettes de sarasin, with savory fillings, reserving the white-flour crepes for desserts. These blintzes are influenced by this healthy habit and are rolled around ratatouille, a French favorite that is quite similar to Sephardi eggplant fillings for pastries.

To reduce the fat and simplify the ratatouille's preparation, I braise the eggplant with the other vegetables instead of frying them the traditional way. I dice the vegetables small so the blintzes are easy to eat. For Shavuot's dairy custom, I enhance the filling with flavorful goat cheese. It complements the vegetables and the hearty blintzes beautifully, and a little goes a long way.

If you don't feel like making blintzes, you can use thin tortillas instead. Choose whole wheat or oat-flour blends for the best nutrition. For breakfast or brunch, you can use the same filling in omelets.

BUCKWHEAT BLINTZES

½ cup buckwheat flour

¼ cup plus 2 tablespoons all-purpose flour

½ teaspoon salt

2 large eggs

2 large egg whites

About 1¼ cups milk, preferably nonfat or low-fat

1 or 2 tablespoons canola oil or olive oil, plus a few
    teaspoons for pan

FILLING

3 fresh thyme sprigs

1 bay leaf

2 fresh rosemary sprigs

4 to 5 tablespoons olive oil, preferably extra virgin

1¼ pounds ripe tomatoes, peeled, seeded, and
    chopped, or one 14-ounce can tomatoes,
    drained and chopped

Salt and freshly ground black pepper

1 large onion, halved and chopped

1 small green bell pepper, cut into thin strips

1 small red bell pepper, cut into thin strips

6 to 8 ounces zucchini (3 small), diced small

1 pound thin eggplant, peeled and diced small

3 large garlic cloves, minced

6 to 8 ounces fairly creamy goat cheese

2 tablespoons chopped fresh basil leaves

Small basil sprigs for garnish (optional)

To make the blintzes: Sift together buckwheat flour, all-purpose flour, and salt. In a blender combine eggs, egg whites, 1 cup milk, and flour mixture. Blend on high speed for about 1 minute or until batter is smooth. Strain batter if it is lumpy. Cover and refrigerate for 1 hour or up to 1 day.

When you're ready to cook blintzes, stir batter well. Gradually whisk in 1 to 2 tablespoons oil. Batter should have consistency of whipping cream. If it is too thick, gradually whisk in more milk, about 1 tablespoon at a time.

Heat a 6- to 6½-inch crepe pan or skillet or an 8- to 9-inch skillet over medium-high heat. Sprinkle pan with a few drops of water. If water immediately sizzles, pan is hot enough. Brush pan lightly with oil. Remove pan from heat and hold it near bowl of batter. Working quickly, add 2 tablespoons batter to small pan or 3 tablespoons to large pan; add batter to edge of pan and tilt and swirl pan until base is covered with a thin layer of batter. Immediately pour any excess batter back into bowl.

Return pan to medium-high heat. Loosen edges of blintz with a metal spatula, discarding any pieces clinging to sides of pan. Cook blintz until its bottom browns very lightly. Slide blintz out onto a plate, with uncooked side facing up. Top with a sheet of wax paper or foil if you want to freeze them. Reheat pan a few seconds. Continue making blintzes, stirring batter occasionally with whisk. Adjust heat and brush pan with more oil if necessary. If batter thickens on standing, gradually whisk in a little water, about 1 teaspoon at a time. Pile blintzes on plate as they are done.

To make the filling: Make a bouquet garni by wrapping thyme, bay leaf, and rosemary in a piece of cheesecloth. Heat 1 tablespoon oil in a heavy stew pan. Add tomatoes, salt, pepper, and bouquet garni and cook over medium-high heat, stirring often, for 15 minutes.

Heat 1 to 2 tablespoons oil in a large sauté pan. Add onion and cook over medium-low heat for 5 minutes. Add green and red peppers and cook, stirring often, for 10 minutes; cover pan and add 1 to 2 tablespoons water if pan becomes dry. Add zucchini and cook over low heat for 3 minutes or until barely tender. Remove from pan. Pat pan dry.

Heat remaining 2 tablespoons oil in sauté pan. Add eggplant, salt, and pepper and sauté over medium-high heat for 5 minutes. Add tomato sauce, cover, and simmer for 10 minutes or until eggplant is tender.

Remove bouquet garni. Add garlic and zucchini-pepper mixture. Bring to a boil. Cover and cook over low heat for 2 minutes or until all vegetables are tender. If mixture is too thin, cook, uncovered, over medium-high heat for 3 minutes to evaporate excess liquid. Crumble in three-quarters of goat cheese. Stir in chopped basil. Taste and adjust seasoning.

Preheat oven to 425°F. Oil a large shallow baking dish or 2 medium baking dishes. Set aside a few tablespoons of filling for garnish. Spoon 3 tablespoons filling onto browned side of each blintz, across blintz's lower third. Roll up in cigar shape, beginning at edge with filling. Arrange blintzes, seam side down, in one layer in oiled dish. Brush blintzes with oil.

Bake blintzes for 10 minutes or until filling is hot. Serve immediately, garnishing each with a small spoonful of reserved filling, topped with a little crumbled goat cheese and small basil sprigs, if you like.

Makes 6 servings

For this Sicilian-inspired entrée, the fish is crowned copiously with lightly cooked vegetables. The colorful mixture of broccoli, carrots, zucchini, and red peppers has a lively taste, due to a small number of bold flavorings: olives, olive oil, balsamic vinegar, fresh basil, and cayenne pepper.

According to food historian Clifford Wright, Jews in Sicily used olive oil more than other Sicilians did in the Middle Ages, as they did not cook with lard, and Jewish merchants exported Sicilian olive oil.

When spooned over the fish, the tasty vegetables play a double role, acting both as accompaniment and as sauce, keeping the fish moist and succulent. Grilling the fish and serving it with a vegetable sauté makes for an entrée that is lower in calories than flouring the fish, frying it in oil, and stewing it with the vegetables the old-fashioned way.

There are plenty of variations you can easily prepare, depending on what you feel like eating. The vegetable sauté is almost like a warm salad and can be served as such, even without the fish. Or you could combine the vegetables with vermicelli or other pasta, either as an entrée or as a substantial side dish to serve with a grilled or broiled fish. Whichever way you choose to go, the result is a light but satisfying dish, perfect for Shavuot, when the weather is often warm. You can either grill or broil the fish fillets for this dish.

1½ pounds fish fillets, such as sea bass, cod, halibut, haddock, or salmon

1 carrot, cut into diagonal slices

2 cups large broccoli florets, cut into thick lengthwise slices

3 tablespoons extra virgin olive oil

1 pound zucchini, halved and cut into ⅜-inch slices

Salt and freshly ground black pepper

1 red bell pepper, cut into strips

1 garlic clove, chopped (optional)

¼ to ⅓ cup sliced flavorful olives, green or black

¼ teaspoon cayenne pepper or hot red pepper flakes, or to taste

2 tablespoons chopped fresh basil

1 to 2 tablespoons balsamic vinegar

Run your fingers over fish and carefully pull out any bones with aid of tweezers or a sharp paring knife. Pat fish dry. If using grill, brush or spray it lightly with oil to prevent sticking. Preheat grill or broiler.

Add carrot and broccoli to a saucepan of enough boiling salted water to cover them and cook, uncovered, over medium-high heat for 5 minutes or until just crisp-tender. Drain well.

Heat 1 tablespoon oil in a large, heavy sauté pan or stew pan. Add zucchini, salt, and pepper. Sauté over medium heat, stirring often, for 2 minutes or until not quite tender. Remove to a plate with a slotted spoon.

Add 1½ tablespoons oil to pan and heat it. Add red bell pepper and sauté over medium heat for 5 minutes or until barely tender. Stir in garlic (if using) and add carrot, broccoli, zucchini, salt, and pepper. Heat through. Add olives, cayenne, basil, and vinegar and mix well. Taste and adjust seasoning.

Brush fillets with remaining oil and season lightly with salt and pepper. Arrange fish on grill or broiler pan. Broil or grill fish for 4 minutes on each side, or just until fish turns opaque. Transfer fish to plates. Heat vegetable mixture briefly and serve over fish. Serve hot or warm.

Makes 4 servings

❧ SESAME SALMON WITH SPINACH

Fish dishes are a great choice for Shavuot entrées because a dairy dessert can be served as the kosher meal's festive finale. This colorful, nutritious dish makes a savory Shavuot starter or entrée. It can also be served cold as an easy summertime lunch.

A double dose of sesame—toasted oil and toasted seeds—is what makes this Japanese-seasoned dish so flavorful, along with mirin (sweet Japanese rice wine), soy sauce, and sugar. You can add grated ginger or cayenne pepper for a touch of spice. If you don't have mirin, use sake (rice wine), sherry, or white wine, and add an extra teaspoon of sugar. You can also omit the salmon and serve the spinach as a partner for other grilled, baked, or braised fish, broiled chicken, or tofu.

1 to 2 tablespoons soy sauce

4 teaspoons mirin (sweet Japanese rice wine)

2 teaspoons Asian sesame oil

2 teaspoons sugar

1 teaspoon grated peeled ginger (optional)

Pinch of cayenne pepper (optional)

1 to 1½ pounds salmon fillet

3 pounds fresh spinach, stems removed, or
*   two 10-ounce bags of cleaned spinach leaves*

2 tablespoons sesame seeds, toasted (page 380)

Preheat oven to 450°F. In a small bowl, whisk soy sauce, mirin, sesame oil, sugar, ginger, and cayenne (if using). Set salmon in a heavy roasting pan. Sprinkle fish with 1 teaspoon of soy sauce mixture and rub it over fish. Roast salmon, uncovered, for 12 to 15 minutes or until fish can just be flaked with a fork and has changed color in its thickest part. Keep warm or set aside to cool.

Thoroughly rinse spinach leaves. Boil spinach leaves in a saucepan of boiling salted water, uncovered, over high heat for 2 minutes or until just tender. Drain in a colander, rinse with cold water, and drain well. Gently squeeze dry by handfuls. Gently separate squeezed clumps of spinach and put on a serving platter or on plates in a fairly thin layer. Arrange salmon next to spinach.

Drizzle 1 teaspoon soy sauce mixture on salmon, and pour remaining mixture over spinach. Taste and adjust seasoning. Just before serving, sprinkle salmon and spinach with toasted sesame seeds. Serve at room temperature.

Makes 4 servings

WHOLE WHEAT BLUEBERRY BLINTZES WITH CITRUS RICOTTA FILLING

Blueberries—one of the joys of summer—flavor the filling and the sauce for these luscious blintzes. Nutritionally, they are a "superfood," one of the best foods you can eat. They are higher in antioxidants, or substances that protect the body's cells from damage, than almost any fruit or vegetable. They have plenty of fiber too. In these blintzes fresh blueberries are best, but when they're out of season, you can use frozen berries.

Low-fat sour cream mixed with ricotta makes a creamy filling that seems richer than it really is, and nicely complements the blueberries. For an elegant presentation, spoon a little blueberry sauce over each blintz and top it with a small dollop of lemon or orange yogurt and a few blueberries.

WHOLE WHEAT BLINTZES

¾ cup whole wheat flour

¾ teaspoon salt

3 large eggs

About 1⅓ cups milk

2 tablespoons vegetable oil, or 1 tablespoon butter and 1 tablespoon oil

A few teaspoons vegetable oil for pan

RICOTTA BLUEBERRY FILLING

1 cup fresh or frozen blueberries

3 to 5 tablespoons sugar, or to taste

2 cups ricotta, low-fat or nonfat (about 15 ounces)

¼ cup low-fat or nonfat sour cream or lemon- or orange-flavored yogurt

1 large egg, or 1 egg white

1 teaspoon grated lemon zest

1 teaspoon grated orange zest

2 to 3 teaspoons butter (optional)

1 tablespoon vegetable oil

Lemony Blueberry Sauce (page 125), or 1 cup fresh blueberries

To make blintzes: Sift flour with salt. In a blender combine eggs, 1¼ cups milk, and flour mixture. Blend on high speed about 1 minute or until batter is smooth. Strain batter if it is lumpy. Cover and refrigerate about 1 hour or up to 1 day.

When you're ready to cook the blintzes, heat oil or mixture of oil and butter in microwave or in a very small saucepan over low heat. Stir batter well. Gradually whisk oil into batter. It should have consistency of whipping cream. If it is too thick, gradually whisk in more milk, about 1 teaspoon at a time.

Heat a 6- to 6½-inch crepe pan or skillet or an 8- to 9-inch skillet over medium-high heat. Sprinkle pan with a few drops of water. If water immediately sizzles, pan is hot enough. Brush pan lightly with oil. Remove pan from heat and hold it near bowl of batter. Working quickly, add 2 tablespoons batter to small pan or 3 tablespoons to large pan; add batter to edge of pan and tilt and swirl pan until base is covered with a thin layer of batter. Immediately pour any excess batter back into bowl.

Return pan to medium-high heat. Loosen edges of blintz with a metal spatula, discarding any pieces clinging to sides of pan. Cook blintz until its bottom browns very lightly. Slide blintz out onto a plate, with uncooked side facing up. Reheat pan a few seconds. Continue making blintzes, stirring batter occasionally with whisk. Adjust heat and brush pan with more oil if necessary. If batter thickens on standing, very gradually whisk in a little more water, about 1 teaspoon at a time. Pile blintzes on plate as they are done.

To make filling: Sprinkle blueberries with 1 tablespoon sugar and let stand for 5 minutes. Mix ricotta with sour cream, egg, remaining sugar, and lemon and orange zests until well blended. Stir in blueberries.

Spoon 2½ tablespoons filling onto brown side of each blintz near one edge. Fold over edges of blintz to right and left of filling so that each covers about half of filling. Roll up blintz, beginning at edge with filling.

Preheat oven to 400°F. Arrange blintzes in one layer in a shallow, lightly oiled baking dish. Melt butter (if using) in a small dish in microwave and mix with oil. Lightly brush blintzes with mixture. Bake for 20 minutes or until heated through and lightly browned.

Serve blintzes with sauce or with fresh blueberries.

Makes 6 servings, about 12 large or 15 small blintzes

✸ LEMONY BLUEBERRY SAUCE

Pureed and whole berries form this tasty sauce. Serve it over Whole Wheat Blueberry Blintzes (page 123) with their ricotta filling, with plain cakes like angel food cake, or spoon it over yogurt or sundaes.

Brown rice syrup is a mild-tasting sweetener that is less sweet than sugar. You can find it at natural foods stores.

1 cup fresh or frozen blueberries
½ cup water
½ teaspoon grated lemon zest
1 to 2 tablespoons maple syrup, honey, or brown
*   sugar, or 2 to 3 tablespoons brown rice syrup*

2 teaspoons cornstarch
1 to 2 teaspoons fresh lemon juice

Puree ¼ cup blueberries in a blender or mini-food processor. Transfer to a small saucepan. Add water, lemon zest, syrup, and cornstarch. Bring to a simmer over medium heat, stirring. Stir in ½ cup blueberries and simmer for 1 or 2 minutes or until thickened. Stir in lemon juice and remaining ¼ cup berries. Taste, and add more syrup or lemon juice if you like.

Makes 1 cup, about 6 servings

🔯 LIGHT AND LUSCIOUS VANILLA CHEESECAKE WITH ALMONDS

People often describe a specific dessert as healthy because it is low in this or low in that. But this delicious cheesecake is healthy due to its beneficial ingredients. The yogurt and ricotta cheese contribute calcium. Almonds add richness and a pleasing crunch to the crust and the topping, and from a health standpoint, possess monounsaturated fat as well as fiber and vitamin E. Raspberries have everything going for them—a star companion to creamy cheesecake because of their fine flavor and lovely color, they are also nutritional superfoods.

Vanilla bean seeds and vanilla yogurt give the cheesecake a good vanilla flavor. Choose trans fat–free cookies or graham crackers for the crust. Roasted almond oil is a great choice in the almond crust, but if you don't have it, use light olive oil; it has the healthy fat profile of olive oil, but its flavor is neutral like that of vegetable oil and it will not give the cake an "olive" taste.

For a variation, make the crust with low-fat cocoa cookies. If you like, substitute a calorie-free sweetener such as sucralose for the sugar in the crust, and for 1/4 cup of the sugar in the filling.

ALMOND CRUMB CRUST

5 ounces plain low–fat cookies or low–fat graham crackers (to obtain 1 1/4 cups crumbs)

3 tablespoons slivered almonds

1 1/2 tablespoons sugar

2 to 3 tablespoons almond oil, light olive oil, or vegetable oil

VANILLA CHEESE FILLING

3/4 cup sugar

One 15–ounce container fat–free ricotta (1 3/4 cups)

1/2 cup nonfat sour cream

2 large eggs, separated, or 1 egg, separated, and 1 egg white

2 tablespoons whole wheat or all-purpose flour

1 1/2 teaspoons grated lemon zest

Seeds scraped from 1 split vanilla bean, or 1 teaspoon pure vanilla extract

1/4 cup low–fat or nonfat vanilla yogurt

CREAMY TOPPING WITH ALMONDS

3/4 cup low–fat or nonfat vanilla yogurt or plain yogurt

3/4 cup nonfat sour cream

2 to 3 tablespoons sugar

1 teaspoon pure vanilla extract

3 to 4 tablespoons sliced almonds

Red Berry Sauce (page 372), for serving

To make crust: Preheat oven to 350°F. Process cookies in a food processor to fine crumbs. Measure 1 1/4 cups. Add almonds and sugar and process to chop almonds. Mix almond mixture with cookie crumbs in a bowl. Add just enough oil to barely moisten the mixture, and mix well. Lightly oil a 9-inch springform pan. Press crumb mixture in an even layer on bottom and about 1 inch up sides of pan. Bake for 7 minutes. Let cool completely. Leave oven at 350°F.

To make cheese filling: Set aside 1 tablespoon sugar to beat into egg whites. Beat ricotta with sour cream at low speed until very smooth. Gradually beat in remaining sugar. Beat in egg yolks, flour, lemon zest, and vanilla. Stir in yogurt. In a small bowl, whip egg whites to soft peaks. Beat in reserved tablespoon sugar and continue beating whites until stiff. Fold them into ricotta mixture. Carefully pour filling into cooled crust. Bake for 50 minutes or until top center is just firm but still shakes when you gently move pan; cracks will form in cake. Remove from oven and cool for 15 minutes. Raise oven temperature to 425°F.

To make topping: Pour off any liquid from top of yogurt. Mix yogurt with sour cream, sugar, and vanilla. Spoon topping evenly over cake in spoonfuls. Carefully spread topping in an even layer, without letting it drip over edge of cake. Bake cake for 4 minutes. Sprinkle evenly with sliced almonds. Bake for 3 more minutes. Remove from oven and cool to room temperature. Refrigerate at least 2 hours before serving. Remove sides of pan a short time before serving. Serve with berry sauce.

Makes 10 servings

CREAMY PEACH PISTACHIO NOODLE KUGEL

To enrich this delicate-tasting dessert kugel, I cook the noodles in low-fat milk. It's amazing how creamy they become. Garnish each portion with extra peach slices and a dollop of peach or vanilla yogurt sprinkled with pistachios.

2½ cups milk
1 cup very fine noodles
Pinch of salt
1 teaspoon finely grated lemon zest
4 to 6 tablespoons sugar

1 tablespoon butter (optional)
¼ cup chopped unsalted pistachios
2 peaches, peeled and chopped, or 2 nectarines, chopped
2 large eggs

Bring milk to a simmer in a heavy, medium saucepan. Add noodles and salt, and cook over low heat, stirring occasionally, for 20 to 30 minutes or until noodles are tender and absorb most of milk.

Meanwhile, preheat oven to 350°F. Butter or oil a 4- to 5-cup baking dish and sprinkle a little sugar on sides of dish. Set this dish inside a larger baking dish.

Stir lemon zest and 4 tablespoons sugar into hot noodle mixture. Cool several minutes. Stir in butter (if using), pistachios, peaches, and eggs. Add more sugar if desired.

Transfer to baking dish. Add very hot water to larger baking dish, enough to come halfway up sides of dish containing noodle mixture. Bake for 40 minutes or until a small knife inserted into noodle mixture comes out dry. Serve warm.

Makes 6 servings

Shavuot celebrates the "first fruits" of the land of Israel, and some say we eat dairy foods for the holiday because the Promised Land was known in the Torah as "the land of milk and honey." This festive fruit salad combines both themes. The milk in the topping comes in the form of yogurt or low-fat sour cream. As a finishing touch, sprinkle toasted almonds, another food of the Bible, or a little almond granola.

You can substitute 1 1/2 cups diced cantaloupe for the nectarines. If your family insists on cake for dessert, spoon each serving over a slice of angel food or other light cake, or serve it with Macadamia Orange Cake (page 108).

4 ripe nectarines or peaches, or 2 of each
1½ cups strawberries, rinsed, hulled, and sliced
    lengthwise
1 cup raspberries
½ cup blueberries or blackberries
3 tablespoons honey

1 tablespoon fresh lemon or orange juice
1 cup nonfat or low-fat yogurt, or ¾ cup yogurt
    mixed with ¼ cup nonfat or low-fat sour cream
1 teaspoon pure vanilla extract
2 to 3 tablespoons toasted sliced or slivered almonds
    or almond granola

Cut nectarines in wedges and put in a bowl. Add strawberries, raspberries, blueberries, 1 tablespoon honey, and lemon juice.

In another bowl mix yogurt with remaining honey and vanilla. At serving time, divide fruit among 4 dessert dishes and spoon honey-yogurt sauce on top. Sprinkle with toasted almonds.

Makes 4 servings

When I lived in Paris, I found that homey French semolina puddings made enticing comfort food. Their preparation begins like that of breakfast cereal. You cook semolina in milk, then lightly sweeten the mixture with sugar. To turn it into a dessert, cooks add rum-soaked raisins, beautiful candied fruit, dates, or even prunes softened in tea. For further enhancement of the dessert's flavor, the milk might first be infused with a vanilla bean or with strips of orange or lemon zest.

Often the mixture is enriched with egg yolks. Some people turn it into an even fancier sweet by lining a mold with caramel and baking the semolina pudding inside, then unmolding it so it has a golden-brown sauce like crème caramel. Other elegant versions are enriched with chopped toasted hazelnuts or melted chocolate.

Italian cooks make a similar creamy semolina pudding with raisins and rum or with chopped almonds. Greek semolina pudding might be flavored with cinnamon and enriched with walnuts. In Turkey, semolina is made into helva, a form of halvah that resembles a thick buttery pudding, often flavored with saffron and embellished with pistachios. Tunisian cooks make pine nut semolina pudding garnished with thick cream and nuts.

For Shavuot I like to enhance a lightened version of the French home-style pudding with my own "first fruit"—sweet white and yellow nectarines fresh from my garden. If you like, use peach liqueur instead of orange or, for an alcohol-free pudding, substitute 1 teaspoon pure vanilla extract. Use whole wheat semolina if you like; you can find it at natural foods stores.

3½ cups milk
Pinch of salt
1 vanilla bean, split
¾ cup semolina
½ to ¾ cup sugar, or ¼ cup honey and ¼ to ½ cup
   sugar
Grated zest of 2 oranges
1 or 2 egg yolks (optional)

⅓ cup vanilla yogurt, plus a few more tablespoons
   if needed
2 tablespoons orange liqueur, such as Curaçao or
   Cointreau
2 or 3 nectarines or peaches
2 tablespoons sliced almonds, lightly toasted, or
   chopped pistachios (optional)

Bring milk and salt to a boil. Add vanilla bean, cover, and let stand for 15 minutes; then remove vanilla bean.

Return milk to a boil. Reduce heat to low. Gradually add semolina, stirring constantly. Cook over low heat, stirring, for 5 minutes. Add ½ cup sugar, or ¼ cup honey and ¼ cup sugar, and cook for 2 minutes, stirring.

Remove from heat and add grated orange zest. Stir in egg yolks one by one, if using Cool to room temperature. Stir in ⅓ cup vanilla yogurt, followed by liqueur. If pudding is too thick, stir in more yogurt by tablespoons. Taste, and add more sugar by tablespoons if needed. Transfer pudding to a serving bowl or to individual dessert dishes. Refrigerate for 2 hours before serving. You can refrigerate pudding in a covered dish for 1 day.

To decorate pudding, cut nectarines or peaches in thin wedges. Garnish pudding with nectarine wedges and almonds, if you like. Serve cold.

Makes 6 servings

Shabbat

✳

"Let's buy this for Shabbat!" my mother always said when we shopped together and found something special, whether it was an expensive fish, an exotic fruit, or fine chocolate. She was following a time-honored custom—that Shabbat should be a celebration, a theme that permeates Jewish folklore. As a child, I often heard stories emphasizing that even the poorest of Jews did their best to make Shabbat festive.

According to Martine Chiche Yana, author of *La Table Juive* (*The Jewish Table*), published by Edisud, 1990, "Tradition tells us that the six days of the week (not including Shabbat) are divided in two periods . . .

—during the first period, from Sunday to Tuesday, everyone lives in the atmosphere of nostalgia for the Shabbat that had just passed;

—during the second period, from Wednesday to Friday, everyone is waiting for the upcoming Shabbat." (My translation)

This attitude is shared by observant Jews worldwide. Shabbat is a day to look forward to. It is the time when busy family members make a point of getting together to relax and share a meal. Usually the Shabbat meals on Friday night and Saturday afternoon turn out to be the most festive menus of the week, celebrated on an attractive table set with candles, wine, and braided challah.

The choice of dishes is dictated by the Torah prohibition against working and lighting a fire on Shabbat. Menus feature foods that have been cooked ahead. Often they start with a cold appetizer, such as a fish dish. Gefilte fish is the most famous of these and is a healthy choice. Equally famous is chopped liver; you can improve its nutritional profile by slipping in a secret ingredient (see recipe, page 155). But there's no reason to be limited to old-fashioned first courses. You can start off with an array of colorful, healthful vegetable appetizers, such as Balkan Pepper Dip (page 158), Onion Compote with Pine Nuts and Raisins (page 164), and Spicy Spinach Tahini (page 161), accompanied by whole wheat challah or other whole-grain breads.

Chicken soup with matzo balls and a savory or sweet kugel are staples of the Shabbat menu, as both reheat beautifully. It's easy to boost chicken soup's nutrition by including plenty of fresh vegetables and garnishing it with light, whole wheat matzo balls. Kugels have always been a favorite of mine. Making these casseroles gives cooks a great chance to include produce in the meal in a creative and festive way—for example, by

SHUL FOOD

*N*ot many people think of going to Shabbat services as a gastronomic experience.

Yet, after diligently praying for heavenly goodwill, many appreciate temporal rewards in the form of Jewish soul food. The occasion for the indulgence is the kiddush, which technically means a blessing over wine, but has been extended to refer to a light meal served at the ceremony.

Chabad Web sites advertise this bonus on the Saturday schedule: "Morning prayers, followed by kiddush with hot cholent." For those who are not computer literate, I've often heard the rabbi finish his recitation of upcoming services and classes with the announcement "and we have the best cholent in town."

The tasty, well-seasoned cholent at our local Chabad synagogue contains little cubes of beef, potato chunks, sweet vegetarian kishke (which resembles bread stuffing), barley, and beans. Those who want something lighter than cholent can usually find tuna salad, gefilte fish with horseradish, egg salad, coleslaw, crackers, cookies, and marble cake. Occasionally there might be potato kugel, smoked whitefish salad, and even Chinese chicken salad with a sweet ginger dressing and fried chow mein noodles. And, for a l'chayim, a shot of vodka.

But there's much more to shul food. It varies by location and by congregation. When I was growing up, kiddush at our shul was composed of typical American-Jewish brunch food—bagels with lox and cream cheese, mini-gefilte fish balls, marinated herring, Jell-O molds, and iced white and chocolate sheet cakes.

Several years ago, my mother and I visited Honolulu and found the Shabbat experience at Chabad of Hawaii completely different from any we'd had before. First of all, the shul was in a hotel. The kiddush was a full lunch, for the benefit of tourists searching for a kosher Shabbat meal. On our visit, the Israeli-Moroccan buffet included spicy fish and cooked pepper salad, as well as the islands' sweet pineapple in a fruit salad, and soft, block-shaped Hawaiian sweet rolls.

accenting them with sautéed mushrooms (see page 148) or with apples and apricots (page 50).

For a main course on Saturday afternoon, there often is cholent or hamin, prepared by Jews around the world. Cholent has a reputation for being heavy, but this one-pot meal of grains, beans, and meat can be one of the most healthful of dishes, if you use a modest amount of meat. Choose a low-fat cut; you don't need to worry that perhaps it might be tough, as it tenderizes beautifully from being slowly cooked overnight. (For more on cholent, see page 136.)

When there's a bar mitzvah, shul spreads can become elaborate or even downright fancy, especially if the family brings a caterer into the picture. A shul in Montgomery County, Maryland, where I grew up, offers kiddush dishes that I never heard of as a child, like balsamic four-bean salad, sesame cabbage salad, crisp apple rice salad, and cumin-flavored corn-and-bean salad. A Rhode Island kosher caterer suggests French-style quiches for a kiddush menu: one of mushrooms and caramelized onions, and another of eggplant, roasted peppers, and goat cheese. In Melbourne, Australia, the kiddush food of Passionate Kosher Catering is eclectic. In addition to the usual Ashkenazi-Jewish items, you can have Indian and Japanese vegetables, Moroccan couscous, Persian brown rice, and a sabra cake made of orange and chocolate cake layers, chocolate mousse, and chocolate ganache. With such offerings, going to the synagogue is practically like visiting a gourmet restaurant.

Small shuls have their own selections of tempting kiddush treats. At a neighbor's bar mitzvah kiddush, the shul's caterer happened to be Persian. His menu featured three types of cholent. The one I liked best was vegetarian, consisting mainly of deeply browned rice, carrots, tomatoes, and sautéed onions.

The most memorable shul food I've had to date was in the humblest of surroundings—Yemenite Shabbat services in the converted garage of a Los Angeles house, the rest of which serves as a Moroccan synagogue. There the food was a potluck. Some people brought typical Israeli items like potato burekas (phyllo pastries), spicy carrots, hummus, tahini, pickles, and pita. For me the highlight was the wonderful Yemenite Shabbat cake called **kubaneh,** *made of a rich, slightly sweet yeast dough. The woman who had baked it overnight kept it warm at shul by covering the pot with a blanket.*

A favorite shul food of mine is Jerusalem kugel, which is not well known to American Jews. I often wish it would appear on the kiddush tables at American synagogues to evoke the flavors of Jerusalem. Fortunately, it's easy to make at home. (For my whole wheat pasta version, see page 152.)

CHOLENT—THE JEWISH MOTHER OF CASSOULET

*W*hen I used to walk around my mother's Jerusalem neighborhood on Saturday around noon, I enjoyed the aroma of cholent that filled the air. Perhaps the most universal Jewish dish, this meal-in-one-pot is one of the few cooking formulas with roots in the Torah. Not that you would find a commandment, "Thou shalt eat cholent." It's the prohibition against lighting a fire on Shabbat that led to the prominence of this age-old recipe for overnight stews. Observant cooks prepare cholent faithfully and speak of it with reverence, almost as if it were an ordained ritual.

Called hamin *in Hebrew and* cholent *in Yiddish, this satisfying entrée is known primarily as a casserole of meat and beans. Over the centuries, as Jews migrated to many parts of the world, they came up with countless savory variations. Both my mother, born in Warsaw, and my mother-in-law, born in Yemen, fed their families cholent, but the seasonings and certain elements were different.*

Beef is the most frequently used meat for cholent, usually a long-cooking cut like brisket. Chicken is a close second, but cooks might choose turkey or lamb. Each cook has his or her favorite beans. They might be large or medium white beans, pink beans, brown beans, chickpeas, or a mixture of these. My mother added barley and occasionally a big matzo ball, which was sliced for serving. Whole wheat berries are another favorite grain, as are rice and, in some families, kasha (buckwheat). Potatoes are a frequent addition, and some cooks add sweet potatoes.

A healthy habit of many nutrition-conscious Jews is to enjoy a piece of cake only on Shabbat. In my family, a cake flavored with dark chocolate and nuts has always been the favorite. Today nutritionists tell us that both are beneficial. You can combine them in Almond Applesauce Cake with Chocolate Chips and Honey (page 21). Another elegant dessert for Shabbat is cookies served with Ginger-Scented Plum Sorbet (page 340) and Holiday of Love Fruit Salad (page 336).

When my husband and I visited Languedoc in southern France, we were struck by the similarity of cassoulet, the region's celebrated meat-and-white-bean casserole, to our parents' Shabbat stew. We wondered whether hamin might have been the precursor of the French specialty. Larousse Gastronòmique, the standard reference work on French cooking, suggests that cassoulet might be a descendant of Spanish or Roman fava bean stews. Could it be that Mediterranean Jews introduced their stews to Languedoc? After all, Jews had made this French province their home since the early Middle Ages and had a long history of residing in neighboring Spain.

I wasn't a big cholent fan until I tasted my mother-in-law's cumin-scented rendition. Added appeal came from the appetizing eggs that slowly baked in their shells on top of the casserole.

Kurdish Jews sometimes put in quinces, and Moroccans might sweeten their cholent, called schina, with raisins or make it fiery with hot pepper paste. Not everyone sticks to tradition. A spoonful of jam, says one of my sisters-in-law, turns the sauce a nice, deep brown. I've seen a recipe calling for a bottle of beer. Another recipe specifies to add chocolate; I guess you could consider it cholent mole!

Cholent might be very simple, like a Greek one made only of beef, cracked wheat, and onions, or elaborate, like an Iraqi-Jewish rendition that features a stuffed chicken cooked with rice, carrots, and squash and seasoned with cinnamon and cardamom. I serve the substantial stew when the weather is cool, but for many families it's the Shabbat midday dinner year-round. The usual finale to the copious feast is a good long nap!

Israeli Salad for Holidays

Easy and Healthy Gefilte Fish

Salmon and Halibut Salad with Peppers and Tomatoes

Mushroom Edamame Soup

Chicken Soup with Kasha, Bow Ties, and Carrots

Shabbat Chicken with Potatoes, Capers, and Olives

Cheaters' Chicken Cholent

Cauliflower and Potato Kugel with Mushrooms

Shabbat Chayote Squash with Onions

Chile-Garlic Stuffed Eggplant

Zucchini Mushroom Stuffing with Pecans

Whole Wheat Jerusalem Kugel

To add a festive touch to the standard tomato-cucumber-onion trio, I stir in a pungent ingredient like olives, capers, pickles, or oil-packed sun-dried tomatoes, or I scatter nuts over the top. Quality cheese is a good addition for Shavuot or for special-occasion meatless meals and, together with the olives and almonds, makes this salad a celebration. A wonderful choice is braided string cheese, especially a type with herbs or seeds.

5 ripe but firm tomatoes, diced small

2 or 3 small slim cucumbers, preferably Persian or Middle Eastern, or ½ hothouse cucumber, diced small

¼ red or mild onion, finely chopped

½ small red or yellow bell pepper, diced small

1 cup chopped romaine (optional)

2 tablespoons chopped flat-leaf parsley (optional)

2 to 3 tablespoons extra virgin olive oil

1 to 2 tablespoons fresh lemon juice

¼ teaspoon dried oregano or thyme

Salt and freshly ground black pepper

Pinch of cayenne pepper (optional)

¼ cup good-quality green or black olives, pitted and halved or quartered

3 to 4 ounces braided string cheese, Bulgarian feta, or fresh mozzarella, crumbled or cut small (optional)

3 tablespoons slivered almonds, toasted (page 379)

Mix tomatoes, cucumbers, onion, bell pepper, romaine, and parsley (if using) in a shallow bowl. Add olive oil, lemon juice, oregano, salt, pepper, and cayenne, if you like. Taste and adjust seasoning. Serve topped with olives and sprinkled with cheese, if desired, and almonds.

Makes 4 servings

My mother was known in our family for her tasty gefilte fish. She bought whole fish, filleted them, and made fish stock with the heads and bones. When she lived in the United States, she used the time-honored trio of carp, whitefish, and pike. During the years she lived in Jerusalem, she used carp, which you can buy live at the supermarket, and combined it with mullet, which is readily available in Israel.

Over the years we both experimented with making the dish more easily. When my mother was in a hurry, she purchased fish fillets or even packaged ground fish and was satisfied with the results. I find that a flavorful vegetable broth, even a canned one, makes a fine substitute for the fish stock.

Gefilte fish is a wholesome dish, but to boost its nutrients even more, I use salmon, which is rich in healthy omega-3 fatty acids. To preserve the delicate taste of the dish, I like to combine the salmon with a mild-flavored fish. Whether or not gefilte fish should be sweet is a subject of ongoing controversy. I find the natural sweetness of vegetable broth makes the fish sweet enough, but add the optional sugar to the fish and the broth if you like sweet gefilte fish.

Serve the fish the traditional Ashkenazi way, with each piece topped with a carrot slice (cooked in the broth alongside the fish) and accompanied by beet-red horseradish. Or follow the custom of Sephardi Jews who have adopted gefilte fish, and serve it with Easy Green Chile Garlic Relish—Zehug (page 363). A Sephardi student at a cooking class of mine told me she has been serving it this way for years, and her children grew up thinking that everyone serves gefilte fish with Yemenite zehug!

1 pound salmon fillets, free of skin
1 pound halibut or sole fillets
2 large eggs, or 3 egg whites
2 medium onions, finely chopped
1½ teaspoons salt

½ teaspoon ground black pepper
1 teaspoon sugar (optional)
3 tablespoons matzo meal
4 cups vegetable broth
1 carrot, sliced (optional)

Run your fingers carefully over fish fillets and remove any small bones. Cut fish into large pieces.

Grind salmon in a food processor until very fine; remove from processor. Grind halibut fillets in processor until very fine. Remove about half of ground halibut and return half of ground salmon to the processor. Add 1 egg, half the chopped onions, ¾ teaspoon salt, ¼ teaspoon pepper, and ½ teaspoon sugar if you like. Process to mix thoroughly. Transfer to a large bowl. Repeat with remaining fish, egg, onions, salt, pepper, and sugar. Transfer to bowl and mix thoroughly with first batch. Stir in matzo meal.

Combine broth and 2 cups water in a large saucepan and bring to a simmer. With moistened hands, shape fish mixture into ovals or balls, using about ⅓ cup mixture for each. Carefully drop fish balls into simmering broth. If necessary, add enough hot water to barely cover them, pouring it carefully into broth near edge of pan, not over fish. Return to a simmer, cover, and simmer over low heat for 45 minutes. Add carrot slices, if you like, cover, and simmer for 15 more minutes. Taste broth, and add salt and sugar if desired. Let fish cool in broth. Refrigerate fish in broth for at least 4 hours before serving. At serving time, remove fish pieces from broth and serve cold.

Makes about 8 servings

✿ SALMON AND HALIBUT SALAD
WITH PEPPERS AND TOMATOES

To best highlight the delicate flavor of fresh fish, I keep the additions simple—diced fresh tomatoes, yellow or green peppers, green or red onions, and a touch of thyme or oregano in the olive oil dressing. Capers provide a zesty finishing touch, or you can use black olives or toasted pine nuts instead. Serve this colorful salad while the fish is still warm or let it cool to room temperature. If you like, spoon it onto a bed of green-leaf or romaine lettuce.

Vary the vegetables to your taste and, if you like, add cooked ones. Favorites of mine are lightly cooked asparagus and slim green beans.

One ¾-pound piece salmon fillet, about
    1 inch thick
One ¾-pound piece halibut fillet, about
    1 inch thick
2 to 2½ tablespoons strained fresh lemon juice
4 to 5 tablespoons extra virgin olive oil
Salt and freshly ground black pepper

1 teaspoon chopped fresh thyme leaves, or
    ½ teaspoon dried thyme or oregano
4 small ripe tomatoes, diced
1 small yellow or green bell pepper, diced
1 green onion, chopped
2 tablespoons chopped parsley
2 teaspoons capers, drained

Preheat oven to 450°F. Lightly oil a heavy roasting pan; or line pan with foil and lightly oil the foil. Set both kinds of fish in roasting pan. Mix 1 tablespoon lemon juice and 1 tablespoon oil in a bowl. Pour mixture over salmon and halibut and lightly rub it into fish flesh.

Sprinkle fish with salt and pepper. Bake fish about 10 minutes; when tested, fish should just flake and should have changed color in thickest part. Let fish cool and flake it into large pieces, discarding any skin or bones.

In a small bowl, whisk remaining lemon juice with salt and pepper. Whisk in remaining oil and thyme. Taste and adjust seasoning.

Lightly mix tomatoes, yellow pepper, green onion, and parsley. Add salmon and halibut pieces and mix gently. Toss lightly with dressing and sprinkle with capers.

Makes 4 to 6 main-course or 7 to 8 appetizer servings

❖ MUSHROOM EDAMAME SOUP

This light, flavorful soup is a perfect beginning for springtime Shabbat meals or for a Purim feast. The quick-cooking soup makes a pleasant change from chicken soup, but if you would like to add an element of tradition, you can serve it with Whole Wheat Matzo Balls (page 201).

½ large celery root, or 3 celery ribs

1 large onion, chopped

2 cups vegetable or chicken broth

2 fresh thyme sprigs, or ½ teaspoon dried thyme

2 to 3 cups water

2 carrots, halved and sliced

6 to 8 ounces frozen shelled edamame
    (green soybeans)

2 pale green Mexican zucchini (also called white
    or Tatuma squash) or zucchini, halved
    and sliced

4 ounces white mushrooms, halved and sliced

1 garlic clove, minced

Salt and freshly ground black pepper

2 tablespoons chopped parsley

If using celery root, peel it thoroughly, rinse it, quarter it, and cut it into thin slices, forming rough cubes. If using celery ribs, peel them if they are stringy and slice them thin.

Combine onion, broth, thyme, and 2 cups water in a saucepan and bring to a boil. Cover and cook over low heat for 5 minutes. Add carrots and celery, cover, and cook for 3 minutes. Add edamame and bring to a boil. Add squash, mushrooms, garlic, and more water if soup is too thick. Bring to a boil. Cover and cook over low heat for 5 minutes or until vegetables are just tender. Discard thyme sprig. Season to taste with salt and pepper. Add parsley just before serving. Serve hot.

Makes 4 servings

✠ CHICKEN SOUP WITH KASHA, BOW TIES, AND CARROTS

Kasha, or roasted buckwheat groats, is a healthy whole grain that has long been part of the Ashkenazi kitchen. Often it's matched with caramelized onions so their sweetness balances its earthy flavor, or with pasta. Sometimes it's cooked in soup. For soup, I find the kasha is best cooked separately and flavored with onions, then served alongside the soup so it keeps its fluffy texture. In the soup I like to include kasha's traditional partner, pasta bow-ties, as well as sweet carrots.

½ cup tiny bow-tie noodles
1 cup medium kasha (roasted buckwheat groats or kernels)
1 egg, or 1 egg white, beaten
2 cups chicken or vegetable broth or water (for cooking kasha)
1 tablespoon canola oil

1 medium onion, chopped
5 to 6 cups chicken broth, preferably homemade (for soup)
2 large carrots, sliced about ¼ inch thick
2 teaspoons chopped fresh dill, or ½ teaspoon dried dill
Salt and freshly ground black pepper

Cook noodles according to package directions, rinse, and drain.

Combine kasha with beaten egg in a wide bowl and stir with a fork until grains are thoroughly coated. Set a dry, heavy sauté pan over medium heat. Add kasha mixture and heat it over medium heat about 3 minutes, stirring to keep grains separate. Meanwhile, heat 2 cups broth nearly to boiling.

Add hot broth to kasha and stir. Cover and cook over low heat for 15 minutes or until liquid is absorbed.

Heat oil in a skillet, add onion, and sauté over medium-low heat, stirring often, about 7 minutes or until soft and well browned. Stir kasha with a fork to fluff it. Lightly stir onion into kasha. Season to taste with salt and pepper.

In a large saucepan, bring 5 to 6 cups chicken broth to a simmer. Add carrots, cover, and cook over medium heat until just tender, about 7 minutes. Add dill. Season to taste with salt and pepper. At serving time, add noodles to soup and heat through. Serve soup hot, with kasha on the side for spooning into each bowl.

Makes 4 servings

❧ SHABBAT CHICKEN WITH POTATOES, CAPERS, AND OLIVES

The first time my neighbor Valerie Alon cooked this dish for Friday night dinner, she just put in "all the good ingredients that everyone loves." In addition to capers and olives, she added cumin, garlic, and lemon juice, as she knew how fond her family is of Mediterranean flavors. The dish quickly became a family favorite, and it is a great way to enjoy boneless chicken. For the potatoes, use Yukon golds, or red or white boiling potatoes.

1½ pounds boneless, skinless chicken breasts, thighs, or some of each
2 tablespoons extra virgin olive oil
1 large onion, chopped
3 garlic cloves, chopped
½ teaspoon turmeric
1 teaspoon ground cumin
1½ teaspoons paprika

Salt and freshly ground black pepper
3 carrots, sliced (optional)
3 boiling potatoes, peeled and diced
1 to 1½ cups water
2 tablespoons fresh lemon juice
2 to 3 tablespoons capers, rinsed
¼ cup green or black olives, pitted and sliced
¼ cup chopped flat-leaf parsley

Cut each chicken piece into 2 or 3 chunks. Heat oil in a stew pan. Add chicken in batches and brown lightly over medium heat, removing each piece after it browns. Add onion and garlic and cook over medium-low heat, stirring often, for 5 minutes or until onion begins to turn golden.

Return chicken to pan and sprinkle with turmeric, cumin, paprika, and salt and pepper to taste. Mix well. Add carrots (if using), potatoes, and 1 cup water and bring to a boil. Cover and simmer over low heat, stirring occasionally, until chicken is tender; breasts will need 20 to 25 minutes, thighs 30 to 40 minutes; check water once or twice during simmering and add 3 to 4 tablespoons if needed so that ingredients are moist.

Add lemon juice, capers, and olives and heat through. Taste and adjust seasoning. Stir in parsley. Serve hot.

Makes 4 to 6 servings

❧ CHEATERS' CHICKEN CHOLENT

Cholent is the time-honored Shabbat stew. Instead of spending about 16 hours in a low oven or slow cooker, from Friday before sundown until serving time on Saturday, this "speedy" cholent breaks with tradition—it needs "only" about 4 hours.

Spiced in my mother-in-law's Yemenite style, the healthy cholent is made with two kinds of beans, in addition to the whole wheat. You can find wheat berries in kosher, Middle Eastern, and natural foods stores. I tie the wheat in cheesecloth so it is easier to serve. To keep the amount of saturated fat low, I use a relatively high proportion of beans and grains, and I remove the chicken's skin before cooking the cholent.

To make this cholent the old-fashioned way, see the Notes following the recipe. Be sure to serve cholent very hot.

1 tablespoon olive oil

2 large onions, coarsely chopped

2 to 2½ pounds chicken quarters (legs with thighs attached)

2 teaspoons salt (see Notes)

1½ teaspoons ground black pepper

1 tablespoon ground cumin

1 teaspoon turmeric

1½ cups dried chickpeas (garbanzo beans), picked over and rinsed

1 cup dried white beans, such as great Northern, picked over and rinsed

8 large garlic cloves, coarsely chopped

1 cup whole wheat berries, picked over and rinsed

1½ pounds small boiling potatoes

About 7 to 8 cups water

3 to 6 eggs in shells, rinsed (optional)

Heat oil in a heavy 6-quart or larger stew pan. Add onions and sauté over medium-high heat for 7 minutes, stirring often, or until beginning to brown; add water by tablespoons if pan becomes dry. Let cool.

Preheat oven to 250°F. Pull off skin and excess fat from chicken. Mix salt, pepper, cumin, and turmeric. Add chicken pieces to stew pan and sprinkle with half the seasoning mixture on both sides. Add chickpeas, white beans, and garlic. Wrap wheat berries loosely in a piece of cheesecloth and put in pan. Add potatoes, remaining seasonings, and 7 cups water or enough to just cover the ingredients. Bring to a boil. Cover and cook over low heat for 30 minutes. Remove from heat. Set eggs (if using) gently on top and push them slightly into liquid. Cover tightly.

Bake stew, without stirring, for 3½ hours or until ingredients are very tender. Taste and adjust seasoning. Serve stew steaming hot, from pan or a deep serving dish. Serve eggs, if desired, in a separate dish; or shell and halve them and set on top of stew for garnish. Serve hot stew in shallow bowls, adding spoonfuls of wheat berries to each one.

NOTES: If you prefer to cook with little salt or if you are using kosher chickens, which vary in saltiness, instead of adding salt before cooking, taste liquid after stew has baked for 1 hour and add salt to taste at that time.

Old-fashioned overnight-baked cholent: Follow first two paragraphs, adding 1 extra cup water. Bake cholent at lowest oven setting overnight.

Makes about 6 servings

✠ CAULIFLOWER AND POTATO KUGEL WITH MUSHROOMS

Even reluctant cauliflower eaters will enjoy this savory, nutritious kugel accented with sautéed onions, mushrooms, and paprika. Use a food processor to quickly puree the cauliflower, but mash the potatoes with a potato masher or food mill; a food processor would make them gluey. To reheat the kugel, cover it with foil and heat it in a 300°F oven.

¾ pound baking or boiling potatoes, unpeeled
Salt and freshly ground black pepper
1 small cauliflower (about 1¼ pounds)
2½ tablespoons vegetable oil
1 onion, chopped

4 ounces medium or small mushrooms, quartered
½ teaspoon paprika
2 large eggs
1 tablespoon matzo meal

Put potatoes in a large saucepan with water to cover and a pinch of salt, and bring to a boil. Cover and simmer over low heat for 30 minutes or until very tender. Remove with a slotted spoon. Peel when cool enough to handle. Mash potatoes in a large bowl.

Divide cauliflower in medium florets. Cut peel from large stem and slice stem. Return potato cooking liquid to a boil and add cauliflower. Add hot water to cover if needed. Simmer, uncovered, for 12 minutes or until stems are very tender. Drain well and cool. Puree cauliflower in food processor, leaving a few chunks. Add to mashed potatoes.

Preheat oven to 375°F. Heat 2 tablespoons oil in a medium skillet, add onion, and sauté over medium heat for 7 minutes. Add mushrooms and ¼ teaspoon paprika and sauté for 3 minutes or until mushrooms and onions are light brown.

Add eggs and matzo meal to cauliflower mixture. Season well with salt and pepper. Lightly stir in mushroom mixture and any oil in pan.

Oil a shallow 8-inch square baking dish. Add cauliflower mixture and smooth top. Sprinkle with ½ tablespoon oil, then with ¼ teaspoon paprika. Bake for 30 minutes or until set. Serve hot or warm.

Makes 4 to 5 servings

Chayote squash, a green pear-shaped squash, can be used like zucchini, but has a firmer texture and holds its shape well during cooking. Baking gives the chayote a wonderful sweet flavor, even better than frying. Besides, baking is a more healthful method because it uses much less fat.

In this dish the onions become sweet as they bake with the squash and further enhance its flavor. This casserole is ideal for Shabbat because it can be kept warm in a low oven and it reheats beautifully. I like to bake this dish at the same time as the Shabbat chicken and serve it as an easy-to-prepare, tasty complement for the bird. For a light meal, it's also good with tofu and rice.

Use red and yellow pepper strips if you prefer a more colorful dish. If you're using young, tender squashes, you don't need to peel them.

2 chayote squash (total 1 pound), peeled and halved lengthwise

½ green bell pepper, cut lengthwise into thin strips

1 large onion, sliced lengthwise

1 tablespoon extra virgin olive oil

1 tablespoon water

1 teaspoon dried oregano

Salt and freshly ground black pepper

Preheat oven to 400°F. Cut each squash half into 4 lengthwise wedges. Cut each bell pepper strip in half crosswise. Combine chayote, onion, and pepper strips in a shallow 2-quart casserole. Add oil, water, oregano, salt, and pepper. Toss with your hands to distribute seasonings. Cover and bake for 40 minutes, stirring once and adding another 1 or 2 tablespoons water if necessary to prevent burning, or until squash are crisp-tender. Stir, then bake, uncovered, for 20 minutes or until squash are tender and slightly browned. Serve hot.

Makes 3 to 4 servings

❊ CHILE-GARLIC STUFFED EGGPLANT

Chopped garlic and a peppery Yemenite relish accent this stuffing of roasted pepper, oven-sautéed onion, and tomato sauce mixed with the eggplant pulp. This flavorful dish is lower in oil and easier to prepare than most stuffed eggplant dishes. Once you have roasted the eggplants and pepper, which I usually do ahead, it takes little time to put together. Serve it as an attractive side dish or appetizer for Shabbat or any holiday.

If you are using purchased hot sauce rather than homemade relish, start with a smaller amount, in case it's potent.

2 eggplants (total 2 to 2¼ pounds)
1 onion, halved, sliced thin crosswise
4 to 6 teaspoons extra virgin olive oil, or
    a little more to taste
Salt and freshly ground black pepper
1 green bell pepper

4 garlic cloves, chopped
½ cup thick, chunky tomato sauce
1 to 2 teaspoons Easy Green Chile Garlic Relish
    (page 363) or bottled zehug, hot Turkish-style
    pepper paste, Asian chili garlic paste, or
    Mexican hot sauce

Preheat oven to 450°F. Prick eggplants several times with a fork, set on a foil-lined pan, and bake for 30 minutes, turning once, or until just tender.

Meanwhile, put onion in a heavy, medium (about 8-inch) casserole with 2 teaspoons oil, 2 teaspoons water, and salt. Toss with your fingers, separating the onion into half rings. Cover with foil. Bake for 5 minutes. Stir, then bake, uncovered, for 7 more minutes or until softened and just beginning to brown. Transfer to a bowl.

Reduce oven temperature to 400°F. Set green pepper on a foil-lined tray and roast for 20 minutes, turning a quarter-turn every 5 minutes, or until mostly brown on all sides. Remove from oven and enclose it in its foil. Let stand for 10 minutes. Peel with paring knife, discarding any liquid from inside and removing core and seeds. Dice pepper. Leave oven on.

Remove eggplant caps. Halve eggplants lengthwise. Drain off any liquid inside. Carefully remove about half of pulp, leaving rest attached to skin. Sprinkle pulp left in eggplant with salt. Put shells in casserole used to bake onions or in any baking dish in which they just fit.

Coarsely chop removed eggplant pulp and transfer it to the bowl of onions. Add diced green pepper, garlic, tomato sauce, salt, pepper, and relish and mix well. Taste and adjust seasoning. Mixture should be thick. Spoon into eggplant shells. Sprinkle each with a little olive oil, about ½ to 1 teaspoon per eggplant half.

Add 1 to 2 tablespoons water to baking dish. Cover with foil. Bake for 15 minutes or until heated through. Serve hot or warm, drizzled, if you like, with a little more olive oil.

Makes 4 servings

ZUCCHINI MUSHROOM STUFFING WITH PECANS

In our family, when I was growing up, baked stuffing often came with the Shabbat chicken. You can bake this savory stuffing inside a chicken, turkey, or Cornish hen, but I prefer to bake it as an accompanying casserole so it won't absorb the fat that drips from the bird. Baking the stuffing separately is a time-saver for a couple of reasons: (a) an unstuffed bird roasts much faster and (b) spooning the mixture into a baking dish takes less time than putting it inside the bird. You can make this stuffing with French or Italian bread, but whole wheat bread is a healthier choice.

3 tablespoons extra virgin olive oil or vegetable oil
12 ounces mushrooms, halved and cut into
    thick slices
Salt and freshly ground black pepper
2 large onions, chopped
¾ cup chopped celery
3 garlic cloves, chopped
½ pound zucchini, coarsely grated

½ pound day-old bread, preferably whole wheat,
    cut into ½-inch cubes
½ cup pecans, coarsely chopped
¼ cup chopped parsley
1 teaspoon dried thyme
2 teaspoons chopped fresh sage, or
    ½ teaspoon dried sage
About 1 cup chicken or vegetable broth

Heat 1 tablespoon oil in a large skillet. Add mushrooms, salt, and pepper and sauté over medium-high heat until lightly browned, about 3 minutes. Transfer to a bowl.

Heat remaining oil in skillet. Add onions and celery and cook over medium-low heat, stirring, until softened, about 7 minutes. Add garlic and cook for a few seconds. Remove from heat.

Put grated zucchini in a colander and squeeze out excess liquid. Stir zucchini into onion mixture.

In a large bowl, combine bread cubes, zucchini mixture, mushrooms, pecans, parsley, thyme, sage, and a pinch of salt and pepper. Toss, using two large spoons, until ingredients are mixed thoroughly and bread is moistened. Gradually add ¼ cup broth, tossing lightly. Most of bread should be very lightly moistened; if most of it is dry, gradually add up to ¼ cup more broth by tablespoons. Season to taste with salt and pepper.

Preheat oven to 325°F. Oil a 2½-quart casserole and spoon stuffing into it. Cover casserole and bake for 20 minutes. Baste stuffing by pouring ¼ cup broth evenly over top. Bake for 20 more minutes and repeat with another ¼ cup broth. Bake for 20 minutes more; uncover for last 10 minutes if you would like a slightly crusty top. Serve hot.

Makes 6 to 8 servings

✦ WHOLE WHEAT JERUSALEM KUGEL

This kugel is unusual in two ways: It is spicy from a generous amount of black pepper and is lightly sweetened with a caramel made of sugar cooked in oil. While baking all night, the kugel turns deep brown. Nutritious whole wheat noodles, which are tan in hue, give you a head start on achieving the kugel's desired brown color. In addition, the hearty flavor of the whole-grain pasta complements the peppery kugel well.

This old-fashioned kugel is not rich in eggs and thus is dense rather than light and fluffy, but the noodle pudding is welcoming on a cold winter day. You can cut it in its baking dish and serve it in wedges, or run a knife around it and turn it out like a cake. If you have any left over, you can wrap it in foil and heat it in a toaster oven, or microwave uncovered slices on a plate.

I've seen variations made with apples, raisins, walnuts, cinnamon, and orange juice, but most Jerusalemites enjoy the pure taste of the peppery caramelized noodles without embellishment.

12 ounces thin whole wheat spaghetti	*2 large eggs*
⅓ cup vegetable oil	*1 teaspoon salt*
¼ cup sugar	*1 teaspoon ground black pepper, or more to taste*

Generously grease a 2-quart round casserole. Cook noodles in a large pot of boiling salted water, uncovered, over high heat about 8 minutes or until barely tender. Drain, return to pot, and toss briefly with 1 tablespoon oil. Keep on stove so noodles remain warm; do not cover.

Pour remaining oil into a heavy saucepan, then add sugar. Heat over low heat, shaking pan gently from time to time; do not stir. Cook 15 to 20 minutes or until sugar turns deep brown. Add mixture to noodles, mixing well with tongs.

Beat eggs with salt and pepper. Add to noodles and mix well. Transfer to greased casserole. Cover with foil and with a lid. You can refrigerate kugel for several hours at this point.

Put kugel in oven set at 180°F to 200°F (or see Note). Bake kugel overnight or about 14 hours. Serve hot, in slices.

NOTE: To bake kugel faster, bake it uncovered at 350°F for 1 hour. The kugel will not brown as much but will still taste good.

Makes 10 servings

Appetizers

I find the best appetizers for healthy, delicious cooking are those made from vegetables. Picture an antipasti table in Italy, or a Middle Eastern meze, full of colorful salads, dips, and roasted marinated vegetables.

At Israeli eateries I go for the eggplant appetizer platters that feature the vegetable prepared in several ways. One of my best restaurant eating experiences was in Istanbul, where the appetizer buffet table was covered with such items as roasted eggplant puree, stuffed peppers, and a grand variety of other salads.

Most vegetables can be made into salads and dips, even some you may not think of, like pumpkin and carrots. Such appetizers are much healthier than batter-coated fritters and fried pastries. Besides, they are easy to prepare and convenient, as you can make them in advance.

Some vegetables are best grilled, like the eggplants and peppers in Balkan Pepper Dip (page 158), while others can be stewed or sautéed, like the onions in Fava Bean Canapés with Saffron Onions (page 167).

You can match the vegetables with interesting accents, such as capers, olives, grilled chiles, toasted nuts, and sesame seeds, or with spices, like the cumin and jalapeño peppers in Peppery Pumpkin Carrot Dip (page 162). Small amounts of smoked fish and cheeses can act as a garnish and enhance the vegetables' flavors, as in Mushroom Mozzarella Crostini (page 166). When the occasion calls for a traditional starter like chopped liver, there are tricks for making it more nutritious, for example by slipping in an untraditional ingredient, like lentils.

When served with healthy whole-grain breads, vegetable dips, spreads, and salads make enticing, wholesome beginnings to a meal. With bakeries providing so many healthy bread choices, it's fun to set out several kinds at a festive dinner.

Vegetarian Chopped Liver in Cucumber Boats

Marinated Peppers and Cucumbers with Olives and Capers

Balkan Pepper Dip—Ajvar

Provençal Eggplant Salad

Spicy Spinach Tahini

Peppery Pumpkin Carrot Dip

Fresh Tomato Basil Dip

Onion Compote with Pine Nuts and Raisins

Plum Tomatoes Stuffed with Shallot Cream

Mushroom Mozzarella Crostini

Fava Bean Canapés with Saffron Onions

Sephardi Spinach and Cheese Burekas

Double Salmon Salad

VEGETARIAN CHOPPED LIVER IN CUCUMBER BOATS

In my family, mock liver (as my mother called it) has long been a regular Shabbat starter, and it remains one of my favorite appetizers. There are dozens of formulas, but basically it's composed of vegetables or legumes—from eggplant to canned peas—combined with nuts. Over the years, mine has been evolving. I especially like to use a mixture of chickpeas, fresh green beans, and mushrooms.

The most important element is a generous amount of well-browned onions. I suppose the onions' caramelized flavor, and my addition of a little hard-boiled egg, are the reasons why some students at my cooking demonstrations swear my version tastes just like chopped liver. But I love it as a dish in its own right. Probably this traditional spread developed as a pareve, frugal alternative to chopped liver.

If your friends or family members are squeamish about chopped liver, call this vegetable pâté. Serving it in vegetable containers, such as cucumber boats, hollowed plum tomatoes, or lightly roasted peppers, or using it to top a light green salad, makes the spread into a lighter appetizer; but of course you can simply serve it with fresh bread or crackers. Often I double or triple the recipe to have extra pâté on hand. It keeps well and is great in sandwiches with sliced tomatoes, cucumbers, lettuce, or smoked turkey.

6 ounces green beans, broken in two, ends removed

1 to 2 tablespoons vegetable oil

1 large onion, chopped

3 ounces mushrooms, diced

1½ cups cooked chickpeas (garbanzo beans), or one 15-ounce can chickpeas, drained and rinsed

¼ cup walnuts or pecans

1 hard-boiled egg, or white of 1 or 2 hard-boiled eggs, coarsely grated

Salt and freshly ground black pepper

8 to 10 very small cucumbers (sometimes called Persian or Middle Eastern cucumbers), or 2 to 3 long, hothouse cucumbers

Cook green beans in a saucepan of enough boiling salted water to cover them for about 10 minutes or until very tender. Reserve ¼ cup bean cooking liquid. Drain beans, rinse with cold water, and drain well.

Heat oil in a large, heavy skillet. Add onion and sauté over medium heat for 5 minutes or until beginning to brown. Raise heat to medium-high, add mushrooms, and sauté, stirring often and covering pan if mixture begins to look dry, for 2 minutes or until mushrooms and onions are well browned. Let cool.

Chop green beans in a food processor. Add chickpeas, onion and mushroom mixture, walnuts, and 2 tablespoons bean liquid. Process until smooth. If spread is too thick, add more bean liquid, 1 tablespoon at a time, processing after each addition. Transfer to a bowl. Lightly stir in hard-boiled eggs. Season to taste with salt and pepper. Refrigerate for 1 hour or until ready to serve.

Peel cucumbers if desired, or peel them in stripes for a decorative effect. Halve them lengthwise. With a small, pointed spoon, scoop out seeds. Use a spoon to fill cucumbers with vegetable pâté. If using long cucumbers, cut them into 2- or 3-inch lengths. You can serve them immediately or refrigerate them for 2 to 3 hours so the pâté becomes firmer. Serve cold.

Makes 4 to 5 servings

❊ MARINATED PEPPERS AND CUCUMBERS WITH OLIVES AND CAPERS

All around the Mediterranean, appetizers of grilled marinated peppers appear on the table during the pepper season. They make a healthy, and irresistible, appetizer. At serving time I like to add strips of cucumber, which benefit from the flavor of the marinade. This dish also makes a good accompaniment for cubes of feta cheese or slices of smoked turkey or smoked tofu, served with whole wheat flatbread for a quick, tasty lunch.

If using olives with pits, be sure to mention it to your guests when serving this appetizer.

4 large red bell peppers, or 2 red and 2 green
*   bell peppers*
2 to 3 teaspoons extra virgin olive oil
1 garlic clove, minced
1 teaspoon chopped fresh thyme, or ½ teaspoon
*   dried thyme*
Salt and freshly ground black pepper

2 to 3 teaspoons strained fresh lemon juice or
*   wine vinegar*
2 or 3 Persian cucumbers, cut into thin strips
1 tablespoon capers, drained
⅓ cup good-quality black or green olives, such as
*   Kalamata, niçoise, Moroccan, or Israeli spicy*
*   green olives*

Grill and peel bell peppers (see page 376). Remove cores. Cut peppers into quarters and put them in a shallow serving dish. Pour oil over peppers, add garlic and thyme, and sprinkle lightly with salt and pepper. Mix gently. Let stand at room temperature, turning occasionally, 30 minutes; or refrigerate overnight.

To serve, cut peppers in strips. Add lemon juice to marinade. Put peppers and cucumbers in marinade and mix gently. Taste, adjust seasoning, and add more oil or lemon juice if needed. Sprinkle with capers and garnish with olives. Serve at room temperature.

Makes 4 to 6 servings

This savory red pepper puree is the perfect appetizer for Sukkot, when red peppers are at their peak. I first came across it at an Eastern European market and bought a jar, which came from Bulgaria. Later, Yugoslavia-born Israelis told me that ajvar is part of their culinary heritage and that it's pronounced "ayvar." Serbians, Croatians, and Macedonians all claim this delicious dip as their own. Depending on what kinds of peppers the cook uses, it can be mild or hot. Although the dip is sometimes made only of ground roasted peppers, oil, and vinegar, it generally contains other vegetables too—occasionally carrots and tomatoes, but most frequently, eggplant.

A similar tasty red salad from Croatia calls for blending roasted green peppers (instead of red ones) with the eggplant and adding an equal weight of roasted tomatoes. A related Turkish salad also includes tomatoes, but they are fresh ones that are diced and mixed with diced roasted peppers and chopped roasted eggplant. An Armenian variation calls for adding sautéed onions as well. Ground walnuts and olives embellish a similar eggplant dip, also from Bulgaria. A technique favored in Georgia requires roasting only the eggplant and adding the chopped peppers raw, along with olive oil, lemon juice, garlic, green onion, and cilantro. All of these are healthy ways to modify the appetizer according to your mood and the ingredients you happen to have.

Generally this thick dip is used as a spread for fresh bread—country bread or flatbread are the traditional favorites. For a light lunch or supper, you can make a sandwich of it with a hard-boiled egg or a little feta cheese. You can also serve it as an accompaniment for grilled chicken. Some people add a spoonful or two of this puree to vegetable soups or goulash-type stews to thicken and flavor them. Instead of a portion of the red bell peppers, you can use red Anaheim chiles.

This healthy dip consists mainly of vegetables, with little fat. Red peppers and chiles are rich in vitamin A, and eggplant is a good source of soluble fiber.

2 medium eggplants (total about 2 pounds)	1 onion, minced (optional)
2 pounds red bell peppers	3 garlic cloves, minced
3 red or green jalapeño peppers, or 1 poblano chile (called pasilla in California) (optional)	Salt and freshly ground black pepper
	Hot paprika or cayenne pepper
2 to 3 tablespoons extra virgin olive oil	1 tablespoon white wine vinegar or lemon juice

Grill or broil eggplants, then peel them; for instructions, see Light and Easy Eggplant Dip (page 360).

Broil or grill bell peppers, turning them often, for about 15 minutes or until their skins blister all over. Transfer them to a bowl and cover tightly; or put them in a plastic bag and close bag. Broil or grill jalapeño peppers (if using) the same way, turning them often; they will need only about 5 minutes; be careful, as they burn rapidly. Transfer them to a bowl or bag as well.

Leave sweet and hot peppers in bag for about 10 minutes. Peel peppers, using a paring knife. Remove caps, seeds, and ribs. Be careful; there may be hot liquid inside them. Drain them well.

Chop eggplant and peppers very fine with a knife or in a food processor with a pulsing motion; do not overprocess, so mixture won't become too soupy. Transfer to a bowl.

Heat 2 tablespoons oil in a skillet. Add onion (if using) and cook over medium-low heat for 7 minutes or until softened. Add garlic and cook for ½ minute. Add to eggplant mixture and mix well. Season to taste with salt, pepper, and hot paprika. Mix well. Stir in vinegar and remaining oil. Taste and adjust seasoning. Serve cold or at room temperature.

Makes 6 to 8 servings

✿ PROVENÇAL EGGPLANT SALAD

Cooks in southern France flavor eggplant with a Provençal caper-olive paste called *tapenade*, which complements the eggplant well because of its salty taste. I dice the olives and capers instead of pureeing them to a paste and leave the eggplant chunky for a better texture and color. If you want to add anchovies, a classic component of tapenade, use 2 or 3 olive oil–packed fillets and chop them very fine.

Spoon this salad in the center of a bed of romaine lettuce leaves and garnish it with ripe tomato wedges or cherry tomatoes; or serve it in a bowl as a relish and top it with parsley sprigs and olives. Crusty French bread is the perfect partner. Recently my husband came up with a new use that might raise a few eyebrows among Riviera residents—he spreads this Provençal eggplant on grilled soy burgers and sprinkles it with Mexican hot sauce.

2 medium eggplants (total about 2 pounds)
2 large, very fresh garlic cloves, finely minced
2 to 3 tablespoons extra virgin olive oil
1½ to 2 tablespoons strained fresh lemon juice
2 teaspoons chopped fresh thyme, or ¾ teaspoon dried thyme
Salt and freshly ground black pepper

¼ to ⅓ cup black olives, pitted, quartered, or cut into large dice
¼ to ⅓ cup green olives, pitted, quartered, or cut into large dice
1 tablespoons capers, drained, left whole if small, chopped if large
3 tablespoons chopped flat-leaf parsley

Roast eggplants, then peel them and drain them (see page 360).

Chop eggplants with a knife, leaving pieces a bit chunky. Transfer eggplant to a bowl. Add garlic and mix well. Stir in oil, lemon juice, thyme, salt, pepper, black and green olives, capers, and parsley. Taste and adjust seasoning. Serve in a shallow bowl or on a plate.

Makes 6 servings

❧ SPICY SPINACH TAHINI

Israelis sometimes spice up their favorite dip, tahini, by adding hot pepper relish, which is guaranteed to chase away blandness. For this recipe I blend spicy tahini with lightly cooked spinach and a little of its cooking liquid, similar to the French technique for making green mayonnaise. The result is a flavorful, pale green appetizer dip that also makes a good sauce for poached or baked fish, grilled chicken breasts, or firm tofu.

Since part of the dip is spinach puree, it is lower in fat and in calories than traditional tahini. Unlike mayonnaise, it is cholesterol free. You can use other chopped cooked greens, such as chard or mustard greens, the same way. If you are serving the dip the same day, you can make it with raw spinach instead of cooked greens. For a dairy meal, stir in 1/4 to 1/2 cup low-fat or nonfat plain yogurt if you like.

1/2 pound spinach, stems removed, rinsed well
1/3 cup tahini paste, stirred before being measured
2 garlic cloves, minced
2 to 3 tablespoons strained fresh lemon juice
Salt

*1/2 teaspoon Easy Green Chile Garlic Relish
    (page 363), or purchased zehug, or hot sauce
    to taste*
*Fresh pita breads, preferably whole wheat
    (for serving)*

Boil 2 cups water in a saucepan and add spinach leaves. Boil, uncovered, over high heat for 2 minutes or until just tender. Transfer to a colander with a slotted spoon, reserving cooking liquid. Rinse spinach with cold water and drain well. Puree spinach in a food processor. Measure 1/2 cup spinach cooking liquid and let cool.

In a medium bowl, combine tahini and garlic. Stir in 2 tablespoons lemon juice, 1/4 cup spinach cooking liquid, and salt to taste. Stir in spinach puree. If dip is too thick, gradually stir in more lemon juice or spinach cooking liquid. Taste, and add more salt or lemon juice if desired. Stir in relish.

Serve dip in a shallow bowl, with pita bread.

Makes 4 to 6 servings

PEPPERY PUMPKIN CARROT DIP

This tasty, nutritious appetizer is based on a salad I enjoyed at Sassi, a kosher Israeli-style restaurant in Encino, California. Usually the thick, chunky puree is made of pumpkin or winter squash, but some cooks make it from carrots. I like combining both vegetables, as they did at Sassi.

At the restaurant the puree is served as a spicy topping for their Tripolitan couscous, but it also makes a tasty dip for scooping up with whole wheat pita bread or tortillas. For Thanksgiving, it makes a healthful, change-of-pace accompaniment for roast turkey. Garlic, chiles, and the vitamin A–rich vegetables make it one of the most nutritious of appetizers.

For the best flavor, choose a rich-textured squash or pumpkin, such as butternut squash or kabocha (Japanese pumpkin) or, if you frequent Hispanic markets, calabaza. I microwave the squash for this recipe, as this is the easiest way to prepare it. If you have harissa (North African hot relish) or packaged or homemade zehug (Yemenite hot relish, see page 363), you can substitute it for the garlic and the hot pepper—start with ½ teaspoon and add more to taste.

*1½ to 2 pounds hard-shelled squash, such as
    butternut or kabocha (Japanese pumpkin)*
1 pound carrots, sliced
*1 or 2 jalapeño peppers, minced, or
    ¼ teaspoon cayenne pepper, or to taste*
4 to 6 garlic cloves, minced

1 teaspoon ground cumin
¼ to ½ teaspoon paprika
2 tablespoons fresh lemon juice
*1 to 3 tablespoons extra virgin olive oil or
    vegetable oil*
Salt

Halve squash and set in a baking dish or other shallow microwave-safe dish. Cover and microwave on high for 10 minutes or until very tender. Remove seeds. Scoop out flesh; it will be soft. Drain in a colander to be sure it's not watery, and transfer to a bowl.

Put carrots in a saucepan, cover with water, and add a pinch of salt. Bring to a boil. Cover and cook over medium-low heat for 7 minutes or until very tender. Remove with a slotted spoon and drain well in a colander.

Mash squash and carrots with a fork or potato masher in a bowl; or puree squash and carrots in a food processor, pulsing so there will still be chunks, then transfer to a bowl. Stir in jalapeño peppers, garlic, cumin, paprika, lemon juice, and oil. Season to taste with salt. Serve at room temperature.

Makes 6 to 8 servings

✿ FRESH TOMATO BASIL DIP

At a neighborhood Italian ristorante, this simple mixture of diced tomatoes, garlic, basil, and olive oil is served with the bread. It makes a tasty replacement for butter, especially if you use top-quality fruity extra virgin olive oil and ripe tomatoes. Use it to dip your bread but be sparing; a little goes a long way. Instead of serving it in a ramekin, try it as a topping for small slices of toast to make bruschette.

6 ripe plum tomatoes, diced
Salt
2 to 3 tablespoons extra virgin olive oil

1 garlic clove, minced
1 tablespoon fresh basil strips

Sprinkle tomatoes lightly with salt to taste, put in a strainer, and drain for 5 to 10 minutes. Transfer to a bowl. Add oil, garlic, and basil and mix gently. Taste, and add more salt if needed. Serve at room temperature.

Makes 4 servings

ONION COMPOTE WITH PINE NUTS AND RAISINS

Compote d'oignons is what the French often call slowly stewed onions like these. French chefs serve onion compote alongside meat, but it has many other uses. The idea for serving it as an appetizer came to me when I enjoyed it at a casual Santa Barbara café, where it was set on the table with the bread as a butter re-placer. The addition of pine nuts and raisins makes the compote festive enough for a holiday table. Serve the compote in small ramekins with fresh, crusty bread, preferably whole-grain bread. It also makes a tasty topping for cooked brown rice, quinoa, or bulgur wheat. Remember that although it's much lower in fat than butter or oil, it's still rich.

2 to 3 tablespoons extra virgin olive oil, or
    1 tablespoon butter and 1 to 2 tablespoons oil
1½ pounds onions, halved and thinly sliced
Salt and freshly ground black pepper

2 to 3 tablespoons raisins
1 to 2 teaspoons wine vinegar (optional)
1 to 2 teaspoons honey (optional)
2 to 3 tablespoons pine nuts, lightly toasted

In a heavy stew pan, heat oil. Add onions, salt, and pepper. Cover and cook over low heat, stirring often, for 20 minutes. Uncover and cook, stirring very often, for 15 minutes longer, or until onions are golden and tender enough to crush easily with a wooden spoon; do not let them burn. Stir in raisins and heat briefly. Taste, and add vinegar or honey if you like. Stir in pine nuts. Taste and adjust seasoning. Serve warm or at room temperature.

Makes 4 to 6 servings

PLUM TOMATOES STUFFED WITH SHALLOT CREAM

In Paris at La Varenne Cooking School, I learned to make a luscious puree of butter-braised shallots enriched with crème fraîche. To make it healthier, I braise the shallots with a little extra virgin olive oil and enrich it with milk and yogurt. I love the puree spooned into baked tomatoes, as their slight tartness complements its lovely rich flavor. Serve these stuffed tomatoes as a starter or an accompaniment for fish or meatless entrées. You can also use the puree on its own as a spread for crackers or pita crisps, or spoon it into broiled large mushroom cups.

½ pound shallots, peeled and cut in half
1 tablespoon plus 2 teaspoons extra virgin olive oil
Salt and freshly ground black pepper
8 ripe plum tomatoes (about 12 ounces)

2 tablespoons milk, fat-free or low-fat
2 tablespoons plain yogurt or low-fat sour cream
About 1 teaspoon thinly sliced chives, or a few small
 parsley sprigs (optional)

Preheat oven to 400°F. In a saucepan cover shallots with water, bring to a boil, and cook 2 minutes. Drain well.

In a heavy sauté pan, heat 1 tablespoon oil over low heat, add shallots, a pinch of salt, and pepper. Cover and cook, stirring often, for 20 minutes or until shallots are very tender; be careful not to let them burn.

Meanwhile, cut tomatoes in half lengthwise and scoop out interiors with a small melon-ball cutter. Oil a shallow baking dish in which tomatoes can fit in one layer. Put tomato halves in baking dish. Season with salt and pepper, then sprinkle lightly with oil. Bake for 10 minutes or until just tender. Carefully pour out juices from inside tomato halves. Pat dry with a paper towel.

Puree shallots in a food processor. Put puree in a small, heavy saucepan and stir over low heat. Add milk and continue to stir until absorbed; do not boil. Remove from heat and stir in yogurt or sour cream. Taste and adjust seasoning.

Spoon shallot puree carefully into tomatoes, using 2 or 3 teaspoons puree for each tomato half.

Return tomatoes to oven. Bake for 7 minutes or until heated through. If desired, garnish with chives or parsley sprigs. Serve hot or warm. If any shallot puree remains, reheat it gently and serve it separately.

Makes 4 servings

❧ MUSHROOM MOZZARELLA CROSTINI

Crostini, crowned with a slice of fresh mozzarella sitting on a quick mushroom pâté, make an easy, festive appetizer. Serve the crostini for Shavuot or to start off a meatless dinner. Choose good-quality crusty bread, preferably whole grain.

Using mozzarella in this fashion is a good way to enjoy the luscious cheese in a healthy menu. You can substitute a slice of another cheese of similar texture, such as braided Middle Eastern string cheese; try to choose one made with part-skim milk. For a pareve appetizer, substitute a thin slice of smoked tofu for the mozzarella.

6 to 8 ounces mushrooms, rinsed, patted dry
2 to 3 teaspoons extra virgin olive oil
1 garlic clove, minced
Salt and freshly ground black pepper
1 tablespoon chopped basil

Cayenne pepper
12 thin slices of whole-grain baguette
12 thin slices of fresh mozzarella
12 small basil leaves (optional)

Chop mushrooms in a food processor in fine pieces until they are almost a puree. Heat 2 teaspoons oil in a medium skillet. Add garlic and sauté over medium heat, stirring, for a few seconds. Add mushrooms, salt, and pepper. Cook over medium-high heat, stirring, for 3 minutes or until mixture is dry. Off heat, stir in chopped basil. Add cayenne to taste; taste and adjust seasoning.

Preheat broiler with rack about 5 inches from heat source. Toast bread about 2 minutes per side or until lightly browned. Turn off broiler; set oven at 450°F.

Put toasted bread slices on a baking sheet. Spread them with mushroom mixture and top with mozzarella. Return to oven and heat just until warm, about 3 minutes. Drizzle with olive oil if you like. Top each with a basil leaf, if desired, and serve.

Makes 6 servings

This recipe is an easy adaptation of a delicious hors d'oeuvre created by chef Suzanne Goin of Luques restaurant in Los Angeles. It looks and feels like a light, colorful form of hummus, with a green hue that makes it perfect for spring.

You can use fresh fava beans, which you need to shell, or buy frozen ones. After you cook the beans, you still have to remove their thick skins if you want the puree to be smooth and bright green, except in the case of already peeled frozen fava beans, which are available in some markets. The quickest solution is to use frozen shelled green soybeans, or edamame, which don't need peeling. You'll find them at natural foods stores, Asian markets, and many supermarkets. These delectable beans make a vivid green puree. Frozen lima beans are another good substitute.

Spread the fava puree on small pieces of fresh or toasted pita, Italian focaccia, or other flatbreads, or on a sliced baguette or good-quality crackers.

*1 pound shelled fresh or frozen fava beans,
    edamame, or lima beans*
1 or 2 garlic cloves, minced
*1½ teaspoons minced fresh rosemary, or
    ½ teaspoon minced dried rosemary*
Salt and freshly ground black pepper
3 to 4 tablespoons extra virgin olive oil

*Pinch of pure chile powder, hot red pepper flakes, or
    cayenne pepper*
Pinch of saffron threads or turmeric
1 large onion, diced small
*Fresh or toasted pita wedges, focaccia squares,
    or baguette slices*

Cook fresh fava beans for 10 minutes or until tender. Cook frozen beans according to package directions or until done to taste. Drain beans. If using fava beans, for a bright green puree, press the end of each bean to pop it out of its thick skin.

Puree beans in a food processor with garlic, rosemary, salt and pepper to taste, and 2 tablespoons oil, pulsing to make a chunky puree or blending if you prefer a smooth puree. Transfer puree to a bowl. Add chile powder and 1 more tablespoon oil if you like. Taste and adjust seasoning.

In a small cup, soak saffron threads (but not turmeric) in 3 tablespoons hot water for 5 minutes. Meanwhile, heat remaining tablespoon oil in a skillet. Add onions and cook over medium-low heat, stirring often, for 5 minutes or until light golden. Add salt, pepper, and saffron in its liquid or turmeric. Cover and cook, stirring occasionally, for 5 minutes or until onions are tender. If any liquid remains in pan, uncover and cook briefly over medium heat to evaporate it.

Serve bean puree and onions at room temperature. Spread bean puree on bread and top with a small spoonful of saffron onions.

Makes 8 to 10 hors d'oeuvres or appetizer servings

SEPHARDI SPINACH AND CHEESE BUREKAS

You may think that the luscious pastries known as burekas would not be appropriate for a healthy diet, but the Sephardi way to prepare them, coupled with a modern phyllo technique, enables them to fit in very well.

Spinach burekas resemble mini-versions of Greek spanakopita. The phyllo dough used to make them contains no fat, but must be brushed with fat so it won't be too dry. Yet when I asked several Sephardi friends whether they used butter on their phyllo, they seemed shocked at the idea. Olive oil is the best choice for giving these pastries their traditional taste, and is healthful too. For best nutrition, you don't want the burekas to be dripping with oil, but use just enough to prevent them from being dry. A technique developed at *Eating Well* magazine, which has become popular among health-conscious bakers, calls for mixing the oil with egg whites to help accomplish this, and to keep the pastry crisp.

1 pound phyllo sheets (about 20 sheets)
One 10-ounce bag of cleaned spinach leaves
About 5 tablespoons extra virgin olive oil
1 garlic clove, chopped
3 green onions, chopped
⅔ cup cottage cheese, low-fat or nonfat

⅓ cup crumbled feta
Salt and freshly ground black pepper
Freshly grated nutmeg
2 eggs, or 1 egg and 1 egg white
2 egg whites (for brushing)
About 2 teaspoons sesame seeds (for sprinkling)

If phyllo sheets are frozen, thaw them in refrigerator 8 hours or overnight. Remove sheets from refrigerator 2 hours before using and leave them in their package.

Add spinach to a saucepan of boiling water to cover spinach by half. Cover and cook over medium-high heat, stirring occasionally, for 2 minutes or until wilted. Drain, rinse with cold water, and squeeze to remove as much liquid as possible. Chop spinach fine.

Heat 1 tablespoon oil in a skillet. Add garlic, followed by spinach, and cook over low heat for 2 minutes. Remove from heat, transfer to a bowl, and let cool slightly. Add green onions, cottage cheese, and feta and mix well. Season to taste with salt, pepper, and nutmeg; filling should be highly seasoned. Stir in eggs.

Lightly grease a baking sheet. In a small bowl, beat remaining 4 tablespoons oil with 2 egg whites. Remove phyllo sheets from package and unroll them on a dry towel. With a sharp knife, cut stack in half lengthwise, to form two stacks of sheets of about 16×7 inches. Cover phyllo immediately with a piece of wax paper, then with a damp towel. Work with only one sheet at a time and always keep remaining sheets covered with wax paper and towel so they don't dry out.

Remove a pastry sheet from pile. Using a brush, dab it lightly with oil mixture and fold it in half lengthwise, so its dimensions are about 16×3½ inches. Place about 1½ teaspoons filling at one end of strip. Fold end of strip diagonally over filling to form a triangle, and dab it lightly with oil mixture. Continue folding it over and over, keeping it in a triangular shape after each fold, until you reach end of strip. Set filled pastry on greased baking sheet. Dab it lightly with oil mixture. Shape more pastries with remaining phyllo sheets and filling. Sprinkle pastries with sesame seeds.

Preheat oven to 350°F. Bake pastries for 20 to 25 minutes or until golden brown. Serve warm (not hot) or at room temperature.

Makes about 32 turnovers, or 10 to 16 appetizer servings

❧ DOUBLE SALMON SALAD

This appetizer salad is made of smoked and cooked salmon. The smoked fish adds flair to the tried-and-true formula of salmon salad with mayonnaise.

Note that smoked salmon and lox are not the same, although you can use either one for this salad. Smoked salmon is first cured in brine or with a dry rub and then either cold- or hot-smoked. Fish smoked at a low temperature (cold-smoked) retains a silky texture like that of uncooked fish, while the hot-smoked type has the consistency of moist baked fish. Lox and gravlax, the dill-flavored Scandinavian salmon, are not smoked, only cured in brine.

If you prefer an intensely smoky flavor, omit the cooked or canned fish and make the salad entirely from hot-smoked salmon. Spicy cured salmon like salmon pastrami is another tasty choice. Spread or mound the salad on crisp, thin cucumber slices, or on thin slices of cocktail rye or pumpernickel bread or split mini-pita breads. If you prefer crackers, choose salt-free or low-salt ones because the smoked salmon is salty.

Salmon is a great fish to use often, as it is rich in heart-healthy omega-3 fatty acids. So is tuna. For a tuna salad, substitute canned light tuna for the canned salmon and pair it with smoked tuna. For other variations, you can use smoked whitefish and match it with cooked whitefish, or choose other smoked fish such as halibut, cod, or trout. (See "Safe Fish," page 237.)

3 to 4 ounces smoked salmon or lox (about
  ¾ to 1 cup), flaked or finely chopped
1 cup cooked salmon (poached, baked, or broiled),
  or 3 to 4 ounces canned red salmon, flaked
2 green onions, green and white parts, finely
  chopped
2 to 3 tablespoons low-fat mayonnaise

3 to 4 tablespoons plain yogurt, nonfat or low-fat
1 to 2 tablespoons strained fresh lemon juice, or
  to taste
1 tablespoon chopped fresh dill (optional)
Cayenne pepper
Freshly ground black pepper
Salt (optional)

Combine smoked salmon, cooked salmon, and green onions. Stir in 2 tablespoons mayonnaise, 3 tablespoons yogurt, 1 tablespoon lemon juice, and dill (if using). Season to taste with cayenne and black pepper and, if necessary, add more yogurt and lemon juice. Add salt only if needed. Serve cold.

Makes 6 to 8 servings as hors d'oeuvres

Salads

When I get together with my friends, often the salad is the star of the meal. It might be a medley of tender baby greens, thin, crisp apple slices, and toasted walnuts in a rice vinegar vinaigrette or a feta-topped mix of romaine, olives, and tomatoes.

Serving a salad is one of the best ways to start a meal on a bright, positive note. The more colorful the salad, the more nutritious it is. Vegetables of each color contribute a different beneficial element—orange vegetables like carrots are rich in vitamin A, tomatoes are a great source of lycopene, and dark greens are packed with a host of healthy nutrients. Besides, if you eat salad first, when you're most hungry, you'll eat more of the healthful greens and a smaller amount of high-calorie foods.

In my kitchen I usually prepare a vegetable salad as the first course of every meal; yes, even for breakfast. Most often I prepare an Israeli diced salad of tomatoes, cucumbers, and onion, a green salad, or a combination of both.

To vary your meals, expand your salad repertoire. Just about any ingredient can be part of a salad, from raw and cooked vegetables to legumes to grains to fish to meat.

Green salads are so much fun to make these days. With cleaned, ready-to-eat salad greens on display at the supermarket, there is no excuse for serving meals without vegetables. I am delighted that mixed baby lettuces are now easy to find. These pretty greens are a treat. Whenever I serve them, they bring back memories of feasts I enjoyed in restaurants in Paris. With just a sprinkling of vinaigrette dressing, they are perfect as a bed for such ingredients as sautéed wild mushrooms or a favorite goat cheese.

There's another good reason to use these greens rather than iceberg lettuce alone. They are much more beneficial nutritionally than iceberg lettuce. Like intensely colored cooking greens, they contain plenty of vitamins and minerals. Some of them, such as the lovely, round, deep green tat-soi leaves, are mild members of the cabbage family and boast the same nutrients of this valuable vegetable group.

I am surprised that some of my friends and relatives don't like these lovely lettuces. I suppose their palates are not used to the mixtures that contain bitter greens like arugula and chicory. To balance these flavors, I often include some iceberg lettuce in my green salads. Its mild, slightly sweet taste and refreshing, crisp texture makes it an ideal associate for the more assertive greens. Besides, it costs much less and so it stretches the special greens, which can be pricey.

To garnish our salads, nuts are at the top of my list, both for flavor and nutrition. Toasted or raw almonds sprinkled on green salads lend a welcome taste, richness, and crunch. Other favorites of ours are Brazil nuts, walnuts, pecans, roasted peanuts, pine

GOOD FATS

*T*he fact that olive oil is a healthful fat has been highly publicized. Yet, there are other fabulous fats that are not only healthful, but contribute a wonderful flavor to your cooking. You'll find them if you browse the aisles of fine ethnic markets, natural foods stores, and gourmet groceries.

At an exposition of natural foods I attended, this group of ingredients caught my attention—beautiful oils in hues of gold, green, and red. They were made from foods that most of us love, like hazelnuts, macadamia nuts, pumpkin seeds, and avocados.

First I tried the hazelnut oil. It had a nutty aroma and its flavor practically exploded in my mouth—it was pure essence of hazelnut. Roasted almond oil and pumpkin seed oil also were fragrant and flavorful. Next to these, avocado oil seemed almost neutral to my palate. As I tried other oils, I learned that roasting nuts and seeds gives these oils their pronounced tastes. If you've used Asian sesame oil in Chinese cooking, you're familiar with the effect that toasting the seeds has on the oil's character.

Like fine extra virgin olive oil, these luscious oils have many uses in the kitchen. To me, the aromatic, toasted nut oils have the most exciting possibilities; they are so flavorful that a little bit will give you a lovely burst of flavor. Serving them for dipping is a good introduction; simply pour some into a ramekin or a little bowl to accompany bread or raw or lightly steamed vegetables. A small amount of any toasted nut oil also gives a flavor boost to a big bowl of greens.

nuts, sunflower seeds, and black or green olives. Like olive oil, the fat in nuts, seeds, and olives is monounsaturated and therefore they are recommended by nutritionists as foods that are heart healthy. Still, I add them with a light touch, as they are high in calories.

Of course, my husband and I don't eat the same salads every day. That would be too boring for food lovers like us. Our salads change with the seasons and with what is featured at the market. In fact, the only thing they have in common is that I try to include a tasty surprise.

I'm always on the lookout for new wholesome treats for salads. Some of our salad surprises are nutritious snack foods. We especially like roasted chickpeas. We buy them at Israeli and other Middle Eastern stores and Indian grocery shops. They are similar to soy

Years ago, in Perigord in southwest France, I encountered the region's delicious walnut oil, which people are fond of sprinkling on green salads, and found that the oil is fantastic in mashed potatoes too. These days, top chefs use it with enthusiasm. It is delicious with fish and can also perfume desserts.

Such toasted nut and seed oils are a boon to cooks on a hectic schedule. Simply add them to cold dishes or sprinkle them over hot food at serving time.

These unique oils are best showcased in salads, seafood entrées, and simple vegetable dishes. Often I include the same nut for emphasis. Spinach salad is sensational when embellished with pecan oil dressing, pecans, a bit of goat cheese, and a few sautéed mushrooms. Potato salad is terrific with hazelnut oil vinaigrette and toasted hazelnuts, and so is brown rice salad. Make up your own pesto variations by using nut or seed oils with their corresponding nuts. To add pizzazz to a bowl of vegetable soup, drizzle roasted hazelnut or pumpkin seed oil over it.

Mild oils like sunflower oil are ideal for dressing foods when you want their flavors to stand on their own. Combined with a hint of wine vinegar, such oils enhance salads of warm steamed fish with slim green beans, or of baby lettuces with pears. The unobtrusive oils are also good for sautéing subtle fish like sole. For many people's palates, olive oil would overpower these foods, but the mildly flavored oils help to highlight the foods' intrinsic tastes.

These bottles of liquid gold are good news for health-conscious cooks, as they marry fine taste with nutritional benefits. All are low in saturated fat. Like olive oil, certain ones such as hazelnut are high in health-promoting monounsaturated fat.

nuts, which are tasty salad toppers too. They give a nice crunch to salad, and the spicy ones have a bonus of a peppery kick.

A few months ago, we discovered roasted corn kernels at a local natural foods store. They were delicious—sweet, light, and delicately crunchy—and unlike any corn we had ever tasted. Crunchy green peas, carrots, bell peppers and, of course, sliced dried tomatoes also make delightful salad sprinkles. When you embellish your salads this way, remember that crunchy snacks are best when they are not mixed with the other ingredients so they won't become soggy. Simply scatter the goodies over each individual serving to preserve and enjoy their crisp texture.

For appetizer salads you might like to top the greens with a few pieces of smoked fish, sliced mushrooms, strips of roasted peppers, or slices of tangy fruit like kiwi, tart apples, or plums. Strips of grilled fish or chicken or cubes of feta or goat cheese can make the salad substantial enough to serve as a summertime main course.

AVOCADO—BUTTER FROM A TREE

*I*n my college years in Jerusalem, I tasted avocado for the first time. I noticed that most people in this avocado-rich country prepared the fruit by mashing its pulp with salt, pepper, and a squeeze of lemon juice, and spreading it on bread. I immediately loved this simple spread; it reminded me of my favorite food—butter!

Later, during the years I was studying cooking in Paris, I learned that the French import avocados from Israel, but prepare them differently. Chefs use them as containers for salads, serve them with vinaigrette, and turn them into sauces, soups, and mousses. Like cooks in Israel, the French use just enough seasoning to highlight the fruit's fine flavor without overpowering it.

In California, I became acquainted with guacamole. At first I was amazed that anyone would use such strong seasonings as cilantro and chiles, which appeared to compete with the avocado's delicate character. But soon I realized that avocado, like butter, has an affinity for assertive ingredients as well as subtle ones. Maybe that's why it's so popular in the California rolls at sushi bars, in which the fruit is matched with tuna and rice with a little kick of wasabi.

Avocado seems designed for quick, easy summertime dishes because it does not require cooking. In fact, overheating mars its subtle taste. Many avocado dishes are so simple that there is no need to give precise

Fruit can be a nice foil for the lettuces, lending its sweetness to contrast with their sharpness. Almost any fruit—fresh or dried—can fulfill this function. Nectarines, peaches, apricots, mangoes, and papayas add a pretty contrasting color, as do raspberries and orange segments. Apples and Asian pears contribute crunch.

As for dressing, I'm not wild about the commercial concoctions. Making your own vinaigrette is nearly as fast as using prepared dressing and gives you much better control over its taste and its nutritional value. Dressings make salads tasty and can contribute to the salads' healthy nutrients as well. Use a fruity extra virgin olive oil or a flavorful walnut oil, hazelnut oil, or other nut oil and turn it into a vinaigrette-type dressing by blending it with a fine vinegar or a squeeze of fresh citrus juice. Such fluid dressings season the leaves without weighing them down, in contrast to thick mayonnaise-type dressings that can overwhelm the greens. Use just enough dressing to lightly moisten the salad without leaving a puddle at the bottom of the bowl.

recipes for them. I love to embellish the popular Italian insalata caprese (fresh mozzarella cheese, tomato slices, and basil) by alternating avocado slices with the other components to make a red, white, and green salad. Avocado cubes or balls are a delicious addition to the Israeli tomato-cucumber-onion salad.

For sandwiches and sauces, avocado makes a refreshing change from butter, cream cheese, or mayonnaise. Besides, it's cholesterol-free and low in saturated fat. Its fat is mostly the monounsaturated type— the healthful kind found in olive oil. A favorite sandwich of mine is avocado, lox, and bagel, with avocado replacing the customary cream cheese (see page 32). For another tasty sandwich filling, match avocado with smoked turkey and tomato.

Avocado's richness makes it an especially good partner for poultry, fish, vegetables, grains, and tropical fruits. Its pulp can be a base for velvety sauces, in which I use the more healthful avocado instead of adding a large amount of cream.

At the market, select avocados that are heavy, with unblemished skins. They will be ripe when they yield to gentle pressure. If an avocado is still hard, let it ripen for a few days at room temperature. Once it is ripe, you can keep it in the refrigerator for a few days.

To halve an avocado, run a knife lengthwise around the fruit, then twist to separate the two halves. Remove the pit by hitting it with the heel of a chef's knife, using just enough force so that the knife sticks in the pit. Then lift the knife, with the pit attached.

FRUITFUL RESCUES

*O*n his first visit to the United States from Israel, my brother-in-law ordered fruit salad. He was as-
tounded when the waiter asked what dressing he wanted—Thousand Island or Italian.

I understood his reaction perfectly. When I returned to the United States after twelve years in France
and Israel, I considered fruit salad a dessert. Seafood salad with mandarin oranges and syrupy curry
dressing left me cold. Deli chicken salad crowned with strawberries did not appeal. Cantaloupe salad
topped with sugary mayonnaise was even worse.

Warming to the idea of savory fruit combinations—I mean "savory" in the sense of piquant as op-
posed to sweet—took me time. True, I enjoyed such classics as French pears with Roquefort, European
cabbage with apples, and Ashkenazi beef tzimmes with dried fruit. Soon I realized that in spite of some
outrageous pairings I had encountered, there are tasty ways to include fruit in salads for entrées, appetizers, and accompaniments.

Fruit is complex in flavor. Certain ones—tart apples, many plums, citrus fruits, and pineapples—have
an inherent tang and are ideal for salads.

Recipes tend to call for fruit at its peak, but sometimes it has less sugar than it should. Too often we
purchase hard fruit and hope in vain to ripen it in the kitchen. Poaching the fruit in syrup is one option.
When the weather is still hot, I prefer a no-cook solution.

Instead of being disappointed by these fruits, I consider them candidates for vegetable salads. Overly
firm peaches and nectarines, plums, and melons lacking sugar; tart kiwis; very green apples; and hard
pears are fine additions. Naturally, I'm not suggesting that anyone eat bad produce or fruits like avocados and Hachiya persimmons that are inedible when underripe.

Frequently I start with a familiar mixture. Braised red cabbage with apples translates easily into red cabbage and apple salad with sweet onions and ginger vinaigrette. Substituting pears is not much of a stretch.

Fruit can replace specific vegetables, especially tomatoes. Anyhow, the line between fruits and vegetables isn't clear. Botanically the tomato is a fruit, but was classified as a vegetable by the U.S. Supreme Court in 1893 due to a customs dispute.

Kiwi is a terrific tomato stand-in, as both share the traits of juiciness, sweetness, and tang. It plays this role in my Mediterranean chopped salad matched with cucumbers, onion, lemon juice, and olive oil. Other tomato alternatives are plums, peaches, nectarines, pineapple, and papaya. They lend color and good flavor even if they're not sweet. If they lack juice, you can add extra lemon juice or balsamic or rice wine vinegar.

Greens gain pizzazz from fruit, especially when seasoned with light dressings. Quick coleslaw dressed with oil and vinegar benefits from diced underripe nectarines. Plums or peaches are a wonderful accent in a simple mélange of red-leaf lettuce, baby romaine, walnut oil vinaigrette, and toasted walnuts. Butter lettuce, iceberg lettuce, mesclun (mixed baby lettuces), and Napa cabbage work well too. For a more substantial appetizer or light entrée, you can top the medley with small goat cheese chunks or roast chicken strips.

A brief look at other cuisines yields a wealth of ideas. At a reception I attended, a Mexican chef served fruit with jicama. The white-fleshed crunchy tuber with its subtle applelike taste is a great partner for fruit in salads. I love it with peaches and red onion tossed with spinach. Persians add their delicate cucumbers to fruit platters, and together they also make cool salads with baby greens, chives, lime juice, and a touch of olive oil.

There's an unexpected bonus. Less than perfect fruit appears to improve in salads dressed with a slightly tart vinaigrette. From the contrast between the vegetables and the dressing, the fruit seems sweeter. Yet I still wouldn't pour Thousand Island dressing over my bowl of fruit.

MEDITERRANEAN VEGETABLE SALAD WITH SUNFLOWER SEEDS

CRUNCHY CARROT BROCCOLI SLAW WITH PEANUTS

CUCUMBER, JICAMA, AND ORANGE SALAD WITH BLACK OLIVES

DICED VEGETABLE SALAD WITH PEPITAS AND PAPAYA

BABY GREENS WITH TOASTED WALNUTS, FIGS, AND LIGHT ROSEMARY VINAIGRETTE

CALIFORNIA FRENCH PEAR AND BLUE CHEESE SALAD WITH MIXED GREENS

PROVENÇAL GREEN BEAN AND CHICKPEA SALAD WITH TOMATOES AND OLIVES

ASPARAGUS SALAD WITH CARROTS AND SHIITAKE MUSHROOMS

TURKISH CARROTS WITH WALNUTS AND YOGURT GARLIC DRESSING

BEET SALAD WITH FETA, PECANS, AND BABY LETTUCES

BEANS AND GREENS SALAD

NEW WORLD TABBOULEH

MEDITERRANEAN VEGETABLE SALAD WITH SUNFLOWER SEEDS

Sunflower seeds are a very popular snack in Israel. Serving the hulled seeds as a salad topping is an easy way to enjoy their taste and crunchy texture and to benefit from their nutrients. The seeds are a good source of vitamin E, vitamin B₁, magnesium, and selenium, and they are one of the best sources of cholesterol-lowering phytosterols. They also contain protein and fiber.

This is a practical, everyday salad because you can prepare it quickly by adding greens to the typical Mediterranean chopped salad. Whether you opt for romaine, iceberg lettuce, or spinach, the greens add a pleasing textural contrast to the diced vegetables and easily help to increase the volume of the salad. You can use packaged salads to make preparation faster.

1 hothouse cucumber, or 4 Persian
    (Middle Eastern) cucumbers, or
    2 slim pickling cucumbers
3 medium tomatoes, or 4 to 6 plum tomatoes
1 small red, yellow, or green bell pepper,
    cut into ½-inch dice
1 or 2 green onions, chopped
1½ cups chopped romaine, iceberg lettuce, iceberg
    lettuce mix, or spinach

2 tablespoons extra virgin olive oil
1 to 2 tablespoons strained fresh lemon juice
½ teaspoon garlic herb seasoning blend, salad herbs
    seasoning blend, or herbes de Provence
Salt and freshly ground black pepper
1 to 2 tablespoons toasted sunflower seeds

Peel cucumbers if you like, cut into ½-inch dice, and put in a glass serving bowl. Cut tomatoes in similar dice and add to bowl. Add bell pepper and green onions, and mix with vegetables in bowl. Add lettuce and toss mixture. Add oil, lemon juice, garlic herb seasoning, and salt and pepper and toss again. Taste and adjust seasoning. Serve cool or cold, topped with sunflower seeds.

Makes 4 servings

CRUNCHY CARROT BROCCOLI SLAW WITH PEANUTS

People who discard the thick stems of broccoli when they prepare dishes that call for the florets are missing a good ingredient. The stems have a delicate sweetness and a pleasing crunch. For serving raw, I find they taste even better than the florets. You do need to cut off the tough peel, but that is easy to do. For speed and convenience, you can opt for packaged broccoli slaw mix, which is composed of shredded broccoli stalks and a little red cabbage and grated carrot. Roasted peanut oil adds a pleasant flavor to the dressing of this salad, which boasts the nutritional benefits of healthful cruciferous vegetables and peanuts.

1 tender carrot, cut into 2-inch chunks

6 thick broccoli stems

1 pickling cucumber, or ⅓ medium cucumber (optional)

1 cup shredded red or green cabbage

1 cup chopped romaine

2 radishes, halved and sliced thin

1 to 2 tablespoons roasted peanut oil or vegetable oil

1 to 2 tablespoons rice vinegar or other mild vinegar

Salt and freshly ground black pepper

¼ cup roasted peanuts

Cut carrot in very thin, lengthwise sticks. Peel broccoli stems, using a sturdy knife. Cut broccoli stems in thin, lengthwise strips of about same size as carrot sticks. Finely dice cucumber (if using). In a bowl combine carrots, broccoli, cucumber, cabbage, romaine, and radishes. Add oil, vinegar, and salt and pepper to taste. Serve sprinkled with peanuts.

Makes 3 to 4 servings

CUCUMBER, JICAMA, AND ORANGE SALAD WITH BLACK OLIVES

Although jicama is not used in Mediterranean countries, I find it goes well with the region's flavors. This enticing savory-sweet salad is similar to Moroccan salads, and is spiked with black olives, cumin, and cayenne. I like it as an appetizer before grilled chicken and couscous.

1 small jicama (12 ounces)
4 small pickling cucumbers (10 to 12 ounces), halved lengthwise, sliced ¼ inch thick (2⅔ cups slices)
⅔ cup black olives, pitted
2 to 3 tablespoons extra virgin olive oil

2 to 3 tablespoons fresh lemon juice
½ teaspoon paprika
½ teaspoon ground cumin
Salt and freshly ground black pepper
Cayenne pepper
2 navel oranges, peeled

Halve jicama from top to bottom and cut off peel. Put each half, cut side down, on a board and cut it in half through its "equator." Slice about ¼ inch thick. Cut largest slices in half so they are roughly the size of the cucumber slices. (You'll need 2⅔ to 3 cups.) Mix jicama, cucumbers, and olives in a shallow bowl.

In a small bowl, combine oil, lemon juice, paprika, and cumin and whisk to blend. Season to taste with salt, pepper, and cayenne. Add to salad and mix lightly.

Trim excess pith from oranges. Halve oranges from top to bottom. Set, cut side down, on a board and cut in crosswise slices about ¼ inch thick. Cut each slice in half, removing any pits. Gently mix orange pieces into salad. Taste and adjust seasoning. Serve cold.

Makes 4 servings

❧ DICED VEGETABLE SALAD WITH PEPITAS AND PAPAYA

In my kitchen this salad evolved from the standard Israeli salad of tomatoes, cucumber, and onions. The papaya, which is known as Maradol papaya but sold in my local markets as "Mexican papaya," found its way into the salad when I was out of tomatoes. We liked it so much that we often add it when it's in season. It's also a great way to make use of papayas that turn out to be not sweet enough for dessert. When the papaya is mixed with vegetables, it seems to taste sweeter.

Jicama is a delightful addition because of its crisp texture and its sweetness. Some people recommend soaking jicama slices or sticks overnight in cold water, especially if the tuber seems a bit dried out, to revive them and give them a moister texture, but I find this treatment makes the jicama less sweet. Soaking does help to keep jicama from discoloring if you want to peel and cut it in advance. The dressing echoes the traditional Mexican way to eat jicama—sprinkled with lime juice, salt, and pure chile powder (not the American mixture of chile and other spices).

Pepitas, or green Mexican pumpkin seeds, add a nutty flavor and pretty green color. Sometimes I make this salad of only papaya and diced vegetables. At other times I add spinach, other greens, red or green cabbage, or a mixture of these.

One 8- to 12-ounce piece of jicama
1½ to 2 cups peeled, diced Mexican papaya
1 pickling cucumber, ¼ hothouse cucumber, or
   ½ medium cucumber, peeled and cut into
   small dice
1 Anaheim or poblano chile (called pasilla in
   California), cut into thin strips (optional)
4 plum tomatoes, cut into small dice (optional)
1 to 2 cups chopped romaine or iceberg lettuce
   (optional)

⅓ cup chopped green onion
1 to 2 tablespoons extra virgin olive oil
1 to 2 tablespoons strained fresh lime or
   lemon juice
Salt and freshly ground black pepper
Cayenne pepper or pure chile powder
   (not the blend)
2 tablespoons toasted pepitas

To prepare jicama, cut it in half and cut off peel with a sturdy knife, removing fibrous layer below brown skin as well. Cut jicama into thin slices, then in dice. You will need about 2 cups.

In a salad bowl, mix together jicama, papaya, cucumber dice, chile strips (if using), tomatoes, romaine (if using), and green onion. Add oil, lime juice, and salt, pepper, and cayenne to taste. Serve cold or at room temperature, sprinkled with pepitas.

Makes 4 servings

BABY GREENS WITH TOASTED WALNUTS, FIGS, AND LIGHT ROSEMARY VINAIGRETTE

I often use mixtures of assertive and mild greens in salads, like this one, for which I combine radicchio and mixed baby lettuces with delicate butter lettuce or crisp iceberg lettuce. This festive salad is based on one I sampled at a tasting of foods of Italy's Veneto province, including the region's radicchio.

The salad demonstrated what a nice foil dried fruit can be for flavorful baby lettuces, lending a lively, sweet accent to contrast with their sharpness. You need just a few pieces of fruit; you don't want to turn this green salad into fruit salad.

If your dried figs are not moist, plump them up by soaking them briefly in lukewarm water. Be sure the walnuts taste fresh. Keep them in the freezer so they don't become rancid.

¼ red, white, or sweet onion, sliced very thin

2 tablespoons walnut oil or extra virgin olive oil

1 tablespoon balsamic vinegar

1 teaspoon minced fresh rosemary

Salt and freshly ground black pepper

2 cups mixed baby lettuces

½ cup bite-sized pieces of radicchio leaves (optional)

3 cups bite-sized pieces of iceberg lettuce or iceberg-lettuce mix with red cabbage and carrots

8 to 12 moist dried figs, halved

2 ounces feta, crumbled (optional)

¼ to ⅓ cup walnut halves, toasted (page 380)

In a shallow serving bowl, combine onion, oil, vinegar, rosemary, salt, and pepper. Let stand so that onion marinates while you prepare remaining salad ingredients.

Rinse baby lettuces, radicchio (if using), and iceberg lettuce. Drain greens well and pat them dry.

A short time before serving, add greens to serving bowl. Toss to mix well with onions and dressing. Taste and adjust seasoning. Serve salad topped with figs, feta if you like, and walnuts.

Makes 4 servings

CALIFORNIA FRENCH PEAR AND BLUE CHEESE SALAD WITH MIXED GREENS

The partnership of pears and blue cheese is decidedly in the style of the French, who happily pair the fruit with Roquefort cheese. Yet matching this duo with greens is a fairly new culinary custom. When I began studying at La Varenne Cooking School in Paris in 1976, our salade verte (green salad) was plain, or occasionally embellished with nuts, and it was served in the time-honored French way, after the main course. A couple of years later our school chefs began to incorporate goat cheese or other flavorful creamy cheeses into the garnish, and served these more substantial salads as starters. Still later, with the inventiveness encouraged by nouvelle cuisine, pears, apples, or other fruit were added.

This type of salad, combining sweet and pungent flavors, was enthusiastically adopted by California chefs. Mary Sue Milliken and Susan Feniger, for example, the chef-owners of Border Grill in Santa Monica, gave the salad a Spanish-Mexican twist in their grilled pear and endive salad enhanced with spiced pistachios, cabrales blue cheese (from Spain), pickled chiles, and chile honey vinaigrette.

Use any variety of ripe, firm pears, either juicy Comice or drier, sweet Bosc. I like to add peppery watercress or arugula, or Belgian endive for a bit of bitterness, which goes well with the rich cheese, the toasted nuts, and the sweet fruit.

6 to 7 cups baby greens, bite-sized pieces of romaine, or other sturdy lettuce
1 cup arugula, chopped Belgian endive, or watercress tops
2 tablespoons white wine vinegar
1 to 2 teaspoons honey (optional)

Pinch of salt and freshly ground black pepper
4 to 5 tablespoons walnut oil or olive oil
⅓ cup crumbled Roquefort, other blue cheese, or goat cheese
⅓ cup pecans, toasted
1 or 2 large pears, ripe but firm

Rinse and dry baby greens and arugula thoroughly. Combine them in a bowl.

For vinaigrette, whisk vinegar with honey (if using), salt, and pepper in a bowl; whisk in oil.

A short time before serving, toss greens with vinaigrette. Add half of cheese and half of walnuts, leaving a little of each for garnish, and toss. Taste and adjust seasoning. Transfer to a shallow bowl or to individual plates.

Just before serving, slice pears. Garnish salad with pear slices, remaining cheese, and remaining walnuts.

Makes 4 to 6 servings

PROVENÇAL GREEN BEAN AND CHICKPEA SALAD WITH TOMATOES AND OLIVES

When fresh shell beans are in season, follow the custom of Provençal cooks and use them for salads like this one instead of the chickpeas. Another beautiful, tasty addition is fresh green chickpeas. They started appearing recently at my local Mexican market and can be found at gourmet markets too. They need only about 10 minutes to cook, but take time to shell, as there usually are only two beans in each pod. Save them for someone you really want to please!

This colorful salad enlivens any menu with a delicious taste of the Riviera, and is full of healthy ingredients: a generous amount of green beans; nutty-flavored, fiber-rich chickpeas; and vitamin-rich bell peppers and tomatoes. I like it as a first course for Shabbat, as a summertime accompaniment for grilled fish, or with some good feta cheese and whole wheat bread for a light meal. It tastes best at room temperature or slightly warm.

For the finest results, use a flavorful olive oil and make sure your garlic and herbs are fresh. Use the technique favored by French chefs to keep the beans bright green: rinse them in cold running water as soon as they are cooked.

¾ cup dried chickpeas (garbanzo beans), or
    1½ to 2 cups cooked chickpeas, or
    one 15-ounce can chickpeas, drained
1 pound green beans, or ½ pound green beans and
    ½ pound yellow (wax) beans
Salt and freshly ground black pepper
1 to 1½ tablespoons fresh lemon juice
1 large garlic clove, finely minced
2 to 3 tablespoons extra virgin olive oil

1 small red or yellow bell pepper, raw or roasted
    (page 376), or from a jar
3 ripe plum tomatoes, diced
¼ cup black olives, preferably oil-cured niçoise type
    or Greek Kalamata, halved and pitted
1 teaspoon chopped fresh thyme
2 tablespoons chopped fresh basil
1 tablespoon capers, drained

If using dried chickpeas, cook them (see page 378). Put green beans in a large saucepan of boiling salted water and return to a boil. Cook, uncovered, over high heat for 5 minutes or until crisp-tender. Drain, rinse with cold water, and drain well.

In a small bowl, whisk lemon juice with garlic, salt, pepper, and 2 tablespoons oil. Cut pepper into strips, making strips very thin if pepper is raw. Combine green beans with chickpeas, pepper strips, tomatoes, and olives. Add garlic dressing, thyme, and half the basil, and mix well. Taste, adjust seasoning, and add more oil if needed. Sprinkle with remaining basil and capers.

Makes 4 to 6 servings

❧ ASPARAGUS SALAD WITH CARROTS AND SHIITAKE MUSHROOMS

With its simple, Chinese-inspired dressing, this colorful salad is good hot or cold, as an appetizer, or as a partner for meat or chicken. If you like, cook the vegetables ahead. If you're serving them hot, heat them in a little oil for extra richness and shine, then add the dressing directly to the skillet. For serving cold, add the asparagus at the last moment so the dressing won't diminish its vivid hue.

To season the salad the Moroccan way and make it kosher for Passover, see the Note following this recipe.

When you prepare this salad, save the cooking liquid from the asparagus, carrots, and mushrooms; it makes tasty broth. You can also save the shiitake mushroom stems and the asparagus bases for making more broth.

---

8 large dried shiitake mushrooms, rinsed

12 ounces medium asparagus spears, peeled if over
    1/4 inch thick and rinsed

2 or 3 long, slim carrots (about 8 ounces), peeled

Salt

2 teaspoons soy sauce

2 teaspoons hoisin sauce, or more to taste

2 teaspoons rice vinegar, or more to taste

2 to 5 teaspoons vegetable oil

Salt and freshly ground black pepper

Few drops of hot sauce (optional)

1 to 2 tablespoons chopped green part of
    green onions (optional)

1/2 teaspoon Asian (toasted) sesame oil

Put mushrooms in a bowl. Cover them with hot water and let them soak until soft, about 30 minutes. Remove mushrooms, rinse, and cut off tough stems. Halve mushroom caps.

Cut asparagus into 3 or 4 pieces on the bias, cutting off tough white bases (about 1/2 inch from the end). Cut carrots into diagonal pieces about the same length as the asparagus pieces.

Add asparagus to a saucepan of boiling salted water, enough to cover it generously. Boil, uncovered, until pieces are barely tender, 2 to 3 minutes; to check, lift a few on a slotted spoon and pierce them with a knife tip. Drain asparagus, reserving liquid. Rinse asparagus with cold running water and drain it well.

Combine asparagus cooking liquid, carrots, mushrooms, and a pinch of salt in saucepan. Bring to a boil. Cover and simmer until carrots are just tender, about 5 minutes. Drain well.

For the dressing, whisk soy sauce, 2 teaspoons hoisin sauce, and 2 teaspoons vinegar in a small bowl until combined. Whisk in 2 teaspoons oil and a little salt, pepper, and hot sauce, if you like.

To serve salad hot, heat 2 to 3 teaspoons vegetable oil in a skillet over medium heat.

Add all vegetables and a pinch of salt and pepper. Cook until hot, about 30 seconds. Add dressing and heat for a few seconds, shaking pan. Off heat, add green onions and sesame oil and toss to combine.

To serve salad cold or at room temperature, toss dressing with carrots and mushrooms. Just before serving, add asparagus, green onions (if using), and sesame oil.

Taste, and adjust the amounts of salt, pepper, hoisin sauce, and vinegar.

NOTE: To season the salad the Moroccan way, substitute lemon juice for the vinegar and olive oil for the vegetable and sesame oils, and omit the soy and hoisin sauces. Doing this makes the dish kosher for Passover for those who avoid rice- and seed-based foods.

Makes 4 servings

TURKISH CARROTS WITH WALNUTS AND YOGURT GARLIC DRESSING

Lightly sautéing carrots in extra virgin olive oil gives this salad a unique taste and texture. The tangy dressing is a perfect match for the carrots' sweetness. Although you might think yogurt dressings sound like dull diet food, you'll change your mind after you've tasted Turkish ones.

I received this recipe from Ulker Dogan, the wife of the director of Gaziantep's Tourist Office, when I visited their fascinating city in southeast Turkey. For her dressing, Mrs. Dogan recommends strained yogurt, which is thicker and richer than the usual yogurt. You can find it in natural foods stores and Greek and Middle Eastern markets, where it might be labeled labneh or kefir cheese. Note that labneh can be as rich as sour cream; if you are opting to use it for its delicious flavor, it's best to use only a few tablespoons mixed with nonfat yogurt so the salad will not be too high in fat. Goat's milk yogurt is another tasty option. For a healthier version, buy Greek low-fat or nonfat yogurt, which is available at some markets, or any plain yogurt you like.

To save time, use shredded carrots from the market, but chop the garlic yourself. Since it's used raw, pre-chopped garlic from a jar just won't do!

2 tablespoons extra virgin olive oil

3 to 4 cups coarsely grated carrots

1 or 2 garlic cloves, crushed and very finely chopped

1 to 1⅓ cups yogurt, or ¼ cup labneh and 1 cup yogurt

1 tablespoon mayonnaise, preferably low-fat

¼ cup coarsely chopped walnuts

Salt

2 tablespoons whole or coarsely chopped flat-leaf parsley leaves

Heat oil in a medium skillet. Add carrots and cook over medium heat, stirring often, for 5 to 7 minutes or until tender. Transfer mixture to a bowl and let cool.

In a small bowl, mix garlic, yogurt, mayonnaise, half the walnuts, and salt to taste. Mix well. If dressing is too thick, gradually stir in 1 or 2 tablespoons cold water. Gently fold dressing into carrots. Taste and adjust seasoning. Serve cold or at room temperature, garnished with remaining walnuts and parsley.

Makes 3 to 4 servings

BEET SALAD WITH FETA, PECANS, AND BABY LETTUCES

At a Santa Monica beach hotel, I enjoyed a low-carb appetizer salad of roasted baby beets with English peas and warm feta in port vinaigrette. Here is a simpler salad of beets and toasted nuts in Dijon mustard dressing, which evolved from one I learned to make in France. I steam the beets, as this takes less time than roasting them.

5 to 6 small beets (about 1½ inches in diameter), rinsed

2 tablespoons white or red wine vinegar

2 to 3 teaspoons Dijon mustard

Salt and freshly ground black pepper

4 to 5 tablespoons vegetable oil or mild-flavored olive oil

6 cups mixed baby lettuces or bite-sized pieces of romaine

¾ cup crumbled feta

½ cup pecans, toasted (page 380)

Bring at least 1 inch of water to a boil in base of a steamer without allowing boiling water to reach steamer holes. Place beets on steamer top above boiling water. Cover tightly and steam over high heat for 50 minutes or until tender, adding boiling water if water evaporates. Remove beets and let cool. Peel beets while holding them under cold running water.

Whisk vinegar with mustard, salt, and pepper until blended. Gradually whisk in oil.

Dice beets and add to lettuce in large, shallow bowl. Add 4 to 6 tablespoons dressing and toss very gently. Add more dressing if needed. Taste and adjust seasoning. Sprinkle with feta and pecans and serve.

Makes 6 servings

BEANS AND GREENS SALAD

In eastern Mediterranean countries, beans and greens are frequently cooked together, in dishes such as chard with chickpeas or spinach with white beans. I find that this healthy combination makes a tasty, colorful, easy-to-prepare salad as well. In summer such a salad is a more enticing way to enjoy both beans and greens. The salad is also perfect for Purim, when beans are often on the menu to honor Queen Esther's vegetarian diet. Serve it in small quantities as an appetizer or in more generous amounts as a main course for lunch.

You can use any mixture of beans and greens you like. Red beans have a beautiful contrasting color with the deep greens, but chickpeas or pinto beans are good as well. I like cannellini beans or other white beans when combined with baby lettuce mixes that include a little radicchio or baby red greens. If you have time, marinate the beans in part of the dressing before adding the remaining ingredients.

¾ to 1 cup cooked or canned red beans
2 to 3 tablespoons extra virgin olive oil
1 to 2 tablespoons fresh lemon juice
Salt and freshly ground black pepper
½ cup very thin strips of carrot
1 cucumber, peeled, quartered, and sliced thin

1 tomato, diced (optional)
1 green onion, chopped, or ⅓ cup finely chopped
    white or red onion
4 cups chopped spinach or romaine
1 to 2 teaspoons fresh thyme, or ½ teaspoon
    dried thyme

Mix beans with 1 tablespoon oil, ½ tablespoon lemon juice, salt, and pepper. Let stand for 30 minutes at room temperature, or cover and refrigerate for 2 to 3 hours. Transfer beans and their marinade to a large bowl. Add carrot, cucumber, tomato (if using), and green onion. Add spinach and toss until well combined. Add remaining oil, remaining lemon juice, thyme, and salt and pepper to taste. Serve at room temperature.

Makes 4 servings

Tabbouleh is such a tasty, versatile recipe that it's natural to make it with other grains besides the traditional bulgur wheat. French chefs recognized this and for years have been making their tabbouleh with couscous. I've also made a hearty version with barley. For this tabbouleh I use quinoa, which you can purchase at natural foods stores, and corn.

With the high-protein quinoa, this salad can be served as a light main course. Corn kernels add an appealing color and texture, and a pleasant contrasting sweetness to the lemony dressing. In summertime I like to add the corn kernels uncooked. Tabbouleh is a healthy salad, due to the generous amounts of parsley and the seasoning of olive oil and lemon juice, but the lavish amount of oil in classic versions can be too caloric. I use less oil and keep the salad moist by including extra tomato.

To keep with the New World theme, I add cilantro and jalapeño.

¾ cup quinoa
1½ cups vegetable broth or water
Salt and freshly ground black pepper
3 to 5 tablespoons extra virgin olive oil
¾ cup corn kernels, fresh, frozen, or canned
and drained
6 plum tomatoes
½ hothouse cucumber, or 2 small, thin-skinned
(Persian or Middle Eastern) cucumbers

1 jalapeño pepper, minced, or cayenne pepper
to taste
4 green onions, white and green parts,
sliced thin
¾ cup finely chopped flat-leaf parsley
¼ cup chopped cilantro
⅓ cup finely chopped mint
3 tablespoons strained fresh lemon juice, or
more to taste

Put quinoa in a strainer and rinse several times with warm water. Drain well. Bring broth, or water with a pinch of salt, to a simmer in a medium saucepan. Add quinoa and bring to a boil. Cover and simmer over low heat for 15 to 20 minutes or until liquid is absorbed. Fluff quinoa and transfer to a bowl. Add 1 tablespoon oil and let cool.

If using fresh corn kernels cut from a cob, rinse and leave them raw; or cook fresh or frozen kernels for 2 to 3 minutes in boiling water to barely cover. Drain; reserve cooking liquid to add to vegetable broth or soups.

Dice tomatoes and cucumbers very small. Mix diced vegetables with jalapeño pepper, green onions, parsley, cilantro, mint, and corn. Add to cooled quinoa. Add salt, pepper, remaining oil, and lemon juice to taste; salad should be fairly tart. Serve cold or at cool room temperature.

Makes 6 to 8 appetizer or 3 main-course servings

Soups

NOURISHING STANDBYS FOR WEEKDAYS
AND SPECIAL OCCASIONS

A useful cooking custom I learned from my Yemen-born mother-in-law was always to have a pot of soup ready to provide a healthy, sustaining meal. Hers featured a richly flavored cumin-scented broth studded with beef cubes and whole potatoes and accompanied by a chile-garlic relish. This type of hearty soup is loved around the Mediterranean.

Putting soup on the menu every day is a popular custom from the Far East to France. A Thai chef friend of mine stressed the importance of a steaming bowl of noodle soup in her country as the daily lunch dish for most people. And when I studied cooking in Paris, a great French chef told me, describing one of his first jobs, cooking at a hotel, "I made a different soup every day of the year."

I was impressed that anyone could come up with 365 soups, but the chef reminded me that you can make soup out of just about any ingredient, from fish to beef to beans. Vegetables, however, give the cook the greatest scope for creativity. By utilizing each vegetable as it comes into season, on its own or as part of a medley, and seasoning it with a variety of flavorings, you will create a wide and lively range of wholesome soups. To start off, try Cauliflower Barley Soup with Shiitake Mushrooms and Edamame (page 205), Indian-inspired Meatless Mulligatawny Soup (page 206), or Vegetable Soup with Smoked Turkey and Fresh Green Hot Sauce (page 211).

Soup hydrates the body with its beneficial broth, creating a feeling of fullness, without adding many calories.

In light of the ardent advice from nutritionists to eat vegetables, soups made of vegetables deserve a more prominent place on the daily menu. When vegetables are combined with a flavorful broth and a protein element such as chicken or turkey breast, tofu, seitan (wheat gluten), or legumes, the soup can make a satisfying entrée.

A clear broth with a few asparagus tips, carrot slices, and strips of chicken makes a great summertime meal. During the winter months, there are plenty of options to enhance soups so they are warming and filling. Even in sunny lands, people prefer substantial pottages when the weather is cold.

A great example is Italian minestrone. In the cool season, it's better to turn to wintery alternatives instead of using tired basil to make the pesto that graces the classic summer version. Italians have created an array of winter minestrones, some with meat and some meatless, based on legumes, pasta, and aromatic vegetables—onions, celery, and carrots.

TWO-STEP SOUPS

*A*t my cooking classes in Paris, we often made vegetable soups. Even when preparing simple soups, we were taught to take a little extra care so they would be attractive and elegant.

To make creamy broccoli soup, we cooked broccoli florets in broth, then pureed them and added cream to make a pale green pottage. For garnish, the chefs instructed us to lightly cook extra broccoli florets in another pot of boiling water. We had to drain them quickly, rinse them with cold water to keep their color bright, and then drain them again. At serving time, we briefly dunked the broccoli florets in boiling water to reheat them, then drained them once again, and added some to each bowl of soup. The florets stayed on top of the thick soup and made a colorful decoration.

We were training to become professional chefs. To traditional Jewish home cooks, preparing matzo balls for such a soup makes sense, but making a separate vegetable garnish might appear impractical and even frivolous, unless you're serving the creamy soup on a holiday like Shavuot or Sukkot. Yet the vegetable garnish has other benefits besides adding visual appeal. When you cook vegetables long enough to make a tasty soup, they give much of their flavor to the water to turn it into broth, but the vegetables themselves become a bit tired. A garnish of briefly cooked, crisp-tender vegetables gives a lively flavor and provides a pleasing contrast with the smooth texture of the soup.

I have adopted a compromise—a way to make use of the classic technique without having to clean extra pots. This alternative method also conserves the vegetables' vitamins. It is easy to use for both smooth and chunky soups.

Flavor them with plenty of garlic and robust herbs like thyme or rosemary, then enrich them with a drizzle of olive oil, and, if you like, a light dusting of grated Parmesan. Vegetable soup with cannellini beans and green pepper is a quick and easy soup of this type, flavored with garlic, oregano, and hot red pepper flakes.

A chunky vegetable soup requires no thickening, but if you prefer more body, there are many ways to thicken a soup that are more interesting and contribute more nutrients than adding white flour. Oatmeal makes soups creamy. Cooking beans in soup and mashing or pureeing part of them is a popular Italian technique. Easier still, buy canned refried beans; I choose the vegetarian or fat-free varieties. At natural foods stores, you can sometimes find flakes of legumes or grains, like black bean flakes or barley flakes,

If I'm making broccoli soup flavored with onions, celery, and carrots, I cook the broccoli florets in water until they are crisp-tender, and I remove them with a slotted spoon to a dish. The broccoli retains good flavor and texture and stays bright green—not quite as vivid as if I had rinsed it in cold water, but good enough.

I leave most of the broccoli stems in the pot and add the other vegetables. They simmer in the broccoli's cooking liquid, so that the water-soluble vitamins that washed out of the broccoli during cooking are still in the soup. At serving time I reheat the florets directly in the soup or microwave them in their dish. (For an example, see Quick Broccoli-Vegetable Soup with Garlic and Rice, page 38.)

This technique of cooking a portion of the vegetables for a shorter time and removing them is great for green vegetables because their color dulls when they simmer at length. I find that it works even for traditional "soup vegetables." Carrots and turnips have a sweeter, more intense flavor when they're briefly cooked, but it's good to cook a portion of them for longer so they lend their natural sweetness to the broth. Mushrooms, cauliflower, celery, and even sweet onions benefit from this treatment in flavor and texture. Keeping some of the vegetables separate takes a little more attention than simply throwing everything in the pot, but the results are worth it.

Tender, leafy greens need only one step to add a bright green touch to vegetable soups. You simply add the chopped leaves to the soup at the last minute. Adding chopped kale, chard, arugula, or other greens to bean soups or to minestrone for the last few minutes gives such soups a lively taste and color and contributes a wonderful nutritional boost.

which cook quickly. Just sprinkle some into your soup and as it cooks, the broth will thicken. You can use soy granules the same way. Persian cooks often simmer split peas in vegetable or meat soups to thicken them. For a quicker idea, a friend of mine buys split pea soup mix in bulk at a health food store and simmers a little bit of it in her vegetable soups.

Adding vegetable puree is another good way to give vegetable soups body. To do this, cook a higher proportion of vegetables than usual in the soup, along with a few spoonfuls of quick-cooking brown rice if you like. Then puree all or part of the soup in a blender or food processor or with a hand blender. I use this technique in Creamy Broccoli Soup Without the Cream (page 202). It works well with most vegetables.

Instead of making a new soup every day, I usually make enough for several meals. On the second or third day, I sometimes cook frozen vegetables in the soup for a few minutes and finish it with some herbs to freshen it up.

A healthy habit in many Jewish homes is beginning holiday dinners with chicken soup. The simplest way to avoid a fatty broth is to prepare the soup a day ahead. Chill the broth; the fat will rise to the top and congeal and you can easily remove it with a spoon. You'll have less fat to skim if you use skinless chicken and trim off any blobs of fat from the chicken before cooking it. Chicken bones give flavor to the broth, so use pieces on the bone. I find legs and thighs make more flavorful broth than breasts. To make my soup more colorful and flavorful while increasing its nutritional value, I include plenty of vegetables, as in Springtime Chicken Soup with Asparagus, Fava Beans, and Whole Wheat Matzo Balls (page 200).

Main-Course Chicken Soup with Chickpeas, Winter Vegetables, Ginger, and Garlic

Springtime Chicken Soup with Asparagus, Fava Beans, and Whole Wheat Matzo Balls

Whole Wheat Matzo Balls

Creamy Broccoli Soup Without the Cream

Portuguese Kale Soup

Carrot Velouté Soup with Tarragon

Cauliflower Barley Soup with Shiitake Mushrooms and Edamame

Meatless Mulligatawny Soup

Chayote Soup with Corn and Cilantro

Lentil Lovers' Soup, Southern Mediterranean Style

Magic Carpet Noodle Lentil Soup with Tomatoes

Vegetable Soup with Smoked Turkey and Fresh Green Hot Sauce

Green Pozole

MAIN-COURSE CHICKEN SOUP WITH CHICKPEAS, WINTER VEGETABLES, GINGER, AND GARLIC

A touch of fresh ginger gives such good flavor and aroma to Chinese chicken broth that I add a slice or two regularly to other soups as well, like this wholesome supper-in-a-pot, which resembles the popular whole-meal cocidos of Spain. These popular pottages, which some consider one of Spain's oldest national dishes, consist of poultry or meat cooked with winter vegetables and usually chickpeas, along with a spicy sausage or smoked meat for extra pizzazz. Some cocidos might include saffron, while others can be quite peppery from cayenne. Depending on the family's preference, cabbage or turnip greens might be cooked in the soup or in a separate pot.

Although traditional versions of this soup can be fatty, using skinless chicken and a generous proportion of vegetables turns it into a healthy, delicious dish. Buy chicken pieces with bones for a flavorful broth. In Spain, cocido is often served in two courses: first the broth, often with a little white rice or fried bread cubes, followed by the meat and vegetables. I like to serve them together, as the broth keeps the chicken moist. In some homes rice is cooked with the other ingredients, but the soup reheats better if you cook the rice separately. I use brown rice for a more nutritious result.

1½ cups dried chickpeas (garbanzo beans) (about 10 ounces), or two 15-ounce cans chickpeas, drained

About 6 cups water (for soup), plus 6 cups for cooking dried chickpeas

2½ pounds skinless chicken pieces with bones, either all breasts or some breasts and some legs

1 large onion, whole or coarsely chopped

2 to 3 slices of ginger

1 leek, split and rinsed well (optional)

4 large garlic cloves, minced

Salt and freshly ground black pepper

2 large carrots, cut into 2-inch pieces

1 turnip, cut into 6 pieces

One 4- to 6-ounce piece of smoked chicken or turkey (optional)

4 to 6 ounces chicken, turkey, or vegetarian sausages, preferably spicy

2 to 3 cups coarsely shredded cabbage

Cayenne pepper

1½ cups hot cooked rice, preferably brown (see page 362) (optional)

If using dried chickpeas, put them in a large stew pan or soup pot. Add 6 cups water and bring to a boil. Cover and simmer for 1 hour, adding hot water occasionally to keep them submerged.

Add chicken pieces, onion, and ginger slices to pot of chickpeas or to a stew pan. Add about 6 cups water, or enough to cover ingredients by about 1 inch. Bring to a boil, skimming foam from top. If using a leek, slice white and pale green parts and reserve. Cut off green leek tops, tie them together for easy removal, and add to pot. Add garlic and salt and pepper to taste. Cover and cook over low heat for 20 minutes, occasionally skimming off foam and fat.

Add carrots, turnip, leek slices, and canned chickpeas, and bring to a simmer. Cook for 15 minutes. Add smoked chicken (if using), sausages, and cabbage, and cook over low heat for 10 minutes or until chicken, chickpeas, and vegetables are tender. Discard leek greens and ginger slices. Skim fat thoroughly. Add cayenne to broth; taste and adjust seasoning. Leave chicken pieces whole or remove meat from bones in large chunks, discard bones, and return meat to soup. Slice sausages, cut smoked chicken in strips, and return to soup. Serve hot in shallow bowls with rice if you like.

Makes 4 to 6 main-course servings

SPRINGTIME CHICKEN SOUP WITH ASPARAGUS, FAVA BEANS, AND WHOLE WHEAT MATZO BALLS

Fava beans are as much a symbol of spring in Middle Eastern and Mediterranean countries as asparagus is in Europe and America. In the homes of Jews from North Africa and Iran, favas are highlighted on the Passover menu. Here I combine both favorite springtime vegetables to make a colorful soup bursting with taste.

Serve the soup with the vegetables as a light first course, and save the chicken for salads. When you prefer a heartier main-course soup, cut the chicken into strips and add them to the soup. If you have chicken broth on hand, you can make a quicker version of the recipe by cooking the carrots, asparagus, and fava beans in it.

You can find fresh fava beans at farmers' markets and in Middle Eastern, Latino, and many Jewish markets, where they are often available frozen and peeled as well. If you like, substitute lima beans.

1½ pounds skinless chicken breast pieces, with bones
1½ pounds skinless chicken thigh or drumstick pieces
1 large onion, whole or sliced
1 bay leaf
3 tablespoons chopped parsley, stems reserved
*   for soup*
4 fresh thyme sprigs, or ½ teaspoon dried thyme
About 2 quarts water

1¼ pounds fresh fava beans, shelled, or
*   1½ cups frozen fava beans or lima beans*
4 medium carrots (total ¾ pound), peeled and
*   cut into 2-inch lengths*
Whole Wheat Matzo Balls (page 201)
½ pound medium-width asparagus, peeled and
*   cut into 1½-inch pieces*
Salt and freshly ground black pepper

Thoroughly trim any fat from chicken. Put chicken breast and thigh pieces in a large saucepan. Add onion, bay leaf, parsley stems, and thyme sprigs (but not dried thyme), and cover ingredients generously with water. Bring to a boil. Skim excess foam from surface. Cover and cook over low heat for 1 hour.

Put shelled fava beans in a medium saucepan of boiling salted water and cook, uncovered, over high heat for 5 to 7 minutes or until they are done to your taste; some people like to cook them for only 2 minutes, while others prefer as long as 20 minutes. Drain well; peel off the thick skins.

Add carrots and dried thyme to soup, cover, and cook over low heat for 30 minutes. Discard bay leaf and thyme sprigs. Skim fat completely from soup. (This is easier to do when soup is cold.) Remove chicken meat from bones; reserve for other meals or cut into strips and return to soup.

Separately, heat matzo balls. Reheat soup, add asparagus, and cook over medium-low heat for 7 minutes or until asparagus is just tender. Add fava beans and heat through. Add chopped parsley and season to taste with salt and pepper. Serve 2 matzo balls in each bowl.

Makes about 6 servings

❖ WHOLE WHEAT MATZO BALLS

Carrot and parsley give these matzo balls a lively, springtime look. To make them I combine soaked, crumbled whole wheat matzos with matzo meal and eggs. If you wish to go whole wheat all the way, process some whole wheat matzos in a food processor until ground nearly to a powder and use as matzo meal.

I am finding whole wheat matzo on more and more lists of recommended foods by nutritionists—it's lower in fat and the low-carb camp loves it because its fiber brings down the carb content. Besides, it adds more flavor than plain matzo.

1 whole wheat matzo	¼ teaspoon baking powder (optional, see Note)
2 large eggs, or equivalent in egg substitute	½ cup finely grated carrot (optional)
¼ cup matzo meal, plus more if needed	1 tablespoon minced parsley (optional)
¼ teaspoon salt	1 to 2 tablespoons chicken soup or water
Pinch of black pepper	About 2 quarts salted water (for simmering)

Break matzo in a few pieces into a bowl. Cover with water and soak until soft. Drain well and squeeze dry. In a small bowl, lightly beat eggs. Add soaked matzo, matzo meal, salt, pepper, and baking powder, and stir with a fork until smooth. Stir in carrot and parsley, if using. Stir in chicken soup, adding enough so mixture is just firm enough to hold together in rough-shaped balls. Cover and refrigerate for 30 minutes to make matzo balls easier to shape.

Bring salted water to a bare simmer. With wet hands, take about 2 teaspoons matzo ball mixture and roll it into a ball between your palms. Mixture will be soft; if it is too soft to handle, stir in more matzo meal by spoonfuls until you can shape it. Gently drop matzo ball into simmering water. Continue making balls, wetting hands before shaping each one. Cover and simmer over low heat for 30 minutes. Cover and keep them warm until ready to serve. When serving, remove matzo balls with a slotted spoon, add them to soup bowls, and ladle hot soup over them.

NOTE: Omit baking powder if preparing these for Passover.

Makes 18 to 20 small matzo balls, or 4 to 5 servings

CREAMY BROCCOLI SOUP WITHOUT THE CREAM

Use the broccoli stems as well as the florets for this rich-tasting soup, as they give the puree more substance and a pleasant, slightly sweet flavor. I cook part of the broccoli tops separately to give the soup a lively green color, then garnish it with bright green, briefly cooked florets. You can also use chicken broth as the cooking liquid, and enhance the soup with unsweetened soy milk.

2 pounds broccoli, florets and stems
4 cups water
Salt
1½ tablespoons vegetable oil or olive oil
1 large onion, chopped
4 to 5 cups vegetable broth

3 tablespoons white rice, or ¼ cup quick-cooking brown rice
Freshly ground black pepper
2 fresh thyme sprigs, or ½ teaspoon dried thyme
1 bay leaf
⅓ cup milk
Cayenne pepper

Peel broccoli stems by cutting off tough outer skin with a sturdy knife; slice stems. Cut broccoli tops into medium florets and about 20 to 24 small florets for garnish.

Boil 4 cups water in a large, heavy saucepan; add salt. Add small florets and boil, uncovered, over high heat for 3 minutes or until just tender. Remove florets with a slotted spoon. Rinse, drain well, and reserve.

Return water to a boil. Add about half of medium broccoli florets. Boil, uncovered, over high heat for 7 minutes or until tender but still bright green. Drain, reserving liquid. Rinse florets and reserve. If you like, use broccoli cooking liquid as part of vegetable broth for soup.

Heat oil in saucepan. Add onion and cook over medium-low heat, stirring often, for 7 minutes or until soft but not browned. Add broccoli-stem slices and remaining uncooked florets, 4 cups vegetable broth, rice, salt, pepper, thyme, and bay leaf. Stir and bring to a boil. Cover and cook over low heat for 30 minutes or until rice is very tender. Discard thyme sprigs and bay leaf.

Let soup cool for 5 minutes. Pour soup into a blender and puree it until very smooth. Return it to saucepan. Puree cooked medium broccoli florets and add them to soup.

Bring soup to a simmer over medium-low heat, stirring often. If soup is too thick, add about 1 cup broth, or enough to bring soup to desired consistency. Bring to a boil, stirring. Stir in milk and heat gently. Season to taste with salt, pepper, and cayenne.

Just before serving, reheat small florets briefly in microwave. Garnish each bowl with a few florets.

Makes 4 to 6 servings

❧ PORTUGUESE KALE SOUP

Make this soup in winter or early spring, when kale is at its peak. Known as *caldo verde*, or "green soup," this savory, easy-to-make soup is a favorite in Portugal and among the Portuguese living in Paris.

Kale is a vegetable worth getting to know, as it is one of the healthiest of all greens. According to the World's Healthiest Foods Web site (whfoods.com), kale is an excellent source of dietary fiber and vitamins. It has "more nutritional value for fewer calories than almost any other food around. . . . Its combination of vitamins, minerals, and phytonutrients makes kale a health superstar!"

This soup contains few ingredients and cooks in a short time. It is thickened with potato and, like classic bouillabaisse, is boiled with olive oil to emulsify the oil in the broth, thus enriching the flavor. Instead of potato you can make kale soup the Scottish way and thicken it with oatmeal.

Generally the Portuguese add garlic sausage, like linguica or chorizo. In its place you can add turkey franks, spicy tofu hot dogs, or a few slices of soy pepperoni, cut into strips. Traditionally the ingredients are cooked in water, but you can use chicken or vegetable broth.

If you don't have kale, substitute cabbage or other greens.

1½ pounds boiling potatoes, scrubbed and quartered
6 cups water, or half chicken or vegetable broth
Salt and freshly ground black pepper
¾ to 1 pound kale, stalks discarded, leaves
* rinsed well*

1 large onion, finely chopped
2 large garlic cloves, chopped
1 to 2 tablespoons extra virgin olive oil
4 to 6 ounces turkey or soy frankfurters, sliced

Combine potatoes and water in a saucepan and add salt. Bring to a boil, cover, and cook over medium-low heat for 20 to 25 minutes or until potatoes are very tender.

Meanwhile, pile kale leaves on a cutting board and halve lengthwise. With a sharp knife, shred kale in crosswise strips as thin as possible.

With a slotted spoon, transfer potatoes to a bowl. Peel, if desired, and mash them. Return to saucepan.

A short time before serving, bring soup to a boil, stirring. Add onion, garlic, kale, and oil. Boil, uncovered, over medium-high heat for 5 minutes or until kale and onion are crisp-tender. Add turkey franks and simmer to heat through. Taste and adjust seasoning. Serve immediately.

Makes 4 servings

❧ CARROT VELOUTÉ SOUP WITH TARRAGON

This velvety soup makes an elegant starter for festive dinners. To give it a creamy texture, I adapt the traditional French technique of making velouté or "velvet" soup to healthy cooking. In classic versions this method calls for cooking butter and flour to make a roux, adding stock, and enriching the soup with cream and egg yolks. With carrots, lightening up the soup is easy—the puree itself gives the soup a luscious texture, making the cream and egg yolks unnecessary.

Just a bit of flour cooked lightly as a roux with a little oil gives the soup its appealing smoothness and richness, which is enhanced by the addition of milk. It's good even when made with low-fat or nonfat milk or soy milk. Although I generally opt for unsweetened soy milk for soups, with carrots it's okay to use a brand that is slightly sweet. For extra flavor I infuse the carrot's cooking liquid with tarragon stems.

1½ tablespoons vegetable oil or butter
1 onion, chopped
1 tablespoon all-purpose or whole wheat flour
2½ cups vegetable broth or water
1¼ pounds carrots, diced
Salt and freshly ground black pepper

3 tarragon stems, leaves reserved for chopping
1 fresh thyme sprig, or ¼ teaspoon dried thyme
1 bay leaf
1 to 1½ cups low-fat milk or soy milk
Pinch of sugar (optional)
2 teaspoons finely chopped fresh tarragon

Heat oil in a heavy saucepan. Add onion and cook over medium-low heat, stirring often, for 5 minutes or until softened. Reduce heat to low, sprinkle mixture with flour, and cook, stirring, for 1 minute. Pour in broth, stirring constantly, and bring to a boil. Add carrots, salt, pepper, tarragon stems, thyme, and bay leaf. Return to a boil, stirring. Cover and cook over low heat, stirring occasionally to prevent sticking, for 20 minutes or until carrots are very tender. Discard herb sprigs and bay leaf.

Puree soup until very smooth in a blender. If using a food processor, with a slotted spoon transfer vegetables from soup to processor, puree them, and gradually pour in cooking liquid with machine running. Return puree to saucepan.

Stirring often, simmer soup over low heat for 5 minutes or until thickened to taste. Add 1 cup milk and bring to a simmer, stirring. Add more milk if necessary to thin soup to desired consistency and return to a simmer, stirring. Taste and adjust seasoning; add sugar if needed.

Serve garnished with tarragon.

Makes 4 servings

CAULIFLOWER BARLEY SOUP
WITH SHIITAKE MUSHROOMS AND EDAMAME

Cauliflower can be used to make all sorts of wonderful soups. Its flavor is complemented well by the onions, celery, and mushrooms in this mushroom barley soup. Edamame, or green soybeans, add a lively note.

This wholesome soup is replete with good nutrition. Barley, like oatmeal, is a good source of heart-healthy soluble fiber. Shiitake mushrooms contain a compound that strengthens the immune system and are rich in selenium, which helps protect cells from damage. Cauliflower is an excellent source of fiber, folate, and vitamin C. As a cruciferous vegetable, it may help the body fight disease. Edamame is probably the easiest soy food to love. Soy foods are known to be healthy in numerous ways, and even people who don't like tofu or soy milk often enjoy edamame.

1 ounce dried shiitake mushrooms, rinsed
1 large carrot, diced
1 large onion, diced
1 quart vegetable or chicken broth
2 cups water
½ cup pearl barley
3 celery ribs, diced

2 teaspoons sweet paprika
Salt and freshly ground black pepper
3 cups cauliflower florets
1 cup frozen shelled edamame (green soybeans)
¼ teaspoon hot paprika or cayenne pepper
2 to 3 tablespoons chopped parsley

Soak mushrooms in 1 cup hot water for 20 minutes. Remove mushrooms, reserving liquid. Dice any large ones. Discard tough stems.

In a large saucepan, combine carrot, onion, broth, and 2 cups water, and bring to a boil. Skim foam from surface. Reduce heat to low. Add barley, celery, sweet paprika, salt, and pepper. Add mushrooms. Pour mushroom soaking water into another bowl, leaving behind and discarding the last few tablespoons of liquid, which may be sandy. Add mushroom liquid to soup. Cover and cook over low heat for 30 minutes.

Add cauliflower to soup and return to a boil. Cover and cook for 15 minutes or until barley and cauliflower are tender. If soup is too thick, stir in ¼ cup hot water or more if needed. Add edamame and cook for 5 minutes. Season with hot paprika, salt, and pepper. Serve hot, sprinkled with parsley.

Makes 4 to 6 servings

Mulligatawny, like cassoulet, bouillabaisse, and paella, is one of those "big" dishes that are the subject of endless debate as to the authentic way to prepare them. A popular item in Indian restaurants, it is actually a British adaptation of a South Indian recipe. Mulligatawny is a historic example of fusion, evolving from a thin, spicy, hot-and-sour, broth, served as a beverage or with rice, into a hearty soup that today often contains lamb or chicken and can be the basis of a whole meal. Many cooks make it with curry powder, while others add curry spices individually, to taste. Some enrich their soup with coconut milk, ground almonds, or heavy cream; some thicken theirs with chickpea flour or wheat flour. Mulligatawny can be a simple soup of chicken cooked with chiles, onions, and two or three spices, or a more elaborate preparation with a long list of vegetables and herbs. Often it's a smooth puree, but it may also be chunky.

Traditionally the vegetables are fried in ghee (clarified butter), but today many substitute vegetable oil for a healthier soup. In the interest of nutrition, many cooks have gone back in the direction of the original recipe and make vegetarian mulligatawny based on lentils, beans, or vegetables, as in this recipe.

This satisfying soup is a nice starter for Hanukkah or Purim. To make it more substantial for serving as an entrée, I like to add tofu; you can add instead 1 or 2 cups of diced cooked fish, chicken, or turkey.

The spices and flour give the soup a slightly creamy texture. You can find chickpea flour at Indian, Persian, and Middle Eastern grocery stores, or substitute whole wheat or white flour. For a thicker, smoother soup, puree all or part of it in a blender or with a hand blender before adding the tofu. Hot basmati rice is the traditional accompaniment; at some markets you can find more nutritious brown basmati rice.

1½ to 2 tablespoons vegetable oil

1 onion, chopped

3 garlic cloves, chopped

1 tablespoon minced peeled ginger

2 tablespoons chickpea flour, or 1 tablespoon whole wheat or white flour

½ to 1 teaspoon curry powder

1 teaspoon ground cumin

1 teaspoon ground coriander

¼ teaspoon turmeric

5 cups vegetable or chicken broth

1 medium potato, diced

2 medium carrots, diced

Salt and freshly ground black pepper

1 medium zucchini, diced

1 cup frozen peas (optional)

6 to 12 ounces firm tofu, cut into bite-sized cubes (optional)

Cayenne pepper

Lemon juice

2 tablespoons chopped cilantro (optional)

1 cup hot cooked brown or white basmati rice (for serving)

Heat 1½ tablespoons oil in a medium saucepan. Add onion and sauté over medium heat for 5 minutes. Add garlic and ginger, and cook over low heat, stirring, for 1 minute. Add flour, curry powder, cumin, coriander, and turmeric, and stir over low heat to blend well; add remaining oil if mixture is dry. Cook for ½ minute, stirring.

Stir in broth and bring to a simmer, stirring. Add potato, carrots, and a pinch of salt. Cover and cook over low heat, stirring occasionally, for 15 minutes. Add zucchini, peas (if using), and tofu (if using), and cook, covered, for 5 minutes or until vegetables are tender. Season to taste with cayenne and lemon juice. At serving time add cilantro, if you like; top each serving with a few tablespoons of rice.

Makes 4 servings

☒ CHAYOTE SOUP WITH CORN AND CILANTRO

This colorful soup is perfect for wintertime, when chayote squash and cilantro are at their best. Pear-shaped chayote squash, called *mirliton* in Louisiana, has a soft shell, mild flavor, and pale green flesh. Unlike zucchini and other soft-shelled summer squash, chayote keeps its shape and does not fall apart even after long simmering. If the peel is tender, you can leave the chayote unpeeled. Occasionally, the white part near the seed is tough; if it feels hard when you are cutting it, discard this part.

Both tomato puree and a few spoonfuls of cream-style corn give the soup body, and the corn imparts an appealing touch of sweetness as well. To turn this soup into a main course, I add firm tofu. Just before serving, I add 1 1/2 to 2 ounces cubed firm tofu per person, and heat it gently in the soup.

I like to serve this soup for Purim, when vegetarian meals are traditional. It is also good to serve at Hanukkah, as a prelude to the latkes and as a way to inhibit overindulging in them.

5 cups vegetable broth
1 small boiling or baking potato, diced
1 onion, chopped
1 chayote squash, peeled and diced
1 medium carrot, sliced
1/3 cup diced fresh or frozen green beans

1/3 cup canned tomato puree
3/4 cup cooked or canned chickpeas
1/3 cup canned corn, kernels or cream style
1/3 cup chopped cilantro
Salt and freshly ground black pepper
Bottled hot pepper sauce

Bring broth to a simmer with potato and onion. Cover and simmer for 15 minutes. Add chayote squash and carrot and simmer for 15 minutes or until squash is tender. Add green beans and simmer for 3 minutes. Stir in tomato puree, chickpeas, corn, and half the cilantro and heat through. Season to taste with salt and hot pepper sauce. Add remaining cilantro at serving time.

Makes 4 servings

LENTIL LOVERS' SOUP, SOUTHERN MEDITERRANEAN STYLE

Moroccan-born Dvora Cohen, a relative of ours who lives in Paris, has adapted this traditional North African recipe for healthy pareve cooking. Most recipes for this soup call for meat, but it is so flavorful that the meat is not necessary. Serve this restoring soup after the Yom Kippur fast or for Sukkot, or make a big batch whenever you want to have a healthy entrée available. It reheats beautifully. Fresh cilantro added at the last moment is the key to its good flavor.

Dvora sometimes serves the soup with a few tablespoons of rice in each bowl. If you'd like to serve it this way, choose brown rice for optimal nutrition.

Dvora notes that you can use any legumes in this soup, but she opts for lentils and chickpeas, the most popular ones in North Africa. Both are packed with nutrients and fiber and are good sources of protein, folic acid, and iron. She cooks dried chickpeas, but to save time I sometimes use canned ones. To make the soup fat-free, omit the oil and the step of sautéing the vegetables.

1 cup brown or green lentils
1 to 2 tablespoons extra virgin olive oil or
    vegetable oil
1 large onion, chopped
1 carrot, diced
3 celery ribs, chopped
3 small zucchini, diced
5 cups vegetable or chicken broth mixed with water,
    or 5 cups water

½ cup tomato sauce
½ teaspoon turmeric
1½ to 2 cups cooked dried chickpeas (garbanzo
    beans), liquid reserved, or one 15-ounce can
    chickpeas, drained
½ to 1 teaspoon ground cumin
⅓ cup coarsely chopped cilantro
Salt and freshly ground black pepper

Spread lentils on a plate in small batches. Pick through them carefully, discarding any stones; rinse and drain lentils.

Heat oil in a large saucepan and add onion, carrot, and celery. Sauté over medium heat, stirring often, for 7 minutes or until lightly browned, adding 1 to 2 tablespoons water from time to time to prevent burning. Add zucchini and sauté for 3 minutes.

Add broth and lentils and bring to a boil. Cover and cook over low heat for 40 minutes or until lentils are tender. Add tomato sauce, turmeric, and chickpeas and simmer for 5 minutes. If soup is too thick, add 1 cup boiling water and simmer for 5 minutes more. Stir in cumin and all but 2 tablespoons cilantro. Simmer for 1 minute. Season soup to taste with salt and pepper. Serve hot, sprinkled with remaining cilantro.

Makes 4 servings

MAGIC CARPET NOODLE LENTIL SOUP WITH TOMATOES

One of the most memorable noodle soups I ever encountered was the excellent Yemenite lentil soup at Magic Carpet, my favorite kosher restaurant in Los Angeles. Unlike the clear broth with noodles that I grew up with, this soup was a thick, vegetarian lentil soup. The long, slim, linguinelike noodles add a comforting quality to the deep orange soup, which is brightened by the flavors of Yemenite spices, tomatoes, and fried onions. This recipe is based on the one I ate at the restaurant. I use red lentils, available at Indian and Middle Eastern grocery stores, as they turn into a thick puree as they simmer.

Nili Goldstein, the owner of Magic Carpet, sautés the onions ahead of time and drains them in a strainer to remove excess fat. This is a good practice to emulate. She notes that the traditional Yemenite version of the soup does not include noodles, but she prefers the soup this way. I agree!

1½ cups red lentils
2 tablespoons olive oil or vegetable oil
1 large onion, chopped
4 to 5 cups water
One 14-ounce can tomatoes, drained
1 teaspoon ground cumin
¼ teaspoon turmeric

Salt
3 ounces linguine, vermicelli, spaghettini, or
*   extra-fine egg noodles, broken into*
*   3- to 4-inch lengths (about 1 cup)*
Freshly ground black pepper
Cayenne pepper or other hot red pepper (optional)

Spread lentils on a plate in small batches. Pick through them carefully, discarding any stones; rinse and drain.

Heat oil in a large saucepan, add onion, and sauté over medium-low heat for 7 minutes or until deep golden. Remove half of onions and reserve.

To mixture remaining in pan add lentils and 4 cups water. Bring to a boil. Cover and simmer over low heat for 15 minutes. Puree tomatoes in a blender or food processor and add to pan. Add cumin, turmeric, and a pinch of salt. Simmer for 15 more minutes, adding more water if soup becomes too thick, or until lentils are very tender.

Meanwhile, cook linguine in a pot of boiling salted water until just tender, and drain them.

Add reserved onion mixture and cooked linguine to soup and heat gently. Taste and adjust seasoning, adding plenty of black pepper and a pinch cayenne to taste. Serve hot.

Makes 4 servings

VEGETABLE SOUP WITH SMOKED TURKEY AND FRESH GREEN HOT SAUCE

This soup makes use of a healthy habit of Yemenite Jews—including vitamin-rich hot pepper and beneficial raw garlic in meals by serving zehug (hot pepper and garlic relish) with the entrée. Following tradition, people spread a little zehug on pita or bread to "wake up their appetite" and eat it with a hearty meat soup.

For this recipe, I prepare a quick batch of the hot pepper relish, and stir a little of it into an easy-to-make vegetable and chickpea soup enhanced with a little turkey. The bright, fat-free green relish gives the soup a lovely fresh hue, like pesto in minestrone. Blended with the soup, the relish still adds plenty of punch, but is not as aggressive as when you eat it "straight."

To thicken the soup lightly, I cook a diced baking potato in the broth until it begins to fall apart. Smoked turkey breast gives this soup a good meaty flavor with almost no fat.

1 onion, chopped
1 russet potato, scrubbed and diced
4 to 5 cups vegetable broth or water
Salt
1 large carrot, sliced
1 large broccoli stem, peeled and sliced, or
   ½ cup small broccoli florets (optional)
2 slices ginger, chopped
2 to 3 cups chopped cabbage

3 small pale green Mexican zucchini (also called
   white or Tatuma squash) or zucchini, diced
One 8-ounce can chickpeas or ⅔ of 15-ounce can
   chickpeas (about 1 cup), drained
5 to 8 ounces smoked turkey breast, sliced and cut
   into thin strips
Pinch of cayenne pepper
Easy Green Chile Garlic Relish (page 363)

Cook onion and potato in 4 cups broth with salt for 30 minutes or until potato begins to fall apart. Add carrot, broccoli (if using), and ginger and return to a boil. Cook over low heat for 3 minutes. Add cabbage and zucchini and return to a boil. Cook over low heat for 3 minutes. Cover and cook for 4 minutes or until vegetables are tender, adding water if soup becomes too thick. Add chickpeas, turkey breast, and a little cayenne and cook just until heated through. Taste and adjust seasoning. Serve hot with relish for stirring into each bowl.

Makes 4 servings

Pozole is a popular Mexican party soup/stew of meat, vegetables, and hominy, a nonsweet type of corn. I first had it at the home of a Mexican-born friend of mine, Leticia Ortega, who served it for her daughter's birthday party. Like many chile-based dishes, pozole comes in two versions—red and green.

What was most interesting to me was how the soup was served. Guests seemed to be making a salad in their bowls of soup. First they squeezed fresh lemon juice into the soup, then sprinkled it with aromatic dried oregano, and finally added generous amounts of raw vegetables: chopped white onions, sliced radishes, shredded cabbage, and cilantro. (Those who wanted more spice added chiles too.)

The onions, radish, and cabbage retain their appealing crunch, adding a fresh note to enliven the soup's meaty flavor. The soup's heat mellows the onions slightly, but they keep enough pungency to contribute a pleasing bite to the broth.

Serving vegetables with soups at the table can be a useful strategy to get people to eat raw vegetables, even those who don't have the patience to eat salads. In addition, you need no extra oil to help the raw vegetables "go down," so you save on calories. Best of all, providing a selection of chopped vegetables makes eating more fun, as each person participates in "designing" his or her own portion of soup.

This is a light, easy-to-make version of the classic pozole. Its flavor base is a fresh, green puree of jalapeño peppers, cilantro, and garlic; you can add 1 cup of tomatillos (husk tomatoes) to the puree if available. If you don't have hominy, substitute fresh or frozen corn kernels to turn this recipe into a chicken and corn soup. If you like, serve the soup with tostadas, a traditional accompaniment, but choose baked, not fried tostadas.

1 to 3 small fresh jalapeño peppers (see Note)
2 large garlic cloves, peeled
½ cup coarsely chopped cilantro
1 to 1½ tablespoons olive oil or vegetable oil
2 medium onions, chopped
4 cups chicken broth
2 cups water
8 to 12 ounces boneless, skinless chicken breasts, cut into small cubes

One 15-ounce can hominy, drained, or
    1½ cups frozen corn kernels
Salt and freshly ground black pepper
1 lemon, cut into wedges
4 small radishes, sliced thin
4 cups shredded cabbage or iceberg lettuce

Remove seeds and membranes of jalapeño peppers if you want the soup to be less spicy. Combine peppers, garlic, and half the cilantro in a small food processor and chop finely; or chop with a knife.

In a large saucepan, heat oil. Add half of chopped onion (1 onion) and sauté over medium heat for 5 minutes. Stir in garlic—hot pepper mixture, broth, and 2 cups water. Bring to a boil. Add chicken and hominy and return to a boil. Cover and simmer over medium-low heat for 7 minutes or until chicken is tender. Season to taste with salt and pepper.

Serve soup with lemon wedges and bowls containing radishes, remaining chopped onion, cabbage, and remaining cilantro.

NOTE: If you're not used to using hot peppers or you are sensitive to them, wear gloves when handling them. If not using gloves, wash your hands well after handling the peppers. Wash the knife and cutting board also.

Makes 4 servings

Dairy and Egg Dishes

In the Jewish culinary culture, meals are usually bsari or fleishig (including meat), halavi or milchig (including milk), and occasionally pareve, neither meat nor dairy. Dairy foods and eggs play an important role, as they often supply the protein in meatless meals. Of course, fish is an option too, but in most households dairy-based dishes and eggs are a more frequent choice, especially for quick, casual meals. They are also favorites for the holiday of Shavuot and for festive brunches.

Some health-conscious cooks hesitate to use dairy foods and eggs due to concerns about fat and cholesterol, but they have a place in healthy cooking. The key is to use them wisely.

The best choice in eggs is those that are high in omega-3 fatty acids, which are very beneficial to the body. A good strategy to avoid overeating eggs is to combine whole eggs with egg whites in omelets and scrambled eggs. If you like, you can also use egg substitutes, which are usually made of egg whites.

A wide variety of reduced-fat and light dairy products, from soft and firm cheeses to yogurt to sour cream, make it easy to include cheese in menus without consuming much butterfat. In many recipes, they fit the bill beautifully. Even delicious cheesecake can be made with a combination of low-fat cheese, yogurt, and sour cream; see Light and Luscious Vanilla Cheesecake with Almonds (page 126).

There's no need to banish excellent cheeses made the "real" way from the menu either. If you want to enjoy Parmesan, kashkaval, feta, goat cheese, or fresh mozzarella, for example, include them in menus in modest amounts. Used with a light touch, they work beautifully in cooked vegetable, grain, and pasta dishes. A sprinkling of crumbled feta gives a wonderful lift to green salads such as Baby Greens with Toasted Walnuts, Figs, and Light Rosemary Vinaigrette (page 183).

Dust grated Parmesan lightly over cooked vegetables, whole wheat noodles moistened with olive oil, or brown rice. Don't overlook the humble sandwich. Use tasty whole-grain breads, especially those high in fiber and protein, and fill them with roasted vegetables and 1 or 2 thin slices of a savory cheese, such as herbed or seed-studded braided string cheese.

The same is true of eggs, used alone or combined with cheese. Pairing them with vegetables, as in Ricotta Noodle Kugel with Caramelized Onions, and Baked Eggs with Onions, Tomatoes, and Cumin, is a nutritious way to enjoy them.

HEALTHY HEROES FOR THE KOSHER KITCHEN

My mother made my lunch-box sandwiches from egg salad or whatever was in the fridge, and I was perfectly happy. She made them on good bread from a kosher bakery, often on caraway rye, which, it turns out, is a perfectly healthy choice when made the traditional way, with all rye flour.

When my friend Nancy Eisman, who is a vegetarian, told me how much she enjoyed preparing savory submarines, I became curious about these layered sandwiches. Until then I didn't think much of them, having sampled only overwhelmingly salty fast-food subs.

A submarine, also known as a hero sandwich, is made with cold cuts, sausages, cheese, and peppers. Generally the filling features Italian elements, notably salami and provolone cheese. Some rib-sticking versions contain meatballs in tomato sauce and are served hot. The saying goes that you have to be a hero to eat one. In some parts of the country, people call them torpedoes, grinders, hoagies, or po' boys, and the required long white rolls are sold as torpedo or grinder rolls.

Americans may be the submarine sovereigns, but layered sandwiches are part of other culinary cultures too. At the café inside Vallarta, a Mexican supermarket chain in Los Angeles, the signature torta features a long bolillo roll stuffed with shredded meat, guacamole, and salsa. A Tel Aviv submarine I loved in my college days had a creamy eggplant filling in a whole wheat roll, topped with smoked turkey or sharp kashkaval cheese.

But how do you make heroes healthy and kosher? Nancy, who works at Melissa's Worldwide Produce, has plenty of solutions. She designs tempting sandwiches with soy meats and cheeses. Her secret? A sprinkling of oil, vinegar, and oregano, which are also used to perk up deli-meat sandwiches. Nancy might make a soy bologna submarine with two tofu cheeses—provolone- and mozzarella-style—layered with yellow tomatoes, Maui onions, and shredded lettuce on French bread spread with mustard and low-fat mayo. With a soy turkey variation, she includes sweet cipolline onions, heirloom tomatoes, and arugula.

If you're using soy meat, you can also add a modest amount of a tasty real cheese, like fresh mozzarella or goat cheese.

Given the sandwich's name, it's funny that you rarely see seafood submarines. One of my favorite combinations is lox, avocado, and tomato. Tuna also works well in this combination.

Nancy also includes condiments like sun-dried tomatoes, pesto, or roasted peppers. Pickles do wonders too to wake up jaded palates. Follow tradition and add Italian-style pickled hot peppers (peperoncini) or, to avoid assaulting your family's taste buds, slice them thin or serve them separately. I also like a bit of Yemenite hot pepper garlic relish (see page 363).

Good bread is the key to a tasty submarine. If it's too spongy, the sandwich quickly becomes soggy. Twenty years ago I had trouble finding fine bread in my neighborhood. These days most of us are lucky to have plenty of crusty, whole-grain choices.

YOGURT REFRESHERS—TART VERSUS SWEET

*T*ake a look at the refrigerator case at the supermarket these days, and you'll find plenty of drinkable yogurts. Sweet, fruity, and filling, they come in such flavors as strawberry, peach, and tropical fruit. They can be quite rich and high in calories; one company, which touts its fluid yogurt as resembling crème anglaise—French custard sauce—recommends the beverage as a dessert sauce. These cultured drinks help feed our ever-increasing appetite for yogurt. In the past thirty years, consumption of yogurt among Americans has quadrupled.

Yogurt is a basic staple in Mediterranean countries known for their healthy diet. Such dairy drinks have long been important in the lands of the Bible and beyond. In contrast to the yogurt drinks in our standard supermarkets, which imitate thick smoothies, in other regions of the globe many are designed as savory thirst-quenchers for hot weather. Popular in areas where people enjoy yogurt's natural taste, they are often tart rather than sweet.

If you're feeling adventurous, stroll through a Persian grocery store and try the yogurt soda called **doogh**. The first time my husband and I tasted it, we both reacted differently. Being from the Mideast, Yakir liked it right away. Since I grew up in the United States, where sweet drinks are the norm, the fizzy, tangy, slightly salty beverage seemed odd to me. But I quickly acquired a taste for this cooling drink.

In Israel and in Turkey, we enjoyed the popular Turkish **ayran**, which some call Turkish buttermilk. Smooth, creamy, and rich-tasting, it went down easily in the sultry late-summer weather. Like the Persian version, it was tangy and slightly salty, but wasn't carbonated. We loved it as an energy-restoring snack, and soon discovered that the Turks don't limit it to between-meal pick-me-ups. Ayran is frequently served with main courses and rice pilaf as an accompanying beverage. In Armenian markets you'll find a similar drink called **tahn**.

Recipes for these three yogurt drinks—ayran, tahn, and doogh—are as simple as can be. They are just yogurt diluted with ice-cold water, with salt to taste. For a bubbly beverage, you use sparkling water. Frequently they are made from cow's milk yogurt, but depending on regional preferences, goat's or sheep's milk yogurt might be used instead. You blend the ingredients in a bowl or, for a frothy glass of ayran prized by many aficionados, use a blender.

You can make your drink light or luscious, according to the ratio of yogurt to water, to obtain a viscosity like that of buttermilk or thicker. As a basic recipe, many mix yogurt with an equal amount of water, while others prefer twice as much water as yogurt, especially for serving with a meal. Obviously you need more yogurt than water for a satisfying, milkshake-like drink. It all depends on your mood and on how thick your yogurt is. For a sweeter taste, substitute fresh milk for part of the yogurt. The drink is always served cold, often over a few ice cubes. A favorite garnish is a sprinkling of dried or chopped fresh mint, a common Middle Eastern partner for yogurt, which accentuates its refreshing quality. Afghans enhance the cooling effect by adding a little grated cucumber.

At a Russian deli, we discovered kefir, a related beverage with a creamy consistency and a slightly sour taste. It is made from milk fermented with kefir cultures, which are different from yogurt cultures. Like doogh, kefir sometimes has a slight carbonated effervescence. Kefir connoisseurs claim that this cultured beverage, which originated in the northern area of the Caucasus Mountains, is even higher in health-promoting probiotics (beneficial microorganisms) than yogurt. Kefir also comes in sweetened fruit flavors.

Many consider tart, liquid yogurt more refreshing on a sizzling summer day than a sweet drink, which makes you thirstier.

Cooks in India have developed the greatest number of yogurt beverages, called lussi or lassi. For savory versions, they spice the yogurt, notably with toasted ground cumin and black pepper. They make sweet yogurt drinks as well, adding nutmeg, cardamom, or fruit as well as sugar. Mango lassi is the best known, but you can use other fruit as well.

NINE DAYS TOMATO MOZZARELLA PASTA SALAD

MEDITERRANEAN BEAN SALAD WITH BABY GREENS, FETA CHEESE, AND OLIVES

CREAMY GREEN VEGETABLE SOUP WITH BULGUR WHEAT

COLD SPINACH AND CORN SOUP WITH YOGURT AND MINT

THREE-WAY SUBMARINES

RICOTTA NOODLE KUGEL WITH CARAMELIZED ONIONS

ISRAELI OMELET AND ROASTED VEGETABLE SANDWICH

BAKED EGGS WITH ONIONS, TOMATOES, AND CUMIN

SCRAMBLED EGG WHITES WITH HUNGARIAN SPICED MUSHROOMS

GARLICKY PERSIAN EGGPLANT WITH EGGS

LOX, EGGS, AND SPINACH BURRITOS

Between the first and the ninth day of the Hebrew month of Av, dairy foods are on the menu of Orthodox Jews who observe the "Nine Days." The custom is to abstain from eating meat as a sign of mourning for the destruction of ancient Jerusalem. When I was a child, I particularly enjoyed the meals during this period because I loved dairy foods.

Usually this period in the lunar calendar occurs in August, when ripe, garden-fresh tomatoes are abundant. When you get really excellent tomatoes, the simplest recipes are the best for showing off their flavor. One of my favorites is the Italian insalata caprese, named for the beautiful island of Capri. The salad needs only four ingredients: tomatoes, mozzarella cheese, basil, and olive oil. What makes it outstanding is their quality—perfect tomatoes, soft, fresh mozzarella, fragrant basil, and aromatic extra virgin olive oil. You just alternate the cheese and tomato slices on a plate, scatter the whole basil leaves, and drizzle everything very lightly with the olive oil. It's so delicious, who wouldn't gladly eat it during every one of the Nine Days?

For a more substantial course, you can put the caprese salad on good-quality pita or fresh Italian ciabatta bread to make a delicious summer sandwich. Or turn the combination into a delightful warm-weather entrée salad by dicing the ingredients and mixing them with cooked brown rice or, as in this colorful salad, with whole wheat pasta. If you prefer, instead of mozzarella use diced Bulgarian feta, a favorite cheese in Israel, or a soft Middle Eastern string cheese with nigella seeds.

8 ounces whole wheat or tomato–flavored
    pasta spirals
3 to 6 tablespoons extra virgin olive oil
8 ounces fresh mozzarella

¼ cup basil leaves, or more to taste
1 pound ripe tomatoes, diced
Salt and freshly ground black pepper
Cayenne pepper (optional)

Cook pasta, uncovered, in a large pot of boiling salted water over high heat, stirring occasionally, for 7 minutes or until tender but firm to the bite. Drain well and toss with 3 tablespoons oil. Slice half the cheese; dice the remainder. Cut half the basil into thin strips; leave remaining leaves whole or, if they are large, tear each into a few pieces.

Add tomatoes, diced cheese, and basil strips to pasta. Season to taste with salt, pepper, and cayenne, and add 1 more tablespoon oil if desired. Serve at room temperature, garnished with mozzarella slices and whole or torn basil leaves, and drizzled with a little more oil.

Makes 4 servings

MEDITERRANEAN BEAN SALAD WITH BABY GREENS, FETA CHEESE, AND OLIVES

My green salads often turn into French-style composed salads, made of vegetables and other ingredients attractively arranged on the plate, like this one enhanced with tomatoes, olives, and zucchini and dressed with thyme vinaigrette. It is based on a lovely salad created by chef Anne Cooper at the Getty Museum, where she passionately promoted the virtues of organic, sustainable food and of teaching children to prepare and enjoy healthy dishes. The beautiful, simple salad was made of heirloom tomatoes, aged goat cheese, and baby lettuces dressed with a little olive oil and balsamic vinegar and garnished with fresh olive breadsticks.

I embellish Anne's salad with fresh shell beans, a seasonal treat and a delicious addition to all sorts of vegetable salads. At some farmers' markets, you can buy the beans already shelled to save time. You can substitute frozen baby lima beans or green soybeans (edamame), which are sold shelled or in their pods. If your market doesn't have heirloom tomatoes, buy vine-ripened ones, or the best tomatoes you can find.

Instead of goat cheese, I sometimes use feta or very thin strips of Gruyère or Eastern European sheep's milk kashkaval.

1⅓ cups fresh or frozen lima beans or frozen shelled
    green soybeans (edamame)
1⅓ cups fresh or frozen corn kernels
½ pound zucchini or other summer squash,
    cut into 1-inch dice
1½ to 2 tablespoons balsamic vinegar
Salt and freshly ground black pepper
1½ teaspoons fresh thyme, or ½ teaspoon
    dried thyme (optional)

4 to 5 tablespoons extra virgin olive oil
3 cups mixed baby lettuces
½ hothouse cucumber, cut into thin slices, or
    ½ red or yellow bell pepper, cut into strips
4 ripe tomatoes, preferably heirloom or
    vine-ripened, cut into thin wedges
⅓ cup good-quality black or green olives
½ cup crumbled feta or goat cheese

Cook beans in a saucepan of boiling water, allowing 15 minutes for fresh beans or 5 minutes for frozen beans. Add corn and zucchini and boil for 2 minutes or until vegetables are just tender. Drain well and put in a bowl.

For the dressing, whisk vinegar with salt, pepper, and thyme in a small bowl; whisk in oil. Reserve 1 tablespoon dressing. Add remaining dressing to bean mixture and toss lightly. Taste and adjust seasoning.

Combine lettuce with cucumber in a shallow serving dish, sprinkle with reserved dressing and a little salt and pepper and toss lightly. Spoon bean salad over lettuce mixture. Arrange tomato wedges on top of or around salad. Garnish salad with olives and cheese.

Makes 4 servings as an appetizer or light main course

CREAMY GREEN VEGETABLE SOUP WITH BULGUR WHEAT

This tasty soup is full of healthy foods—greens, lots of fresh herbs, garlic, and wheat—and is inspired by a traditional dish I sampled at an Assyrian food festival: a peppery pottage of chard and bulgur wheat. It owes its creamy texture not to high-fat cream, but to yogurt.

The Assyrians' language, Neo-Aramaic, is related to Hebrew. Those in North America are originally from Iran, Iraq, and Russia. They utilize yogurt and grains liberally in their cuisine. Some cooks make soups like this with barley or with light-colored peeled wheat berries instead of bulgur.

Hearty and easy to prepare, the soup is perfect for a vegetarian meal when the weather is cold, during Hanukkah, or for Purim. Instead of chard, you can use spinach or follow a Turkish variation and add mushrooms. Utilize a green pepper for a mild soup, or poblano or jalapeño chiles for a slightly hotter result. For additional heat, season the finished soup with cayenne pepper. Serve it with whole wheat lavash, pita, or other flatbread.

1½ to 2 tablespoons extra virgin olive oil or
    vegetable oil
6 celery ribs, sliced thin
1 poblano chile (pasilla in California), or
    3 jalapeño peppers, chopped, or
    1 diced green bell pepper
6 green onions, chopped
3 garlic cloves, chopped
¾ to 1 pound chard (about 1 bunch), rinsed and
    chopped

½ cup chopped flat-leaf parsley or cilantro, or
    ¼ cup of each
2 tablespoons chopped mint (optional)
1¾ cups vegetable broth or one 14½-ounce can
    broth, or a mixture of broth and water
½ cup bulgur wheat
Salt
1½ cups plain yogurt, at room temperature
1 tablespoon plus 1½ teaspoons cornstarch
Freshly ground black pepper

Heat oil in a large saucepan. Add celery, chile, green onions, and garlic, and cook over medium-low heat for 2 minutes. Add chard, half of parsley, and half of mint (if using). Cover and cook, stirring often, for 5 minutes. Add broth and 1 quart water and bring to a boil. Add bulgur and a pinch of salt. Cover and simmer over low heat for 10 to 15 minutes or until vegetables and bulgur wheat are tender.

Mix yogurt with cornstarch in a bowl until blended. Slowly stir in 2 cups of the hot soup. With pan of soup off heat, stir in yogurt mixture and mix very well. Return to medium-low heat and cook, stirring constantly, until soup is hot but not boiling. Continue cooking over low heat for 3 minutes, stirring, until soup thickens. If soup is too thick, slowly stir in ½ cup hot water, or more if needed to obtain the consistency you like. Stir in remaining parsley and mint. Season to taste with salt and pepper. Serve hot.

Makes 4 servings

✣ COLD SPINACH AND CORN SOUP WITH YOGURT AND MINT

Fresh corn kernels add interest and color and make this cool, refreshing, creamy soup more satisfying than typical Mediterranean yogurt cucumber soups. Choose a flavorful yogurt, such as Greek style, and for the best nutrition, opt for one that's nonfat or low-fat. This pale green soup is a delicious way to enjoy yogurt, which has long been esteemed in the eastern Mediterranean for its health-promoting properties, and spinach, a source of many vitamins and phytochemicals.

1½ pounds fresh spinach (weight including stems),
  or one 10-ounce bag of cleaned spinach leaves
1 tablespoon extra virgin olive oil
1 large onion, halved and sliced thin
2 large garlic cloves, chopped
Salt and freshly ground black pepper
1 cup fresh corn kernels

1 to 2 cups chilled vegetable broth or ice water
3 cups plain yogurt, regular, low-fat, or nonfat
2 tablespoons finely chopped mint
Cayenne pepper
Lemon juice (optional)
Small sprigs of mint

Discard spinach stems, rinse leaves well, and coarsely chop them. Add spinach to a large sauté pan with the water clinging to its leaves. Cover and cook over medium heat, stirring often, for 3 to 5 minutes or until wilted. Drain in a colander and rinse briefly with cold water. Squeeze gently to remove excess water.

Dry pan used to cook spinach. Heat oil in pan over medium heat. Add onion and sauté over medium-low heat, stirring occasionally, for 7 minutes until tender and golden brown. Add garlic and sauté for ½ minute. Stir in spinach, sprinkle with salt and pepper, and cook for 2 to 3 minutes to evaporate excess moisture. Transfer mixture to a bowl and cool.

If corn is tender, you may want to leave it raw. Otherwise, add it to a small saucepan of boiling water, cover, and cook over medium heat for 1 to 2 minutes. Drain, reserving liquid. Cool corn and cooking liquid. Use cooking liquid as part of vegetable broth.

Puree spinach mixture and 1 cup vegetable broth or ice water in a blender or food processor. Transfer to a bowl. Stir in yogurt, corn kernels, and chopped mint. Slowly add more vegetable broth or water if you'd like a thinner soup. Taste and adjust seasoning, adding cayenne and lemon juice (if using) to taste. Serve cold, garnished with mint sprigs.

Makes 4 servings

For these kosher submarines, you can use all sorts of combinations: (a) real deli meats and nondairy cheeses, (b) soy meats and real cheeses, or (c) soy or other pareve substitutes for both. Whichever you choose, adding a creamy dip makes the submarines extra delicious. Either prepare your own light hummus or eggplant dip, or for a quick meal, buy ready-made eggplant dip or plain or flavored hummus and use it sparingly.

I prefer the taste of soy cheeses made with canola oil, which has healthy monounsaturated fat, rather than the fat-free types.

4 long whole wheat, French, sourdough, or other fresh, crusty rolls

½ cup Light and Easy Eggplant Dip (page 360), Healthy Hummus (page 361), or prepared eggplant dip, or flavored hummus, such as red pepper hummus or spicy hummus

8 to 12 thin slices of smoked turkey breast, soy turkey, or soy salami

8 to 12 thin slices of soy cheese, such as jalapeño-flavored or Swiss-style, other nondairy cheese, or (if using soy meats) low-fat provolone or low-fat mozzarella

2 roasted, peeled red bell peppers, homemade or from a jar, or pickled sweet red peppers, cut into thick strips

1 or 2 large ripe tomatoes, sliced

1 cup shredded romaine or coarsely chopped arugula

1 tablespoon seasoned rice vinegar

1 tablespoon extra virgin olive oil

¼ teaspoon dried oregano

Salt and freshly ground black pepper

2 to 3 tablespoons low-fat mayonnaise, or to taste (see Note)

1 tablespoon Dijon mustard (optional)

Halve rolls lengthwise and remove part of crumb from bottom half of each one. Fill hollow in roll with eggplant or hummus dip. Top with turkey or soy meat, cheese, roasted pepper strips, tomato slices, and romaine. Whisk vinegar with oil, oregano, a pinch of salt, and pepper to taste in a very small bowl, and sprinkle lightly over filling. Spread top half of roll lightly with mayonnaise and mustard (if using) and set it on sandwich.

NOTE: If making sandwich without meat, you can substitute pesto for mayonnaise; in this case, omit mustard.

Makes 4 servings

RICOTTA NOODLE KUGEL
WITH CARAMELIZED ONIONS

My mother taught me that a generous amount of well-browned onions gives noodles great flavor. Browning the onions takes patience; do it carefully, so they will be tender but not burned. To make this kugel creamy, use either ricotta or cottage cheese and combine it with low-fat sour cream or yogurt. Be sure to season the kugel mixture well before baking it so it will not be bland. Chopped pecans give the kugel a festive touch.

3 tablespoons extra virgin olive oil
3 large onions, halved and sliced thin
1 teaspoon paprika
7 to 8 ounces whole wheat noodles, either medium
   or wide
Salt
¾ cup low-fat ricotta

½ cup low-fat sour cream or plain yogurt
⅓ cup finely chopped pecans
Freshly ground black pepper
Cayenne pepper
2 large eggs or equivalent in egg substitute, or
   1 egg plus 2 egg whites

Preheat oven to 350°F. Heat 2 tablespoons oil in a large skillet. Add onions and cook over medium heat, stirring often, for 5 minutes. Stir in ½ teaspoon paprika. Cover and cook over medium-low heat, stirring often, for 15 minutes or until tender and golden brown; add water by tablespoons if pan becomes dry. If onions are tender but not brown, uncover and sauté over medium-high heat, stirring, to brown them.

Add noodles to a large saucepan of boiling salted water and boil, uncovered, over high heat for 5 minutes; they should be nearly tender but firmer than usual. Drain, rinse with cold water, and drain well. Transfer to a large bowl. Add onions and toss with noodles. Add ricotta, sour cream, and half of pecans; mix well. Season to taste with salt, pepper, and cayenne. Beat eggs, add to noodle mixture, and mix well.

Lightly oil a 6- to 8-cup baking dish and add noodle mixture. Sprinkle with remaining tablespoon oil, then with remaining pecans; dust lightly with remaining paprika. Bake, uncovered, for 30 to 40 minutes or until set; if top appears to be browning too quickly, cover and continue baking. Serve from baking dish.

Makes 4 to 6 servings

ISRAELI OMELET AND
ROASTED VEGETABLE SANDWICH

When I moved to Israel at the age of eighteen, I was surprised to see that people commonly whipped up omelets for quick suppers. Until then I considered them a complicated gourmet dish for special occasions.

Unlike the French, Israelis don't make a big deal out of omelets. Usually they make simple flat ones and sauté them in oil instead of butter. Like Americans, Israelis might eat omelets for breakfast or lunch, but most often they are a supper dish, accompanied by a diced vegetable salad. For a delicious sandwich, the omelet is slipped into a pita along with some fried vegetables; I use sautéed or roasted vegetables instead.

Even after tasting the delightful omelets of Paris, an Israeli-style sandwich of an omelet in a fresh pita remains one of my favorite suppers. There's something so satisfying about eating these basic foods together—fresh eggs, pita baked that day, and good olive oil. To make it a healthy dish, I go easy on the oil and include plenty of vegetables. Israeli salsa or Easy Green Chile Garlic Relish (page 363) makes a lively, fresh accompaniment, or serve any hot sauce you like.

½ pound zucchini
2 tablespoons extra virgin olive oil
Salt and freshly ground black pepper
4 eggs, or 2 eggs and 3 egg whites
1 garlic clove, minced
1 tablespoon chopped flat-leaf parsley

1 Japanese, Chinese, or small Italian eggplant,
*   thinly sliced and broiled (page 375)*
1 bell pepper, any color, roasted, either homemade
*   (page 376) or from a jar, cut into strips*
2 pita breads, preferably whole wheat, halved

Scrub the zucchini but do not peel them. Halve them lengthwise, then cut them in crosswise slices about ¼ inch thick. Heat 1 tablespoon oil in a heavy, medium skillet. Add zucchini and sauté over medium-high heat, stirring often, for 3 minutes or until just tender; cover pan during cooking if zucchini become dry. Season to taste with salt and pepper.

Beat eggs with garlic, parsley, salt, and pepper. Transfer zucchini to egg mixture and mix gently. Dry frying pan.

Add remaining oil to pan and heat over medium heat. Swirl pan slightly so oil coats sides as well. Add egg mixture to hot oil. Cook without stirring, but occasionally lift edge of omelet and tip pan so uncooked part of egg mixture runs to edge of pan.

When top is nearly set, carefully slide a wide utensil such as a pancake turner under omelet to free it from pan. Cut omelet in half and turn it over. Cook for ½ minute over low heat to brown second side. Serve omelet with broiled eggplant slices and roasted peppers in pita.

Makes 2 servings

BAKED EGGS WITH
ONIONS, TOMATOES, AND CUMIN

Recently some nutritionists seem to have relaxed the egg taboo, because eggs provide many useful nutrients. All agree that if you're eating eggs, combining them with vegetables is a good idea. This has long been the practice in Mediterranean countries. In this dish, slow-cooked golden onions combined with a spiced tomato sauce provide a tasty bed for the baked eggs. Popular in Israeli homes, this dish is also on the menu at lunch counters and other casual eateries. You can either bake the eggs briefly so that the yolks remain soft in the French manner, or bake them until well done, according to the Israeli taste. Serve them with fresh pita, baguette, or other good crusty bread, preferably whole grain.

You can cook the onions and tomato sauce in advance and reheat them when you're ready to bake the eggs.

3 to 4 tablespoons extra virgin olive oil
2 large onions, halved and sliced
2½ pounds ripe tomatoes, peeled, seeded, and chopped; or two 28-ounce cans plum tomatoes, drained and chopped

1 teaspoon ground cumin
Salt and freshly ground black pepper
Pinch of paprika, Aleppo pepper (semihot red pepper), or cayenne pepper
4 eggs

Preheat oven to 425°F. Heat 2 to 3 tablespoons oil in a heavy, large skillet. Add onions and cook over medium-low heat for 15 minutes or until tender and golden brown; cover pan if it becomes dry. Transfer to a bowl.

Add tomatoes, cumin, salt, and pepper to skillet. Bring to a boil. Cook over medium heat, stirring often, for 15 minutes or until sauce is thick. Stir in onions. Add paprika; taste and adjust seasoning.

Reheat tomato mixture if necessary. Grease 4 individual 6-inch shallow baking dishes or a shallow 5-cup baking dish. Spread tomato mixture in dishes. With a spoon make a depression in mixture in each small dish, or make 4 depressions in large dish, each large enough for 1 egg. Break egg carefully into each one. Drizzle a little oil over each egg and sprinkle it lightly with paprika.

Bake for 12 minutes or until eggs are done to taste. Set individual baking dishes on plates, sprinkle eggs lightly with paprika, and serve.

Makes 4 servings

SCRAMBLED EGG WHITES
WITH HUNGARIAN SPICED MUSHROOMS

Paprika is valued in Jewish cooking, both Ashkenazi and Sephardi, and in the Balkans, the Mideast, and India. In Israel and around the Mediterranean, hot and sweet paprika accent tomato sauces, bulgur wheat salads, and eggs scrambled with vegetables.

According to the experts, paprika peppers originated either in Mexico or South America. The Spanish took the red peppers to Spain and Morocco, and paprika is liberally used in both lands, as in Turkey, where it is proudly labeled according to its Turkish growing areas. The spice is most strongly associated with the cuisine of Hungary. Specific regions of Hungary are known for their top-quality paprika and were officially defined as paprika-growing areas back in 1934.

Most people think of paprika as mild and consider chile powder hot, but all peppers come from the capsicum plant, and there is a range of pungency in both. Some forms of hot paprika are hotter than certain chile powders. Paprika connoisseurs might blend sweet and hot paprikas together or use Aleppo pepper from Syria, which is both sweet and pungent.

When used generously, sweet paprika's subtle fruity flavor becomes distinctive and is compatible with mild and spicy dishes. Due to the natural sugars in the red peppers, paprika enhances browning and thus enables you to sauté foods with less fat. When you sauté onions and mushrooms with paprika, they acquire a wonderful hue and the browning intensifies the spice's aroma and taste. This is a favorite technique of cooks from Hungary to India. Sauté the spice only briefly, however, as it burns easily.

Instead of combining the mushrooms with eggs in this recipe, you can spoon them over tofu or sautéed chicken or toss them with pasta. For an Israeli accent, add cumin as well.

1 1/2 to 2 tablespoons extra virgin olive oil or
    canola oil
1 medium onion, finely chopped
8 ounces small mushrooms, sliced
Salt and freshly ground black pepper
1 teaspoon Hungarian sweet paprika

Pinch of hot paprika, cayenne pepper, or other
    hot red pepper, or 1/4 teaspoon Aleppo pepper
1/2 teaspoon ground cumin (optional)
6 egg whites, or 4 eggs
2 teaspoons chopped fresh dill, or 1 tablespoon
    chopped flat-leaf parsley

Heat oil in a medium skillet. Add onion and sauté over medium heat for 5 minutes; cover skillet if it becomes dry. Add mushrooms, salt, pepper, sweet and hot paprikas, and cumin (if using). Sauté, stirring often, for 5 minutes or until tender and lightly browned.

Beat egg whites with a pinch of salt and hot paprika. Reduce heat under skillet of mushroom mixture to low. Add egg whites and scramble them, stirring often, until they are set to taste. Remove from heat and stir in dill. Taste, adjust seasoning, and serve.

Makes 2 to 3 servings

❧ GARLICKY PERSIAN EGGPLANT WITH EGGS

This dish is my interpretation of a vegetarian entrée I enjoyed at Shoomal, a Persian restaurant in Tarzana, California, which specializes in the cuisine of the Caspian region of northern Iran. It resembled Middle Eastern salads of roasted eggplant, but was served warm and was scrambled with eggs and tomatoes. A generous amount of sautéed garlic gave the dish a lovely aroma and flavor. My husband gave it the ultimate compliment, saying it tasted like an eggplant version of a childhood favorite—shakshuka, or Israeli scrambled eggs with tomatoes. Unlike many egg dishes, it has a high proportion of vegetables to a small amount of eggs. Serve it with fresh whole wheat lavash or pita or with white or brown basmati rice.

Persians normally use neutral vegetable oils. You can use grapeseed oil or canola oil, or substitute mild olive oil.

1 large eggplant (about 1 to 1¼ pounds), or 3 or
    4 Japanese eggplants, roasted (page 360)
2 tablespoons vegetable oil or olive oil
4 to 6 garlic cloves, minced

2 large tomatoes, peeled, seeded, and chopped
¼ teaspoon turmeric
Salt and freshly ground black pepper
4 eggs, or 2 eggs and 3 egg whites

Halve roasted eggplant, scoop out pulp, and chop it. Heat 1 tablespoon oil in a large skillet, add garlic and sauté over medium-low heat, stirring, until just beginning to brown. Add eggplant and sauté, stirring, for 2 minutes. Add tomatoes, turmeric, salt, and pepper and cook uncovered, stirring often, for 5 minutes or until mixture is thick.

Beat eggs with salt and pepper, using a fork. Push eggplant mixture to edges of pan and add remaining tablespoon oil to center. Add beaten egg to center of pan and cook without stirring until beginning to set, as if making a flat omelet. Stir in eggplant mixture, leaving egg in pieces, and continue heating for 1 or 2 minutes or until egg is done to taste. Taste and adjust seasoning. Serve hot.

Makes 2 to 3 servings

❧ LOX, EGGS, AND SPINACH BURRITOS

These burritos are filled with eggs scrambled with lox and onions, and with a spoonful of sautéed spinach, which complements the lox. With so many healthy kosher tortillas of different flavors now available, you can vary the flavor of the burritos by using whole wheat, cilantro, jalapeño, or sun-dried tomato tortillas.

1 bunch of spinach (¾ to 1 pound), stems
*   discarded, leaves rinsed well, or*
*   one 10-ounce bag of cleaned spinach leaves*
3 tablespoons olive oil or vegetable oil, or
*   2 tablespoons oil and 1 tablespoon butter*
1 cup chopped onion

Salt and freshly ground black pepper
4 tortillas, preferably whole grain
6 eggs, or 4 eggs and 3 egg whites
¾ cup fine dice or thin strips of lox or
*   smoked salmon*

Add spinach to a saucepan of boiling salted water and boil, uncovered, over high heat for 2 minutes or until just tender. Drain in a colander, rinse with cold water, and drain well. Squeeze spinach by handfuls to remove as much liquid as possible. Chop spinach fine with a knife.

Heat 1½ tablespoons oil in a heavy nonstick skillet. Add onion and cook over medium-low heat, stirring often, for 7 minutes or until tender and light golden. Remove half of onion and reserve for mixing with eggs. Add spinach to pan, sprinkle lightly with salt and pepper, and heat through. Transfer to a bowl and keep warm. Wipe skillet clean.

Warm tortillas in microwave or in steamer; cover and keep warm.

In a bowl beat eggs with a pinch of salt and pepper. Heat remaining 1½ tablespoons oil (or 1 tablespoon butter with ½ tablespoon oil) in skillet. Add egg mixture to skillet and scramble over low heat, stirring often, until eggs are set to your taste. Remove from heat and gently stir in lox. Spoon spinach onto tortillas, top with scrambled egg mixture, and roll up tortillas. Serve immediately.

Makes 4 servings

Fish

On the traditional Jewish table, fish often starts off a feast. Whether it's an Ashkenazi or Sephardi home, a fish first course is likely to appear on Shabbat, Passover, Rosh Hashanah, and most special-occasion dinners. This healthful habit has long been part of the Jewish culinary culture.

When I was growing up, in our typical Ashkenazi home, we ate fish as a main course at least once a week, in addition to our Friday night fish course. It makes me smile to read current health recommendations, such as that of the American Heart Association (americanheart.org), that we eat fish twice a week. My mother was right all along!

In kosher homes, serving a fish entrée is also a welcome opportunity to enjoy dairy foods on the menu. As children, we were happy to eat fish because we hoped there would be ice cream for dessert. Who knows, maybe that's how my mother taught us to like fish!

In the case of fish, fat is good. Fatty fish are rich in heart-healthy omega-3 fatty acids. Eating fish often is a good way to obtain a variety of nutrients from the sea. It's a good idea to eat most often the kinds of fish that are richest in omega-3s: salmon, sardines, mackerel, and tuna, as well as herring, an Ashkenazi favorite. All are good grilled when fresh. Canned fish make tasty additions to salads, like Mackerel and Soybean Salad with Jalapeño Mint Dressing (page 240). When you're in a rush, you can even top salads with sliced gefilte fish from a jar. Salmon also makes great gefilte fish, on its own or mixed with a milder white fish like halibut.

One of the most delicious ways to enjoy fish also happens to be one of the healthiest. Match the fish with its most popular Mediterranean partners—extra virgin olive oil and fresh lemon juice. You can marinate the fish with a splash of olive oil and a squeeze of lemon juice or sprinkle them on the fish after cooking it.

As an extra flavor boost for whole fish, tuck herb sprigs—thyme, rosemary, or sage—or bay leaves inside it before cooking. Garlic is great with fish too. Add it to a marinade or blend it with oil to drizzle on a cooked fish.

When it comes to cooking fish, there are only two rules to keep in mind. First, freshness is the key to tasty fish. Even the best cook cannot restore freshness to an old fish. Choose fish of good color that does not appear dry and does not smell "fishy." If the fish is whole, its eyes should be clear and bright, and its skin moist and shiny. Ask the vendor's opinion too, and, while you're at it, request to have any scales removed. If only wrapped fish is available, notice the "sell-by" date. Refrigerate the fish promptly and try to cook it by the next day. If you're using frozen fish, store it properly, thaw it in the refrigerator, and cook it as soon as possible.

Second, remember that the secret to moist fish is brief cooking. This can be as easy as getting out a ruler. You measure the fish at its thickest point to estimate the cooking

SMOKED FISH FEASTS FROM BROOKLYN TO PARIS

*I*t's difficult to say who are greater lovers of smoked and cured fish—New Yorkers or Parisians. In both communities, these fish are considered treats. Yet people in each city have completely different ways of savoring these delicacies.

In my childhood home, as in many Jewish families on the East Coast of the United States, lox with cream cheese and bagels was a top choice for weekend brunches. The lox-and-bagel brunch custom has since spread throughout the country. Instead of lox, sometimes we had my mother's favorite—smoked whitefish.

When I lived in Paris, I found that the French are equally fond of smoked fish. At home and in restaurants, slices of saumon fumé *(smoked salmon) are a much-loved appetizer, especially for New Year celebrations. Yet Parisian purists never tuck the fish in a bagel spread with cream cheese. They serve thin salmon slices on a plate and eat them with a knife and fork, accompanied by lemon wedges and perhaps some thin toasts.*

Smoked fish is a boon for people with hectic schedules because it's ready to eat as is. It's also a fabu-

time. Ten minutes for each inch is the guideline for roasting most fish, whether they are whole, fillets, or steaks. If you like certain fish such as tuna or salmon medium or under-done instead of cooked through, check them after 7 or 8 minutes.

No matter how you're cooking a fish, check it several times to be sure you don't over-cook it. Remember that it continues to cook from the heat of the pan or baking dish even after you remove it from the heat.

For holiday meals, roasting fish is often more suitable than grilling. If I'm going to serve a fish cold or at room temperature to start off a Shabbat dinner, I find that a roasted fish often retains its moisture better than a grilled one. Baked uncovered at high heat without liquid, the fish roasts rapidly and doesn't dry out. Besides, baking is easier. Unlike grilling, there's no fear that bits of fish might fall between the grill bars. Because you don't have to contend with the barbecue's searing heat, there's less risk of overcooking or scorching the fish.

---

lous ingredient for creating simple, savory starters. Since smoked fish is not cheap, combining it with other ingredients helps you stretch it to make more portions.

Smoked fish is also valuable as a flavoring. In green salads it makes a light kosher substitute for bacon, contributing a smoky flavor. It perks up cooked greens too; using it this way is a custom of African cooks. Either way, it makes a tasty, healthy appetizer.

Strips of smoked fish are terrific with neutral, quick-cooking foods like pasta, grains, and eggs. One of my favorite dishes at deli-type restaurants is lox and eggs; I prepare a nutritious version with spinach (see page 231). Another good combination is whole-grain noodles with smoked fish and roasted peppers. I can get this dish to the table almost instantly, because the pasta is enhanced by ready-made ingredients.

Rice, too, benefits from the addition of smoked fish. In Taiwan, I discovered a way to match fish with rice for breakfast. A bowl of Chinese congee (rice porridge) was accompanied by small plates of savory items, including cured fish and pickled vegetables. It might seem like a curious combination, but it makes as much sense as lox with bagels, as a small amount of fish flavors the bland "starch" food. A delicious rice salad I enjoyed in France featured smoked haddock, tomatoes, bell peppers, capers, and parsley vinai-grette. Depending on the amounts served, such dishes can play the role of appetizers or entrées.

To keep fish moist during grilling, broiling, or roasting, drizzle it with oil or a bit of melted butter mixed with minced garlic, lemon juice, and herbs like thyme, oregano, dill, or rosemary. For extra zip, spice up the oil with ground coriander, cumin, curry powder, or cayenne pepper. Up to three of these flavorings, along with salt and pepper, are enough to gently accent the fish's taste. In the oven the fish acquires a light golden hue, but you might like to powder pale fish with paprika prior to cooking them.

Garnish your fish with lemon wedges. At serving time sprinkle it with a little more flavored oil. Other fine complements are homemade tomato sauce, vinaigrette, homemade salsa, and for a Yemenite-Jewish accent, Easy Green Chile Garlic Relish (page 363).

In the Sephardi kitchen, a favorite cooking technique is to gently simmer fish directly in a sauce. This type of dish is perfect for festive dinners. The fish gains flavor from the sauce as it cooks and, of course, stays moist. Try, for example, Salmon in Leek and Olive Sauce (page 246) or Rosh Hashanah Tilapia in Saffron Sauce (page 13).

Sauced fish is delicious served over brown rice, whole wheat couscous, orzo (pasta shaped like rice), or whole-grain pasta. You don't even have to worry about reducing the sauce, or boiling it to thicken it, as it will be absorbed by the rice or pasta anyway.

SAFE FISH

*D*ue to the unfortunate situation of pollution of portions of the world's oceans, and of many rivers and lakes, certain fish have absorbed dangerous levels of contaminants, notably mercury and toxic compounds called PCBs (polychlorinated biphenyls).

Some fish should not be eaten at all—lists of these are posted at fish markets. Currently the U.S. Food and Drug Administration advises not to eat shark (which is not kosher anyway), swordfish (which Orthodox rabbis consider not kosher), king mackerel, and tilefish.

According to the Food and Drug Administration, it's safe for adults to eat up to 12 ounces (two average meals) a week of a variety of fish that are lower in mercury. Of the fish commonly eaten, they mention canned light tuna, salmon, pollock, as well as shrimp and catfish (which are not kosher).

The wild form of many fish, notably salmon, is safer to eat than the farmed fish, whether fresh, frozen, or canned. In the case of tuna, canned tuna is safer than fresh, and light tuna is safer than white. Other common safe fish are wild herring, sardines, sole, Pacific halibut, Pacific cod, Atlantic mackerel, and whitefish; and farmed tilapia, trout, carp, and striped bass.

Other fish are considered safe for occasional consumption. Experts disagree on whether it's preferable to eat them once or twice a week or less often. Some health professionals feel that the benefits of fish, even if they may contain a small amount of these substances, outweigh their disadvantages.

The FDA, the Environmental Protection Agency, and some environmental advocacy groups have Web sites listing fish that are considered safe.

Halibut Salad with Hazelnuts and Sugar Snap Peas

Mackerel and Soybean Salad with Jalapeño Mint Dressing

Sardine Salad Niçoise

Trout with Spiced Garlic Oil

Nutty Sole

Herb-Marinated Halibut in Pepper Sauce

Baked Salmon Steaks with Quinoa and Grilled Poblano Chiles

Salmon in Leek and Olive Sauce

Marseilles-Style Fish with Saffron and Fennel

Baked Sea Bass and Chickpeas with Hot and Sweet Peppers

HALIBUT SALAD WITH HAZELNUTS AND SUGAR SNAP PEAS

This elegant main-course salad also makes a festive first course to start off a Purim feast. It is rich in flavor and full of healthful elements—plenty of green vegetables, as well as nuts and nut oil, which contain monounsaturated fat. Nutritious halibut is a good source of high-quality protein, B vitamins, and beneficial minerals, and has a modest amount of beneficial omega-3 fatty acids.

You can double the amount of baby lettuces or spinach instead of using a combination of both; or substitute tender lettuce in bite-sized pieces. Asparagus, green beans, or snow peas are good alternatives to the sugar snap peas.

This salad is also delicious and beautiful when made with salmon or red trout. For the dressing use other toasted nut or seed oils, such as walnut, pecan, pumpkin seed, or sesame oil. Instead of hazelnuts, use other toasted nuts.

½ pound sugar snap peas, ends removed
Salt
½ cup dry white wine (optional)
1¼ pounds halibut steaks
Freshly ground black pepper
1½ to 2 tablespoons white or red wine
    vinegar

3 tablespoons hazelnut oil, or 2 tablespoons
    hazelnut oil plus 1 tablespoon canola oil
3 cups mixed baby lettuces
3 cups baby spinach or bite-sized pieces of trimmed,
    well-rinsed spinach leaves
3 to 4 tablespoons toasted hazelnuts (page 379),
    chopped

Add sugar snap peas to a wide saucepan containing 4 cups boiling salted water. Cook, uncovered, over high heat for 2 minutes or until crisp-tender. Remove with a slotted spoon to a strainer, reserving cooking liquid. Rinse peas with cold water and drain well.

Add wine to saucepan of liquid from cooking peas. Bring to a simmer. Add fish, sprinkle with salt and pepper, and return to a simmer. Cover and cook over low heat for 7 minutes or until fish is opaque inside; cut into thickest part of fish to check. Remove with a slotted spoon and let cool. Break fish into large chunks, discarding any bones and skin.

In a small bowl, whisk vinegar with salt and pepper, then whisk in oil. Taste and adjust seasoning. In a large bowl, toss baby lettuces with spinach. Set aside 2 tablespoons dressing. Add remaining dressing to bowl of greens and toss well. Taste and adjust seasoning. Serve salad topped with halibut and sugar snap peas. Sprinkle fish and peas with reserved dressing, then sprinkle salad with chopped hazelnuts.

Makes 4 servings

MACKEREL AND SOYBEAN SALAD WITH JALAPEÑO MINT DRESSING

This protein-packed salad provides a good way to include omega-3-rich fish in your menu. Instead of mackerel, you can use another cooked or canned fish that is a good source of this nutrient, such as tuna, salmon, or sardines; if using herring, choose a type that isn't packed in a sweet sauce.

Dried soybeans deserve to appear on American menus more often. They taste good, have a pleasing, firm texture, and do not fall apart easily, making them ideal for salads. Instead of yellow soybeans, you can use fast-cooking frozen green soybeans (edamame). If you have cooked brown rice and cooked or canned soybeans on hand, the salad is quick and easy to make. For directions for cooking brown rice and yellow soybeans, see pages 362 and 378.

½ to 1 jalapeño pepper
1 small garlic clove
2 teaspoons water
2 tablespoons extra virgin olive oil
2 tablespoons fresh lemon juice
½ teaspoon dried mint, or 2 teaspoons chopped fresh mint
Salt and freshly ground black pepper
1 cup cooked brown rice

1 cup cooked yellow soybeans or edamame, drained
2 green onions, chopped
1 cup diced hothouse or Persian cucumber
2 radishes, quartered and sliced thin
½ cup thin strips of carrot (about 1½ × ¼ × ¼ inch)
1 cup canned mackerel, drained, flaked in large pieces

To make dressing, cut jalapeño pepper into a few pieces; if you prefer less heat, remove core with seeds and membranes. Puree jalapeño with garlic and water in a small food processor or blender, scraping down often, until finely ground. Transfer to a bowl and stir in oil, lemon juice, mint, and a pinch of salt and pepper.

In a serving bowl, combine rice, soybeans, green onions, cucumber, radishes, and carrot. Stir in dressing. Gently fold in flaked fish. Taste and adjust seasoning. Serve cool or at room temperature.

Makes 3 to 4 main-course servings

SARDINE SALAD NIÇOISE

It's not surprising to find relatives of this French-inspired salad on Jewish menus. After all, the Jewish community of southern France has a long history, dating back ten centuries. Besides, the ingredients are kosher and the salad is suitable for meat or dairy meals. I've often enjoyed salmon niçoise at a Jewish deli near my home.

Sardines make for an attractive platter when used in this salad and are rich in healthful omega-3 fatty acids. Use small, fine-quality sardines, preferably canned in olive oil. If you have fresh sardines, grill them and serve them alongside the salad vegetables. In this recipe I omit the classic anchovies, which are very high in sodium.

½ pound French haricots verts or slim green beans, ends trimmed, cut in two
Salt
4 to 6 baby potatoes, unpeeled, halved
1 tablespoon dry white wine
Freshly ground black pepper
1½ tablespoons red or white wine vinegar

3 tablespoons extra virgin olive oil
½ small mild onion, halved, sliced very thin
2 cups mixed tender lettuces
4 to 6 ripe but firm tomatoes, cut into thin wedges
6 ounces sardines, preferably brisling
⅓ cup good-quality black olives (see Note)
2 hard-boiled eggs, quartered (optional)

Cook green beans in a saucepan, uncovered, with enough boiling salted water to cover them over high heat for 5 minutes or until crisp-tender. Remove with a slotted spoon to a colander, reserving liquid. Rinse green beans with cold water and drain well.

Add potatoes to cooking liquid from beans and bring to a boil. Cover and simmer over medium-low heat for 15 to 20 minutes or until tender but not falling apart. Remove with slotted spoon; you can reserve liquid for soups. Peel potatoes while still warm, slice them, and put them in a large bowl. Mix wine with 1 tablespoon water and pour over potatoes. Sprinkle with salt and pepper and mix gently.

For the dressing, whisk vinegar with salt and pepper in a small bowl; whisk in oil.

Add beans and onion to potatoes. Spoon dressing over vegetable mixture and mix gently. Taste and adjust seasoning.

Make a bed of lettuce in a shallow serving dish. Spoon potato-bean mixture over lettuce. Arrange tomatoes, sardines, olives, and egg quarters (if using) on top. Serve cool or at room temperature.

NOTE: If you're using olives with pits, be sure to mention this to your family or guests.

Makes 3 to 4 servings

For this dish I adapted the European technique of crowning baked fish with garlic butter to a healthier cooking method by creating a similar topping from olive oil. Using oil also makes this entrée more convenient for Shabbat because it can be served at room temperature, so you don't have to worry about heating the fish and overcooking it. I make a double batch of the olive oil mixture, and use part of it to marinate the fish for even more flavor.

You can substitute other whole fish for the trout or use fish steaks and drizzle them with a little of the flavored oil before baking. Serve a colorful accompaniment, like green beans, snow peas, sautéed zucchini, or a big, fresh Israeli salad or green salad.

4 trout, each about 10 ounces
4 tablespoons extra virgin olive oil
2½ teaspoons ground cumin (optional)
2 to 3 teaspoons minced garlic

2 tablespoons fresh lemon juice
Salt and freshly ground black pepper
1 tablespoon minced parsley
Pinch of cayenne pepper

Snip trout fins and trim tails straight, using sturdy scissors. Rinse trout inside and out and pat dry. Put trout in a shallow baking dish. For marinade, mix 2 tablespoons oil with cumin (if using), garlic, lemon juice, and a pinch of salt and pepper in a dish. Set aside 1 tablespoon of mixture to use in sauce. Pour remaining mixture over trout and rub it into fish inside and out. Refrigerate for 30 minutes.

To make spiced oil to finish trout: to reserved tablespoon of marinade add remaining oil, parsley, cayenne, and a little salt and pepper.

Preheat oven to 400°F. Bake trout, uncovered, with its marinade, basting twice, until a skewer inserted into thickest part of fish comes out hot, 12 to 15 minutes; or insert a knife in thickest part of fish near the bone—trout's color should have changed from translucent to opaque.

Remove upper trout skin by scraping gently with a paring knife. Spoon a little of reserved spiced oil over each trout and serve immediately.

Makes 4 servings

Nut-crusted fish seems like an upscale version of schnitzel, the popular meat cutlet coated with flour, eggs, and bread crumbs. Israelis often make schnitzel from chicken breasts, but this technique works well with fish fillets too. Using a nut crust is a distinctive, elegant way to enrobe a fish.

Crusting not only provides flavor and texture, but also helps to keep the fish moist. Today's imaginative cooks use all kinds of nuts—almonds, hazelnuts, walnuts, macadamia nuts, cashews, and pine nuts—to add interest to fish. The nuts might be used alone, or blended with bread crumbs, crushed crackers, flour, or seasonings.

How to apply the crust onto the fish is another area for creativity. Some people dip the fish in eggs, as for schnitzel, before pressing it onto the nuts. Others spread the fish with Dijon mustard or garlic butter, or dip it in oil or buttermilk.

When cooking coated fish, the main concern is to keep the coating from burning. To prevent this, some chefs coat only one side of the fish and sauté that side only briefly to crisp it, then finish cooking the fish on its uncoated side. Others sauté the fish just enough to lightly brown the coating, and then bake the fish until it heats through, as in this recipe. Choosing canola or grapeseed oil is helpful, as they burn less readily than olive oil at high temperatures. An even easier method, favored by many home cooks, is to bake the fish without the preliminary sautéing.

¾ cup almonds, macadamia nuts, or pecans
⅓ cup whole wheat flour
2 eggs or egg whites
1 to 1¼ pounds sole fillets

Salt and freshly ground black pepper
3 to 4 tablespoons canola oil or grapeseed oil
Lemon wedges (for serving)

Preheat oven to 400°F with a rack in upper third of oven. Finely grind almonds in a food processor, stopping often to scrape down mixture so that nuts won't become pasty. Transfer to a shallow bowl. Spread flour in a large plate. Beat eggs in another shallow bowl.

Sprinkle a fish piece with salt and pepper and lightly coat it with flour on both sides, tapping to remove excess flour. Dip fish piece in eggs. Last, dip fish in nuts to coat it, pressing lightly so nuts adhere; handle fish lightly. Repeat with remaining pieces. Set them side by side on a large plate.

Heat 2 tablespoons oil in a heavy, large skillet over medium heat. Add enough fish to make one layer. Sauté on one side only for 1 minute. Transfer fish to a baking dish in one layer. Continue with remaining fish, adding oil to pan if needed. Bake in upper third of oven for 10 to 15 minutes or until fish is cooked through; when checked with point of a knife, flesh should be opaque. Serve hot, with lemon wedges.

Makes 4 servings

Fresh dill and cilantro, pungent cumin and tangy coriander seeds give this North African fish entrée its lively flavor. The fish gains a double layer of flavor, first by being marinated with garlic, olive oil, and a portion of the spices, and then by baking slowly in the savory sauce. Some cooks flavor the sauce with cinnamon and cardamom instead of cumin and coriander. Others fry the fish in butter before baking it. I find the olive oil marinade and the tomato-pepper sauce contribute just enough richness and result in a more healthful dish.

With its colorful sauce dotted with sweet peppers, this dish is a good main course for Sukkot. Rice or bulgur pilaf or whole wheat pita make good accompaniments.

1¼ pounds halibut steaks or other firm, lean fish, about 1 inch thick, cut into 4 pieces
1 tablespoon fresh lemon juice
2 tablespoons extra virgin olive oil
¾ teaspoon ground cumin
1½ teaspoons ground coriander
3 large garlic cloves, minced
Salt and freshly ground black pepper
1 small red or yellow bell pepper, diced

One 14-ounce can tomatoes, drained and finely chopped
1 tablespoon tomato paste
¼ cup water
¼ to ½ teaspoon hot red pepper flakes, or to taste (optional)
1 tablespoon chopped dill
2 tablespoons chopped cilantro
Cayenne pepper

Put halibut steaks in a tray in one layer. Mix lemon juice with 1 tablespoon oil, ¼ teaspoon cumin, ½ teaspoon ground coriander, half the garlic, and a pinch of salt and pepper. Pour over fish and turn to coat both sides. Cover and refrigerate for 1 to 2 hours; or, if there isn't time to marinate it, let fish stand at room temperature while preparing sauce.

Preheat oven to 375°F. Heat remaining tablespoon oil in a skillet. Add bell pepper and cook over medium-low heat for 5 minutes or until it begins to soften; cover if pan begins to become dry. Stir in remaining garlic, followed by remaining teaspoon ground coriander, remaining ½ teaspoon cumin, and chopped tomatoes. Bring to a simmer. Add tomato paste, water, and pepper flakes (if using) and mix well. Simmer, uncovered, for 5 to 10 minutes or until sauce is thick. Stir in dill and 1 tablespoon cilantro. Season to taste with salt, pepper, and cayenne.

Spoon half the sauce into a baking dish large enough to hold the fish in one layer. Top with fish and its marinade, then with remaining sauce. Cover and bake for 22 to 25 minutes or until fish can just be flaked with a fork in its thickest part. Taste sauce again for seasoning. Serve sprinkled with remaining tablespoon cilantro.

Makes 4 servings

❦ BAKED SALMON STEAKS
WITH QUINOA AND GRILLED POBLANO CHILES

New World foods matched with salmon make this a flavorful, healthful dish. Chiles are not only tasty, but a good source of vitamins A and C and fiber. The shiny, heart-shaped poblano chiles (which in California are called pasilla chiles) are often characterized as mild, but when grilled, they can be quite pungent. If you prefer, substitute red bell peppers for half or all the poblanos.

Nutty-tasting, high-protein quinoa makes a pleasant change from the usual rice or potatoes. It cooks quickly and can be prepared as pilaf, just like rice. Serve this light and lively dish as a summertime Shabbat entrée or for a get-together of adventurous eaters.

2 poblano chiles (called pasilla in California),
    broiled and peeled (page 376)
2 to 2½ tablespoons extra virgin olive oil
1 small onion, minced
1 cup quinoa, rinsed well and drained
2 cups vegetable broth or water

Salt and freshly ground black pepper
4 small salmon steaks, about 1 inch thick
1 tablespoon strained fresh lime juice
1 teaspoon ground cumin
Pure chile powder or cayenne pepper
Lime wedges

Dice ½ broiled, peeled poblano chile and reserve; cut remaining poblano chiles into strips.

Heat 1½ to 2 tablespoons oil in a wide-bottomed saucepan. Add onion and sauté over medium heat, stirring often, for 5 minutes or until softened. Add quinoa and cook, stirring, for 1 minute or until grains are coated with onion mixture. Add broth, salt, and pepper. Stir once and bring to a boil. Cover and cook over low heat, without stirring, for 12 to 15 minutes. Taste quinoa; if it is not yet tender, simmer 2 more minutes. Cover and let stand for 5 minutes or until ready to serve. Lightly stir in diced poblano chile. Season to taste with salt and pepper.

Preheat oven to 450°F. Set salmon in a heavy roasting pan. Sprinkle fish with lime juice and ½ tablespoon oil and rub over fish. Sprinkle fish with cumin, salt, pepper, and chile powder to taste. Roast salmon, uncovered, for 12 to 15 minutes or until flesh can just flake and has changed color in its thickest part.

Serve salmon hot or at room temperature, with lime wedges. Spoon quinoa alongside salmon and garnish it with poblano strips and lime wedges.

Makes 4 servings

It's not surprising that the cooks of Provence are masters at preparing fish, given their close proximity to the Mediterranean. When the occasion calls for a festive fish, many simmer their fishmonger's catch of the day in a sauce of the region's renowned foods—ripe tomatoes, fresh garlic, and perhaps a sprinkling of white wine. For extra pizzazz, cooks might throw in a few chopped anchovies or capers or a handful of the region's excellent black olives.

This healthful dish, based on omega-3 rich salmon, is inspired by a Provençal fish entrée that I learned in Paris at École de Cuisine La Varenne. There is a wonderful harmony of flavors—the sweet leeks and carrots, the tart-sweet tomatoes, the pungent garlic, the tangy olives, the rich olive oil, and the herbal accents of thyme and bay leaf. Melded together by the action of the gentle heat, these elements beautifully complement the fish.

To streamline the preparation and make the dish more healthful, I skip the steps of flouring and frying the fish that are characteristic of old-fashioned versions and I braise it directly in the sauce. Chefs often strain sauces to make them silky smooth, but I don't mind the pieces of vegetables in the sauce, so I leave them in. Choose flavorful but not too bitter black olives, such as Kalamata. The fish is delicious served cold as a holiday starter or hot as an entrée.

2 large leeks, white and light green parts only,
    halved lengthwise and rinsed well
1½ to 2 tablespoons extra virgin olive oil
Salt and freshly ground black pepper
1 small carrot, finely diced
4 large garlic cloves, coarsely chopped
1 cup Quick Fish Stock (page 371) or water

One 28-ounce can diced tomatoes, with their juice
1 bay leaf
1 large fresh thyme sprig, or ½ teaspoon dried
    thyme, crumbled
1½ pounds salmon fillet, cut into 4 or 6 pieces
⅓ to ½ cup pitted brined olives, black, green,
    or a mixture, drained well

Cut leeks into very thin slices. Heat 1 tablespoon oil in a large, deep, heavy skillet. Add leeks, salt, and pepper. Cover and cook, stirring often, over medium-low heat for 5 minutes or until tender, adding hot water by tablespoons if necessary to prevent burning. Transfer leeks to a bowl; cover and keep warm.

Add remaining oil to skillet and heat briefly. Add carrot and garlic. Cook over low heat for 3 minutes without letting vegetables brown. Add ½ cup stock, cover, and simmer for 5 minutes. Add tomatoes, salt, pepper, bay leaf, and thyme and bring to a simmer.

Add fish pieces, cover, and cook over low heat for 4 minutes per side or until fish pieces become opaque; check with a fork. With a slotted spatula, carefully remove fish pieces. Discard bay leaf and thyme sprig. Stir one-fourth of leeks into sauce.

If sauce isn't thick enough, simmer it, uncovered, over medium-high heat, stirring often, for 3 minutes or until thick. Stir in olives and simmer for 1 minute. Remove from heat. Taste and adjust seasoning.

To serve hot, return fish to sauce, cover, and reheat briefly. Microwave leeks briefly to reheat. Spoon leeks onto a platter or plates and top with fish pieces; or serve leeks alongside fish. Spoon sauce with olives over and around fish. Serve hot, cold, or at room temperature.

Makes 4 main-course or 6 first-course servings

MARSEILLES-STYLE FISH
WITH SAFFRON AND FENNEL

When I first visited the French Riviera, after years of eating subtle butter- and cream-laden dishes in Paris, I found the region's healthy and high-spirited fare refreshing. I loved the way cooks accented their dishes with generous amounts of fresh herbs, tomatoes, and olive oil, known locally as "the butter of Marseilles." Instead of focusing on long-simmered sauces that demand hours of preparation, cooks on France's Mediterranean coast make theirs quickly from fresh produce.

Golden, saffron-flavored bouillabaisse, a specialty of Marseilles, has been imitated around the world. Some chefs combine the soup's signature flavors to create sauces for fish. I learned such a dish from my teacher and good friend, master seafood chef Fernand Chambrette in Paris, who took the usual bouillabaisse ingredients—ripe tomatoes, onions, garlic, and saffron—then enhanced the mix with fresh fennel and basil. He served his *poisson a la marseillaise* cold. It makes a delicious first course for my Shabbat dinners or a refreshing summertime entrée.

This dish is a healthy adaptation from a recipe in *La Cuisine du Poisson*, the book I co-authored with Chef Chambrette (Flammarion, Paris, 1984). The chef prefers rosy-colored fish called rouget (red mullet), and chooses the tiniest ones for this dish. To make preparation easier, I use fish fillets.

3 to 4 tablespoons extra virgin olive oil
6 large tomatoes, peeled, seeded, and chopped
Salt and freshly ground black pepper
1 fennel bulb
1 large onion, chopped
2 large garlic cloves, chopped
¼ cup dry white wine
⅓ cup Quick Fish Stock (page 371) or water

Pinch of saffron
6 large basil leaves, chopped
1¼ to 1½ pounds halibut, sea bass, or sole fillets,
    in 4 to 8 pieces
12 flavorful black olives, such as niçoise or
    Moroccan, pitted (optional)
1 tablespoon chopped flat-leaf parsley (optional)

In a sauté pan, heat ½ tablespoon oil. Add tomatoes and a little salt and pepper. Cook over medium heat, stirring often, for 15 minutes or until almost all liquid evaporates.

Remove fennel stalks and outer layers, which are slightly fibrous. Cut fennel into very thin strips. Rinse and dry strips. In another sauté pan, heat 1½ tablespoons oil and add fennel, onion, and garlic. Cook over low heat, stirring often, for 10 minutes or until fennel is tender but not brown; cover pan during cooking if it becomes dry.

Add wine, stock, salt, and pepper to fennel mixture and simmer for 5 minutes. Add saffron, cooked tomatoes, and basil and cook for 5 minutes, stirring often. Taste and adjust seasoning.

Preheat oven to 425°F. Brush a large baking dish with oil. Arrange fish pieces in it side by side. Spoon hot tomato sauce over fish. Bake, uncovered, for 10 minutes or until fish can barely be flaked and has changed color in its thickest part—check with a small, sharp knife. Cool, then refrigerate until ready to serve, or up to 24 hours.

Just before serving, drizzle fish with remaining oil, if you like, and shake pan slightly to blend it with the juices. Garnish fish with olives and sprinkle with parsley, if you like. Serve cold.

Makes 4 to 5 main-course or 6 to 7 appetizer servings

✕ BAKED SEA BASS AND CHICKPEAS WITH HOT AND SWEET PEPPERS

Jews of North African origin like to combine chickpeas with fish to make spicy dishes like this easy-to-prepare entrée. You occasionally find the fish and chickpea association in other Mediterranean cuisines as well. On a visit to Italy, I enjoyed a simple entrée of poached fish, chickpeas, and olive oil—three of the healthiest foods out there, according to experts. Greeks pair chickpeas with tuna for appetizer salads.

Two 15- or 16-ounce cans chickpeas (garbanzo beans), drained, or 3 cups cooked chickpeas, with ½ cup of their cooking liquid
1 red bell pepper, diced
1 jalapeño pepper, chopped (optional)
6 dried hot peppers, such as chiles de arbol
6 large garlic cloves, chopped

1 teaspoon paprika
Salt and freshly ground black pepper
⅓ cup chopped cilantro
2 to 3 tablespoons extra virgin olive oil
1½ pounds sea bass, cod, or halibut steaks or fillets, about 1 inch thick
Cayenne pepper (optional)

Preheat oven to 400°F. In a 2-quart casserole, combine chickpeas with bell pepper, jalapeño pepper, dried peppers, garlic, paprika, salt, pepper, and all but 1 tablespoon of the cilantro. Add ½ cup chickpea cooking liquid or water. Cover tightly and bake for 10 minutes to blend the flavors.

Spoon half of chickpea mixture into a bowl. Set fish on top of remaining mixture in casserole and sprinkle it with salt and pepper. Return remaining chickpea mixture to casserole, spooning it over fish, then top with 2 tablespoons oil. Cover and bake for 20 to 30 minutes or until fish can just be flaked but is not falling apart.

Discard dried peppers; or leave them for garnish and remind the diners not to eat them. Taste cooking liquid and add cayenne if you like. Serve hot or lukewarm, drizzled with a little more olive oil, if you like, and sprinkled with remaining cilantro.

Makes 4 to 5 servings

Poultry and Meat

A HOLIDAY TRADITION

❈

"Meat and fish and all tasty things" goes a Shabbat hymn. In many observant homes, a main course of meat or chicken is a must for welcoming Shabbat and most holidays. Whether it's Ashkenazi brisket with dried fruit or Tunisian-Jewish couscous topped with meat-stuffed vegetables, meat and poultry are the stars. Friday night chicken is a standard entrée—often roast chicken, sometimes a stuffed bird or, occasionally, chicken in the pot.

When I share a potluck Shabbat dinner with my friends, the menu tends to be wholesome; generally there is fish, rice, and lots of vegetables. But the standout dish is usually the braised beef. A few bites of fork-tender beef and a spoonful of its savory sauce to moisten the rice are all that most guests need in order to feel they have enjoyed the taste of meat. This type of meal illustrates persuasively that a healthy menu can include meat. You simply prepare your favorite meat main course and serve it in small amounts, and fill the rest of your plate with vegetables.

Saving meat for festive meals is a healthy custom, if it is served in moderate portions. Chicken is a lean protein and is good for you, as long as you don't eat the fatty skin. I favor the techniques of cooks from India, who always remove the skin before cooking chicken. This way the fat from the skin doesn't permeate the sauce or roasting juices. Since the skin helps keep the meat moist, if you are baking chicken, it's best to cover it so it won't be dry.

Making good use of small amounts of meat is a well-known Asian culinary custom. Home cooks in Japan, China, and the Philippines might cook thin slices of beef with plenty of vegetables in a light sauce and ladle it over cooked rice or noodles. Often they include healthy greens among the vegetables. For many people, the rice or pasta moistened with the sauce is the best part.

These principles are also true of Sephardi dishes. Many Middle Eastern recipes allow only 4 ounces of meat per person, which is a good amount according to nutritionists' guidelines. North African cooks often make stews with more vegetables than meat. For example, they might stew veal with twice its weight in onions, along with chickpeas, tomatoes, paprika, and ground coriander. Persians make stews of lamb with eggplant, tomatoes, and saffron that include plenty of eggplant and not much meat.

Some of my friends declare they never eat meat, as proof that they are conscientiously following their healthy diets. Many say this with regret, feeling they have no choice. Yet nutrition-conscious people can have the pleasure of eating meat as long as they do so in moderation.

There are three easy ways to include meat in healthy menus:

1. Change the proportions of the ingredients in your stews, sautés, and braised dishes to include more vegetables and less meat;
2. Make your favorite recipes the usual way so they have the flavor you like, but serve smaller portions. You might like to serve stews over brown rice or whole wheat noodles;
3. Try new dishes that include just a little meat.

Meat contributes a unique taste to sauces and adds rich flavor and contrasting texture to noodle medleys and vegetable stews. Fortunately, a little goes a long way.

Honey-Ginger Chicken Breasts

Kosher Tandoori Chicken

Yom Ha'atzmaut Chicken Paillardes with Israeli Tomato Sauce

Grilled Chicken Salad with Beets and Port Vinaigrette

Chile Chicken Salad

Mexican-Inspired Turkey in Tomato Chile Sauce with Raisins

Sweet-and-Sour Pumpkin and Turkey Stew with Wheat Berries

Roast Turkey Breast with Rosemary-Garlic Sauce

Beverly Hills Brisket

Beef and Vegetable Soup, Latin American Style

Spicy Lamb with Red Beans and Mint

Moroccan Lamb Tajine with Cauliflower

❧ HONEY-GINGER CHICKEN BREASTS

Chicken roasted with honey has become a popular Rosh Hashanah dish in Israel, even though the origin of this recipe may be Chinese. Actually, this is not surprising. Jews have more in common with the Chinese than a lunar calendar. We love Chinese food! Some traditional foods for the Chinese New Year are whole fish, which symbolize bounty, and vegetables carved in a coin shape, and tangerines, the New Year's "good fortune" fruit. Fish and coin-shaped carrots are also on the Jewish New Year menu, as are a variety of fruit for a sweet New Year.

As on most Jewish festive occasions, whole roasted birds are favorite feast-day foods among the Chinese. Their technique of glazing poultry with sweetened soy sauce has been adopted around the world, including in Israel. For this recipe, the chicken pieces are baked without their skin so they will be low in saturated fat. Baking the chicken breasts with a honey-ginger glaze and covering them during baking keeps the meat moist. If you prefer to use chicken thighs, increase the baking time by 10 minutes.

2½ pounds chicken breast pieces, with bones

3 tablespoons liquid honey, plus 1 more teaspoon if needed

2 to 4 tablespoons soy sauce, preferably lower-sodium type, or to taste

2 tablespoons rice wine, sherry, or dry white wine

¼ teaspoon freshly ground black pepper, or to taste

¼ teaspoon ground cinnamon

1 tablespoon finely minced peeled ginger, plus 4 thin slices

½ cup chicken broth or water

2 tablespoons sliced almonds, lightly toasted (optional)

Remove skin from chicken pieces. Mix 3 tablespoons honey, soy sauce, wine, pepper, cinnamon, and minced ginger. Reserve 1 tablespoon mixture in a small cup and cover. Rub chicken thoroughly with remaining honey mixture. Let stand for 20 to 30 minutes; or refrigerate for 2 to 4 hours.

Preheat oven to 375°F. Lightly oil a shallow roasting pan just large enough to hold chicken in one layer, and put chicken pieces with their marinade in it. Pound ginger slices with back of a knife and add to pan. Roast chicken for 5 minutes. Cover with foil and bake for 25 minutes. If pan is dry, add 2 to 3 tablespoons chicken broth. Continue baking chicken covered, basting once, for 15 to 30 minutes longer or until it is tender when pierced with a sharp knife; when chicken is cut in thickest part, meat should no longer be pink. For browner chicken, uncover during last 5 minutes of baking.

Remove chicken from pan. Heat remaining broth to a simmer in a small saucepan. Add to chicken pan juices and blend well, scraping in juices from sides of pan. Pour juices into saucepan. Remove ginger slices. Skim off fat. Add remaining honey mixture and bring to a simmer. Cook briefly over low heat until thickened to taste. Taste and adjust seasoning, adding more honey if you like. Brush chicken with juices and serve hot, sprinkled with almonds, if desired. Serve remaining juices separately.

Makes 4 servings

KOSHER TANDOORI CHICKEN

Classic tandoori chicken is not kosher because the marinade contains yogurt. But Jews from India have come up with a solution. Most substitute oil for the yogurt, and some substitute mayonnaise. Some American chefs suggest using soy milk or soy sour cream, but they tend to make the chicken a bit sweet. Oil works fine and the result is a nicely browned, spicy chicken. It's also healthy, as traditionally tandoori chicken is baked without its fatty skin; the marinade keeps it moist.

Using a food processor gives the smoothest marinade, but instead you can chop the garlic and ginger with a knife until very fine, then blend with the remaining marinade ingredients. Kosher chickens have already been salted and therefore there's no need to add salt to the marinade. White or brown basmati rice is the perfect accompaniment.

2 pounds chicken pieces
¼ onion, peeled
2 large garlic cloves, peeled
1 tablespoon coarsely chopped ginger
1 tablespoon fresh lemon juice
2 tablespoons canola oil or other vegetable oil

2 teaspoons paprika
1½ teaspoons ground cumin
½ teaspoon turmeric
¼ to ½ teaspoon cayenne pepper
¼ teaspoon ground cinnamon
Pinch of ground cloves

Remove skin from chicken. Combine onion, garlic, and ginger in a food processor. Process until finely chopped. Add lemon juice, oil, paprika, cumin, turmeric, cayenne, cinnamon, and cloves. Process until combined.

Put chicken in a shallow bowl. Add marinade and rub it all over chicken. Cover and refrigerate for 4 to 8 hours, turning occasionally.

Preheat oven to 400°F. Set chicken and its marinade in a heavy roasting pan. Cover and roast for 20 minutes. Uncover and continue roasting for 20 to 30 minutes, checking chicken occasionally and covering it again if it browns too fast. When done, juices should come out clear when a skewer is inserted into thickest part of meat; if juices are pink, continue roasting a few more minutes.

Makes 4 servings

YOM HA'ATZMAUT CHICKEN PAILLARDES WITH ISRAELI TOMATO SAUCE

In Israel, the way to celebrate Yom Ha'atzmaut (Israel's Independence Day) is by having a barbecue outdoors, like for the Fourth of July.

A great choice for healthy cooking is a paillarde—a boneless slice or cutlet of meat that is pounded until thin, then briefly sautéed or grilled so the meat remains juicy. By being flattened, a piece of meat looks bigger than it really is.

In classic French cuisine, paillardes referred to beef and veal, but now the term is also used for chicken, turkey, lamb, and even thin slices of large fish. Instead of a delicate French sauce, this spicy, bright red sauce features the robust Middle Eastern flavors popular in Israel.

Be sure to thoroughly heat the grill you're using, whether it's a stovetop grill or a barbecue, so that the meat sears quickly. If the grill is not hot enough, the meat will stick. Use a wide spatula or other flat utensil to turn the meat rather than a fork, as pricking it will release the meat's juices and leave it dry. Make the sauce ahead and heat it in a saucepan on the barbecue while you're cooking the paillardes, or serve it at room temperature. Brown rice, whole wheat pita, or lavash are good accompaniments.

2 tablespoons extra virgin olive oil
½ medium onion, minced
3 garlic cloves, minced
1 or 2 jalapeño or serrano peppers, minced
¼ teaspoon turmeric
1½ teaspoons ground cumin
Two 28-ounce cans tomatoes, drained and chopped

Salt and freshly ground black pepper
Pinch of cayenne pepper
1 tablespoon tomato paste
½ teaspoon paprika
4 whole fairly small boneless chicken breasts
    (total 1¼ to 1½ pounds), skinned

To make sauce, heat 1 tablespoon oil in a large saucepan over low heat. Add onion and cook, stirring occasionally, until soft but not brown. Add garlic and jalapeño peppers and cook, stirring, for 30 seconds. Add turmeric and 1 teaspoon cumin and cook, stirring, for 30 seconds. Add tomatoes, salt, pepper, and cayenne and stir well. Bring to a boil over medium-high heat. Cook, uncovered, over medium-low heat, stirring occasionally, for 20 minutes or until sauce is thick and chunky. Stir in tomato paste and heat through.

Mix paprika and remaining ½ teaspoon cumin. Trim chicken breasts of fat and cartilage. Pound them one by one between 2 pieces of plastic wrap to a thickness of ¼ inch, using a flat meat pounder or rolling pin.

Before serving, reheat sauce if it is cold. Taste and adjust seasoning. Cover sauce and keep it warm.

Heat a ridged grill pan over medium-high heat until very hot; or heat barbecue. To check heat of ridged grill pan, when one end of chicken breast is touched to grill, it should make a sizzling noise. Brush chicken with oil. Sprinkle with pepper and with cumin-paprika mixture. Put 1 or 2 chicken pieces on grill, depending on its size. Cook for 1½ minutes per side, brushing lightly with oil before turning, or until color of chicken has changed inside; cut into thickest part of chicken to check. Use two wide spatulas to turn chicken. Serve chicken hot with sauce.

Makes 4 servings

GRILLED CHICKEN SALAD
WITH BEETS AND PORT VINAIGRETTE

Beets make a colorful addition to salads and are nutritious as well—they are a good source of folate and contain fiber, vitamin C, magnesium, and potassium.

This salad of beets and grilled chicken breast on a bed of baby greens makes an elegant summertime entrée. During grilling I leave the chicken skin on to protect the lean meat, and I remove the skin before serving.

5 small beets, about 1½ inches in diameter,
* rinsed*
1 to 2 tablespoons wine vinegar
1 tablespoon port
Salt and freshly ground black pepper

¼ cup plus 2 teaspoons canola oil, grapeseed oil,
* or olive oil*
1½ pounds boneless chicken breast, with skin
6 to 7 cups mixed baby lettuces, loosely packed
½ cup cooked peas, fresh or frozen (optional)

Bring at least 1 inch of water to a boil in base of a steamer without allowing boiling water to reach steamer holes. Place beets on steamer top above boiling water. Cover tightly and steam over high heat for 50 minutes or until tender, adding boiling water if water evaporates. Remove beets and let cool. Peel beets while holding them under cold running water.

Whisk vinegar with port, salt, and pepper until blended. Whisk in ¼ cup oil.

Heat a ridged stovetop grill pan over medium-high heat, or heat broiler. Rub meat side of chicken with oil and sprinkle with salt and pepper. Lightly oil grill pan or broiler rack. Set chicken, skin side down, on pan or rack and grill or broil for 5 to 7 minutes per side or until color in thickest part is white; cut into chicken to check. Remove chicken skin if desired. Cut chicken in diagonal slices crosswise.

In a large bowl, toss lettuce with half of dressing. Taste and adjust seasoning. Divide lettuce among 4 plates. Set chicken and beets on lettuce, spoon peas around them, and top with remaining dressing.

Makes 4 servings

✵ CHILE CHICKEN SALAD

When you have a taste for chili in the summertime and don't feel like heating up the kitchen, try this refreshing, bold-flavored salad of chicken, beans, and fresh vegetables. It takes only minutes to prepare. If you have leftover roast chicken from Shabbat, this is a great way to use it, but any cooked chicken is fine.

For a deeper flavor, combine the chicken, beans, and onion with the dressing and refrigerate for a few hours or even overnight, so the ingredients can absorb more of the seasonings. Add the peppers and tomatoes no more than a few hours before serving so they keep their fresh taste and texture. Set out small bowls of add-ons, like sliced green onions, chopped cilantro, avocado slices, pickled hot peppers, and lemon wedges. And don't forget a bottle of your favorite hot sauce.

1 to 2 tablespoons fresh lemon juice, or more to taste

3 tablespoons extra virgin olive oil, or more to taste

Salt and freshly ground black pepper

1 garlic clove, minced

1 or 2 jalapeño peppers, seeds removed, minced, or ¼ teaspoon hot red pepper flakes

¼ to ½ teaspoon pure chile powder, or equal parts sweet and hot paprika, or more to taste

½ teaspoon ground cumin

1 tablespoon chopped fresh oregano, or 1 teaspoon dried oregano

2 cups thin strips of cooked chicken

½ small red onion

3 cups cooked white beans, or two 15-ounce cans white beans, drained

1 large red, orange, yellow, or green bell pepper, or ½ red and ½ green pepper, cut into thin strips or diced

3 or 4 ripe medium tomatoes, diced

In a medium bowl, whisk lemon juice with oil, salt, and pepper to taste. Add garlic, jalapeño peppers, chile powder, cumin, and oregano. Add chicken to dressing. Let chicken stand to marinate while preparing remaining ingredients.

Cut onion in thin slices. Halve slices and separate them into slivers. Add onions and beans to chicken and mix well. If you have made salad ahead, remove it from refrigerator about 10 minutes before serving.

Add sweet peppers and tomatoes to salad and toss gently. Taste, and adjust the amounts of salt, pepper, cumin, and chile powder. Add more oil and lemon juice, if you like. Serve at cool room temperature.

Makes 3 to 4 servings

MEXICAN-INSPIRED TURKEY
IN TOMATO CHILE SAUCE WITH RAISINS

A common complaint about Thanksgiving dinner is that the turkey is dry. At the holiday table, many seem to eat turkey almost as a required ritual, dousing it with gravy to wash it down, and helping themselves more enthusiastically to the bread stuffing, mashed potatoes, candied yams, and pumpkin pie.

But turkey is often the healthiest part of the festive meal. Steven Pratt and Kathy Matthews, the authors of *Superfoods Rx*, named skinless turkey breast one of the top fourteen healthy foods because it is "one of, if not the leanest meat protein source on the planet." In addition, its highly nutritious meat contains heart-healthy niacin, selenium, vitamins B$_6$ and B$_{12}$, and zinc.

Turkey can be delicious. Because turkey breast is so lean, I opt for a moist-heat cooking method—braising or stewing—so that it doesn't dry out. As it simmers, the turkey turns the cooking liquid into a savory sauce, which makes preparing a separate gravy unnecessary. Serving is much easier as there is no messy last-minute carving. You can cook and slice this turkey ahead and reheat it over low heat.

For the sauce, I use the Mexican technique of adding raisins and sweet spices as a pleasing balance for the chiles' pungency. Remove the chiles' ribs and seeds if you prefer a milder flavor. A roasted mild chile or sweet bell pepper gives additional depth of flavor, but even adding the pepper raw will enhance the sauce.

Festive and easy to prepare, this entrée is good for Thanksgiving or Shabbat. Baked winter squash is the perfect accompaniment. You can also serve the turkey with mashed potatoes, brown rice, or whole wheat or corn tortillas.

2 tablespoons vegetable oil
One 2-pound piece of boneless turkey breast,
    tied in a compact shape, patted dry
1 large onion, chopped
1 medium carrot, coarsely chopped (optional)
2 to 3 jalapeño peppers, chopped
2 large garlic cloves, minced
One 28-ounce can tomatoes, drained and chopped
One Anaheim chile or green bell pepper, roasted
    (page 376) or raw, diced (optional)
Salt

½ teaspoon dried oregano
½ teaspoon ground cumin
¼ teaspoon ground cinnamon
Pinch of ground cloves
½ cup chicken broth or water
3 to 4 tablespoons raisins
⅓ cup mild green olives, plain or stuffed, drained
    (optional)
Cayenne pepper (optional)
1 tablespoon chopped cilantro or parsley (optional)

Heat oil in a heavy stew pan. Add turkey and brown lightly over medium-high heat on all sides. Remove to a plate. Add onion and carrot (if using) to pan and cook over medium-low heat, stirring often, for 7 minutes or until onion softens. Stir in jalapeño peppers and garlic, followed by tomatoes, diced Anaheim chile or green bell pepper (if using), salt to taste, oregano, cumin, cinnamon, and cloves. Bring to a boil. Add broth.

Return turkey to pan. Cover and cook over low heat, turning meat over a few times, for 1 hour or until an instant-read thermometer or meat thermometer inserted into center of turkey reads 170°F, or turkey is tender when pierced with a sharp knife. Remove meat to a board and keep it warm. For a thicker sauce, boil sauce, uncovered, to reduce it slightly. Add raisins and olives (if using) and simmer for 2 minutes. Taste and adjust seasoning, adding cayenne if desired.

Slice turkey and arrange slices on a platter. Spoon some sauce, with olives and raisins, over slices and sprinkle with cilantro, if you like. Serve remaining sauce separately.

Makes 4 servings

SWEET-AND-SOUR PUMPKIN AND TURKEY STEW WITH WHEAT BERRIES

Kurdish Jews make creative use of grains and greens. Years ago I became interested in their food after I attended an exhibition of Kurdish culture and cuisine in Jerusalem. This entrée is a healthy adaptation of a Kurdish pumpkin stew. Generally, beef is used but for this lighter dish, I use turkey.

If you don't have time to cook wheat berries, use medium bulgur wheat or a fast-cooking type of brown rice. Cook them in broth following the package directions, then continue with the recipe.

1 to 1¼ cups wheat berries, rinsed

4 cups chicken, turkey, or vegetable broth or water

Salt

2½ pounds butternut squash, Japanese pumpkin (kabocha squash), or calabaza squash

2 to 3 tablespoons vegetable oil

1½ pounds boneless turkey, cut into 1-inch cubes

2 onions, chopped

1 green bell pepper, diced (optional)

One 28-ounce can tomatoes, drained and chopped

Salt and freshly ground black pepper

1 tablespoon sugar, or to taste

¼ cup raisins (optional)

2 to 3 tablespoons strained fresh lemon juice, or to taste

In a large saucepan, combine wheat berries, broth, and a pinch of salt and bring to a boil. Cover and simmer over low heat for 1½ to 2 hours or until wheat berries are tender.

Peel squash. Remove seeds and strings. Cut squash meat into 1-inch pieces.

Heat 1 to 2 tablespoons oil in a stew pan. Add turkey and sauté lightly over medium heat in two batches, removing each as it changes color. Add onions and sauté over medium heat for 7 minutes or until golden. Remove half of onions and reserve for mixing with wheat.

Return turkey to pan. Add green pepper (if using) and tomatoes and cook, uncovered, for 5 minutes. Add squash, 1¼ cups water, salt, pepper, and sugar. Stir and bring to a boil. Cover and cook over low heat, occasionally stirring gently, for 30 minutes or until turkey is tender; dark meat will take longer than light meat.

Reheat wheat berries in their liquid. If there is too much liquid, drain excess; you can save it for soups. Add reserved sautéed onions. Taste and adjust seasoning.

Finish turkey stew by adding raisins (if using) and 2 tablespoons lemon juice. Cook for 5 minutes or until raisins soften. Taste and adjust seasoning, adding more sugar or lemon juice if needed. Serve stew spooned over wheat berries.

Makes 4 to 6 servings

ROAST TURKEY BREAST
WITH ROSEMARY-GARLIC SAUCE

This entrée is good for Thanksgiving and for Sukkot, which resembles Thanksgiving in many ways. Peppers, olive oil, and Mediterranean herbs enhance the taste of this simple roast and its savory juices. Adding part of the garlic at the last minute gives the sauce extra punch. If you like, roast some small potatoes in the pan around the turkey, first moistening them with a little extra olive oil.

I find that turkey breasts cooked on their own often come out moister than the white meat of a whole roasted turkey. After all, these smaller roasts cook much faster and the breast meat doesn't have to endure prolonged roasting while it waits for the thigh meat to cook through. Usually I opt for turkey breasts with the bone in, because they make more succulent roasts than boneless ones, and I cover the turkey for part of the roasting time.

Zucchini Mushroom Stuffing with Pecans (page 151) makes a tasty partner for the turkey, along with green beans, broccoli, or Brussels sprouts.

5 fresh rosemary sprigs
One 3-pound turkey breast half, skin on, bone in
2 large onions, peeled and quartered
Salt and freshly ground black pepper
3 tablespoons extra virgin olive oil
6 large garlic cloves, minced
1 tablespoon chopped fresh thyme, or
*　　1½ teaspoons dried thyme*
2 teaspoons chopped fresh rosemary

1 teaspoon paprika
¼ teaspoon cayenne pepper
3 bell peppers, green, red, and yellow, quartered
½ cup dry white wine or water
¾ cup turkey or chicken broth, or more if needed
1 tablespoon potato starch or cornstarch, dissolved
*　　in 2 tablespoons water (optional)*
1 tablespoon chopped flat-leaf parsley (optional)

Preheat oven to 400°F. Put rosemary sprigs in a small, heavy roasting pan and set turkey breast on top, bone side down. Add onions to pan. Sprinkle turkey with salt and pepper. Combine oil, 4 minced garlic cloves (about ⅔ of the garlic), half of thyme, 1 teaspoon rosemary, paprika, and cayenne and rub over turkey.

Roast turkey for 15 minutes. Reduce oven temperature to 350°F. Cover turkey loosely with foil and roast for 30 minutes, basting once or twice. Add pepper pieces to pan. Roast for 20 minutes, baste turkey again, and turn peppers over. Uncover turkey if you would like it to brown more. Add ¼ cup wine and ¼ cup broth to pan. Roast turkey for 30 more minutes or until a meat thermometer or instant-read thermometer inserted in thickest part of meat, not touching bone, registers 170°F.

Remove turkey to a board, cover loosely, and let rest for about 15 minutes before carving. Discard rosemary sprigs.

With a slotted spoon, remove pepper pieces from pan, and most of onion pieces, if you want to serve them. Pour pan juices into a measuring cup and skim fat.

Heat remaining wine to a simmer in a saucepan, pour into roasting pan, and scrape browned juices into wine. Return mixture in roasting pan to saucepan. Pour pan juices in cup into wine. Add remaining broth and simmer for 2 minutes. Skim fat again. For a smoother sauce, strain into a bowl and return to saucepan; return to a simmer. Stir potato starch mixture (if using) and whisk into simmering broth. Simmer for 1 to 2 minutes until thickened. If sauce is too thick, slowly stir in a few more tablespoons broth.

Carve turkey into thin slices. Add parsley (if using) and remaining garlic, thyme, and rosemary to sauce. If you like, add juices from turkey board. Taste sauce for seasoning. Serve turkey with peppers, onions, and sauce.

Makes 4 to 6 servings

This is a lighter rendition of Mexican beef tinga, which I first tasted at a celebration introducing Loews' Beverly Hills Hotel's new kosher menu, catered by Nir Weinblut. Originating in Puebla, in Central Mexico, tinga dishes are based on a slightly spicy tomato sauce accented with sautéed onion, garlic, oregano, and smoked chiles.

Brisket may not seem easy to serve at a party, but Chef Weinblut came up with interesting solutions. Instead of slicing his brisket like for pot roast, he shredded the beef and mixed it with the sauce. He gave guests a choice of two ways to enjoy it: on pieces of French baguette or wrapped in soft flour tortillas.

For my interpretation I add mushrooms and substitute tofu for half the usual amount of meat, so there will be plenty of protein in each portion but less fat. During the slow simmering, the brisket contributes rich flavor to the tomato-mushroom sauce and to the tofu. To serve the dish, shred the cooked meat cubes into long, thin pieces for serving on tortillas or on French rolls; or leave the beef in cubes and serve the stew with beans, potatoes, noodles, or rice.

Be sure to thoroughly trim the fat from the brisket. For a leaner dish, you can substitute skinless chicken thighs or legs for the beef; they will need only about 50 minutes of simmering. For extra flavor, you can make the sauce with grilled or broiled fresh tomatoes instead of canned ones: broil 1 1/2 to 2 pounds tomatoes for 5 minutes on each side until charred, then puree them and add them to the pan.

1 pound beef brisket, fat trimmed, cut into
    1 1/4- to 1 1/2-inch pieces
1 1/2 to 2 tablespoons vegetable oil or olive oil
1 large onion, chopped
2 large garlic cloves, chopped
One 28-ounce can tomatoes, drained and chopped
About 2 cups water
1 to 2 teaspoons minced canned drained chipotle
    chile in adobo sauce, or 1 to 2 jalapeño or
    serrano peppers, chopped

Salt and freshly ground black pepper
1 teaspoon dried oregano
8 ounces medium mushrooms, quartered
12 to 16 ounces firm tofu, drained and cut into
    bite-sized cubes or smaller
Hot red chile powder or cayenne pepper
    (optional)
1 tablespoon chopped cilantro (optional)
4 to 6 tortillas, preferably whole wheat, slightly
    warmed

Pat beef dry. Heat oil in a large, heavy stew pan. Add beef in batches and brown cubes lightly over medium heat on all sides. Transfer cubes to a plate as they brown.

Add onion to pan and cook over low heat, stirring often, for 7 minutes or until softened. Add garlic and sauté a few seconds, stirring. Return meat to pan, adding any juices on plate. Stir in tomatoes and 2 cups water, or enough to barely cover beef. Add chile, salt, pepper, and oregano and bring to a boil, stirring often. Cover and cook over low heat, stirring occasionally and adding more water if pan becomes dry, for 3 1/2 hours or until beef is very tender when pierced with tip of a knife. Add mushrooms and tofu to stew and simmer for 5 minutes.

If serving beef in tortillas, remove beef cubes from stew and let stand until cool enough to handle. Shred beef by hand or with two forks.

If sauce is too thick, stir in a few tablespoons water. If sauce is too thin, boil it uncovered, stirring often, until lightly thickened. Return beef to sauce. Taste and adjust seasoning, adding ground red chile powder if needed. Serve sprinkled with cilantro, if you like, and accompanied by tortillas.

Makes 4 to 6 servings

BEEF AND VEGETABLE SOUP, LATIN AMERICAN STYLE

Cumin, garlic, and cilantro are native to Asia, and yet they give this hearty, warming whole-meal soup an enticing Latin American aroma. Serve it with thick slices of crusty bread, preferably whole wheat, or hot cooked brown rice. Accompany it also with wedges of lemon, and if you like, with a hot pepper relish.

Use a heavy knife or a serrated knife to slice the corn. If using frozen ears of corn, thaw or cook them before cutting. If you prefer, substitute $1/2$ to 1 cup corn kernels. Be sure to thoroughly trim any fat from the meat and to skim the fat from the broth.

2 to $2\frac{1}{2}$ pounds beef shank slices, or $1\frac{1}{4}$ to
  $1\frac{1}{2}$ pounds beef for stew, fat trimmed, cut
  into chunks
6 to 8 cups water
1 large onion, peeled, whole
1 bay leaf
Salt
6 small or medium boiling potatoes, peeled if desired
1 large carrot, cut into thick slices
1 turnip, peeled and diced (optional)
2 celery ribs, sliced
2 tomatoes, diced (optional)

4 garlic cloves, chopped
1 to 2 teaspoons ground cumin
$1/2$ teaspoon freshly ground black pepper, or more
  to taste
2 pale green Mexican zucchini (also called white or
  Tatuma squash) or zucchini, halved lengthwise,
  cut into thick slices
1 to 2 cups chopped kale (optional)
2 or 3 ears corn (fresh or frozen), cut into 1- or
  2-inch pieces
3 to 4 tablespoons chopped cilantro

Put beef in a large saucepan and add water to cover. Bring to a boil. Skim foam from surface. Add onion, bay leaf, and salt to taste. Cover and cook over low heat for 1 hour.

Add potatoes and simmer over very low heat for 1 hour more, skimming fat occasionally. At this point, remove from heat and let soup stand for at least 30 minutes; or cool and refrigerate. Skim fat thoroughly.

Reheat soup to a simmer. Add carrot, turnip (if you like), celery, tomatoes (if using), garlic, cumin, and black pepper. Simmer for 20 minutes or until meat, potatoes, and vegetables are tender. Discard bay leaf. Skim fat from broth again. Add squash, kale (if using), and corn and simmer for 10 minutes or until tender. Taste and adjust seasoning. Serve hot, in shallow bowls. Either sprinkle with chopped cilantro or serve cilantro separately.

Makes 4 to 6 servings

SPICY LAMB WITH RED BEANS AND MINT

Although lamb is a rich meat, it is so flavorful that a little goes a long way. In the Sephardi kitchen, it is a favorite. Pairing lamb with beans is a time-honored practice, as the flavors go so well together. In addition, the healthy protein of the beans is a perfect match for the meat, so that even with smaller meat portions the entrée is still satisfying.

Red beans are especially high in heart-healthy soluble fiber, but you can make this stew with any beans you like—pinto beans, white beans, and chickpeas would be good too. This soup gains lively flavor from chiles and a cool finish from fresh mint.

*1 pound dried red beans (about 2½ cups),
    sorted and rinsed*
*2 pounds boneless lamb shoulder, fat trimmed,
    cut into 1-inch cubes, or lamb for stew*
1 tablespoon extra virgin olive oil
1 large onion, chopped
6 large garlic cloves, chopped
One 28-ounce can tomatoes, drained and chopped

1 small carrot, diced
*1 or 2 jalapeño or serrano peppers, seeds and ribs
    discarded if desired, minced*
Salt and freshly ground black pepper
2 tablespoons tomato paste
Cayenne pepper
2 tablespoons chopped mint

Cover beans with 7 cups water in a large saucepan and bring to a boil. Cover and simmer over low heat for 1½ hours or until just tender.

If using lamb for stew that is already cut in cubes, trim fat from each one. Heat oil in a heavy, wide casserole. Add lamb in batches and brown cubes lightly on all sides over medium-high heat. Remove lamb from pan. If necessary, pour off excess fat (which may have come from meat) from pan, leaving only about 1 tablespoon. Add onion and sauté over medium-low heat for 5 minutes or until softened. Add garlic and sauté for ½ minute. Stir in tomatoes and cook 2 minutes.

Return lamb to pan. Add 1 cup water, carrot, jalapeño peppers, and a little salt and pepper. Bring to a boil. Cover and cook over low heat, stirring occasionally, for 45 minutes or until lamb is nearly tender. Skim off excess fat from sauce. Stir in tomato paste.

Remove beans from their liquid with a slotted spoon and add to meat. If stew is too thick, add a few tablespoons of bean cooking liquid. Bring to a boil. Cover and cook over low heat for 10 to 15 minutes or until meat and beans are very tender. Add cayenne to taste and 1 tablespoon mint; taste and adjust seasoning. Serve sprinkled with remaining mint.

Makes 6 servings

MOROCCAN LAMB TAJINE WITH CAULIFLOWER

I like to cook cauliflower with saffron, as the saffron gives it a good flavor as well as an appealing orange-yellow hue. This savory dish features a generous amount of onions and cauliflower and a small amount of lamb. Serve the stew with couscous, preferably whole wheat, or with brown or white basmati rice.

For many tajines, like this one, Moroccan cooks do not brown the meat. This makes them easier to prepare and lower in fat. Still, it's best to prepare the stew in advance so you can thoroughly skim the fat from the sauce. Ground ginger is a traditional seasoning, but I like to use fresh ginger.

1 tablespoon extra virgin olive oil
2 large onions, coarsely chopped
3 garlic cloves, chopped
1 tablespoon chopped peeled ginger, or 1 teaspoon
    ground ginger
2 pounds lamb stew meat, thoroughly trimmed of
    fat, cut into 1-inch pieces
3 plum tomatoes, fresh or canned, diced
2 small dried chiles, such as chiles de arbol

Salt and freshly ground black pepper
Large pinch of saffron threads (about 1/8 teaspoon)
1 large or 2 small cauliflowers (2 pounds), divided
    in medium florets
2 teaspoons paprika
1/2 teaspoon ground cumin (optional)
4 tablespoons chopped cilantro or parsley
Cayenne pepper (optional)

Heat oil in a large, heavy casserole, add onions, garlic, and ginger, and cook over low heat, stirring, for 2 minutes. Add lamb, tomatoes, chiles, salt, pepper, and saffron and mix well. Pour in enough water to barely cover meat, about 2½ cups. Bring to a boil. Cover and simmer over low heat, stirring occasionally, for 1 to 1¼ hours or until lamb is tender. Skim fat throughly from cooking liquid; if possible, refrigerate, then skim fat.

In a large saucepan of boiling salted water, boil cauliflower, uncovered, for 2 minutes. Drain it immediately in a colander.

Stir paprika, cumin (if using), and half the cilantro into stew. Add cauliflower and stir gently; be sure stems are immersed in liquid. Cover and simmer over low heat, without stirring, for 10 minutes or until cauliflower is tender but not falling apart. Transfer meat and cauliflower florets with a slotted spoon to a heated deep serving plate, leaving chiles and most of onions in casserole. Cover to keep them warm.

Boil sauce, including onions, stirring occasionally, until it thickens. Discard chiles. Add cayenne if you like; taste for seasoning. Spoon sauce over lamb and cauliflower. Serve sprinkled with remaining cilantro.

Makes 8 servings

Legume Accompaniments and Pareve Entrées

Ask the average American in what places beans often appear on the table, and the answer might be Boston because of their baked beans, Mexico because of their refried beans, or perhaps India because of their dal (lentil dishes). Those who know that tofu is made from soybeans might mention China and, indeed, all of East Asia. Sushi lovers are probably familiar with Japanese edamame (green soybeans), and Italian food aficionados know pasta e fagioli (pasta with beans). Jewish bean dishes don't immediately come to mind.

Yet beans play a major role in the Jewish kitchen, both Ashkenazi and Sephardi. In many households they appear on the table every Shabbat, as part of the cholent, a special stew of beans and meat. Chickpeas are staples of Israeli snacks and casual meals, as they are the basis for falafel and hummus, but they also are a popular topping for Moroccan-Jewish couscous. Jews of Egyptian origin often eat fava beans. The Middle Eastern lentil and rice dish, majadra, is a Sephardi meatless main course, and has become a popular side dish for meat and poultry in Israeli restaurants.

Like all plant-based foods, legumes are pareve, and thus can be combined with meat-based or dairy foods, or served as the basis for a pareve meal. In recent years a broad range of pareve meat and cheese substitutes have been created from legumes, especially soybeans, from soy salami to tofu cheese to faux ground beef to vegetable burgers to veggie pepperoni to dairy-free ice cream. This makes possible countless interesting dishes, such as a kosher cheeseburger that doesn't have cheese or a burger, but is better from a nutritional standpoint than the real thing. And of course there is soy milk, which means you can prepare creamy sauces and desserts to serve at kosher meals that include meat.

Legumes are a cholesterol-free, virtually fat-free, nutrient-dense source of protein. They are easy to prepare too. Tofu and canned beans are ready to eat. If you have some cooked vegetables ready, you can have a wholesome main course on the table in minutes if you add tofu or canned beans and serve the medley as a salad, soup, or stew. It's so easy to do this that I even prepare such a dish to start the day—Broccoli and Carrots with Edamame (page 284), which uses frozen shelled green soybeans.

You'll find different selections of dried and canned legumes in supermarkets, in health food stores, and in ethnic grocery stores. Although most beans are interchangeable in recipes, they don't taste the same. Using different beans gives you a new taste and can add interest to a tried-and-true dish. In recent years I've enjoyed using peruano beans, for example, which I buy in bulk from my local Mexican market. Their pale green hue reminds me of French flageolets, and so does their delicate flavor. Like great Northern beans, these beans turn creamy when cooked and thicken their cooking broth.

Chickpeas (garbanzo beans) and soybeans retain a pleasing firmness when cooked, making them ideal for salads, and do not thicken their cooking liquid much. Both of them have a somewhat nutty flavor. This is especially true of their fresh, green versions that come in the pod. Fresh chickpeas and green soybeans, or edamame, cook quickly and have an appealing, nutlike texture and taste.

Lentils also differ from each other. Orange-red lentils, the fastest-cooking legume, cook to a puree in 10 to 20 minutes, making them perfect for soups, while brown and green lentils retain a firmer texture and are good in salads. Yellow split peas cook faster than green ones and have a more delicate flavor.

Plain, everyday dishes gain a new twist and become more substantial if you add canned chickpeas or red beans or cooked edamame to them. I use them as a tasty addition to Israeli salad. They make a savory complement for pasta too. For a quick, colorful dish, cook spiral pasta with broccoli florets, drain both together, add chickpeas or other beans, and season with olive oil, salt, and cayenne pepper.

Beans can easily become a hearty casserole. You can simmer them, for example, in tomato sauce spiked with cumin and garlic. Serve this satisfying dish with couscous or rice for a terrific vegetarian entrée.

❧

Sephardi-Style White Bean Salad

Mediterranean Chickpea Salad with Smoked Tofu

Vegetable Salad with Peppery Peanut Sauce

Lentils and Rice with Cashews and Vegetables

Pinto Bean Burritos with Grilled Salsa and Soy Turkey

Catalan Bean and Pareve Sausage Supper Stew

Indian-Style Greens with Tofu and Beans

Broccoli and Carrots with Edamame

Savory Bean and Corn Medley with Tomatoes

Artichoke and Fava Bean Stew

Ethiopian Spiced Vegetables

❧

SEPHARDI-STYLE WHITE BEAN SALAD

Beans of all types, from fava beans to white beans to chickpeas, are popular on the Sephardi menu, which could be described as the kosher version of the healthy Mediterranean diet. Other Sephardi favorites, such as olive oil, garlic, peppers, and tomatoes, are ingredients that Americans often associate with Italian cooking.

This colorful bean salad is enlivened by grilled mushrooms, peppers, and zucchini. You can accent it with a small amount of an Italian cheese such as provolone or scamorza, which is available kosher, or, to take it more in the Israeli–Middle Eastern direction, use feta. For a pareve dish, omit the cheese and add small pieces of oil-cured, sun-dried tomatoes or diced olives for a salty tang.

1½ cups dried white beans such as great Northern,
   sorted and rinsed, or two 15-ounce cans
   white beans, drained and rinsed
Salt
2 red or orange bell peppers
1 zucchini
4 ounces large or medium white mushrooms

2 small tomatoes, diced (optional)
3 tablespoons coarsely chopped fresh basil
1 tablespoon strained fresh lemon juice or wine
   vinegar (optional)
2 to 3 tablespoons extra virgin olive oil
Freshly ground black pepper
3 ounces feta, crumbled

If using dried beans, put them in a large saucepan and add 6 cups water. Bring to a simmer. Cover and cook over low heat for 1 to 1½ hours or until tender, adding salt after 30 minutes. Drain beans; reserve their cooking liquid for making soups.

Preheat broiler with rack 2 to 4 inches from heat source; or heat grill. Broil or grill bell peppers for 15 minutes or until their skins are blistered and slightly charred, turning them every 5 minutes. Transfer peppers to a plastic bag and close bag. Let stand for 10 minutes.

Halve zucchini and mushrooms lengthwise and brush lightly with oil. Set on a foil-lined broiler rack or on grill. Broil or grill for 3 minutes on each side or until zucchini and mushrooms are slightly tender.

Peel peppers using a paring knife. Halve peppers, draining any juice. Discard seeds and ribs. Do not rinse.

Cut peppers into strips. Dice zucchini. Cut mushroom pieces in half if they are large. Combine grilled vegetables in a glass bowl and add beans, tomatoes (if using), basil, lemon juice (if using), 2 tablespoons oil, and salt and pepper to taste. Add remaining oil, if desired. Serve at room temperature, sprinkled with cheese.

Makes 4 to 6 servings

MEDITERRANEAN CHICKPEA SALAD
WITH SMOKED TOFU

This recipe originated with a main-course salad idea of Julia Child's—white or black beans or lentils served with the same dressing and garnishes as the classic salade niçoise. I find it is delicious when made with chickpeas. I like to keep the salad vegetarian and top it with smoked tofu, but you can go with tradition and top it with tuna if you like.

Julia advised seasoning the cooked beans with the dressing while they are warm; even if they are canned, they should be heated and then dressed, as they absorb the flavors much better. Either use pitted olives or, if using olives with pits, be sure the diners know about it.

1 garlic clove, crushed

Salt

1 tablespoon red or white wine vinegar

1 to 2 tablespoons strained fresh lemon juice

2 to 4 tablespoons extra virgin olive oil

1 teaspoon chopped fresh thyme or ½ teaspoon
   dried thyme

Freshly ground black pepper

Two 15-ounce cans chickpeas

2 shallots, minced, or ½ small mild or sweet onion,
   quartered and sliced very thin into slivers

1 small red, yellow, or green bell pepper, diced
   (optional)

2 cups red-leaf or green-leaf lettuce, torn into
   bite-sized pieces

4 ripe but firm tomatoes, cut into thin wedges

4 to 6 ounces smoked tofu, cut into strips

12 to 16 flavorful black olives, preferably pitted

2 hard-boiled eggs, quartered (optional)

3 tablespoons fresh basil leaves, cut into slivers
   (optional)

For dressing: put garlic in a small bowl, add a pinch of salt, and mash together with a spoon. Whisk in vinegar and 1 tablespoon lemon juice, followed by 2 tablespoons oil, thyme, and a pinch of pepper.

Gently heat chickpeas in their liquid in a saucepan. Drain them and put in a bowl. Add shallots. Reserve 1 tablespoon dressing, and add rest to chickpeas. Let stand while preparing remaining ingredients.

Add bell pepper (if using) to chickpea mixture. Taste, adjust seasoning, and add more lemon juice or oil if you like. Make a bed of lettuce in a shallow serving dish. Spoon chickpea mixture on top. Top with tomato wedges and tofu strips, and sprinkle with reserved dressing. Garnish salad with olives, eggs, and basil, if you like. Serve cool or at room temperature.

Makes 4 servings

Great news—peanuts are good for you! Much of their fat is monounsaturated, the type emphasized in the heart-healthy Mediterranean diet. Peanut packagers are permitted by the U.S. Food and Drug Administration to state on the label that eating 1.5 ounces of peanuts per day may reduce the risk of heart disease.

A study at the University of Florida discovered that peanuts are even healthier than previously thought. Researchers found that peanuts are as high in disease-fighting antioxidants as strawberries, and richer in these substances than apples or carrots.

Peanuts present many possibilities for enhancing modern kosher menus. A peanut sauce is the highlight of a Southeast Asian vegetarian specialty known as gado gado. The salad features lightly cooked vegetables and often tofu. The peppery peanut sauce perks up the vegetables, turning them into a lively appetizer or entrée.

Using peanut butter instead of grinding peanuts makes this sauce quick to prepare. The result is a peanut butter sauce that is rich but not sticky. For a healthful dish, use natural peanut butter without hydrogenated fat. Although some versions of the sauce contain coconut milk, I omit it, as the peanuts provide enough richness. If you prefer the coconut flavor, use ¼ cup light coconut milk and reduce the amount of water to ¾ cup.

To vary the salad, you can leave the cabbage raw or substitute spinach or sliced cauliflower. You can also add cooked sliced potatoes. I add the tofu plain, but if you prefer it sautéed, pat the cubes dry with paper towels, then sauté them for 2 to 3 minutes in a little oil in a large, heavy skillet over medium-high heat. Instead of tofu, you can use tempeh, a fermented soybean cake, which is not eaten raw; it should be sautéed the same way as tofu.

2 to 3 teaspoons peanut oil or vegetable oil

2 large garlic cloves, minced

One ¼-inch-thick slice ginger, peeled and minced

1 or 2 fresh red or green Thai bird chiles or other hot peppers, seeded and minced (optional)

½ cup peanut butter, smooth or chunky, preferably natural

1 cup hot water

¼ teaspoon turmeric

1 teaspoon brown sugar

½ to 1 teaspoon anchovy paste (optional)

2 teaspoons fresh lemon juice

Sambal olek (Indonesian hot pepper relish) or other hot sauce or cayenne pepper

2 to 3 teaspoons kecap manis (Indonesian sweet soy sauce) or soy sauce (optional)

Salt

8 ounces green beans, ends removed, broken in 2 or 3 pieces

6 cups coarsely shredded cabbage

1 cup bean sprouts, ends removed

2 carrots, coarsely grated

1 cake firm tofu, cut into bite-sized cubes (optional)

2 or 3 hard-boiled eggs, quartered (optional)

½ cucumber, cut into thin sticks

2 tomatoes, cut into wedges (optional)

Heat oil in a saucepan. Add garlic, ginger, and chiles and cook over low heat for 2 minutes, stirring. Add peanut butter, water, turmeric, brown sugar, and anchovy paste (if using) and mix well. Cook over low heat, stirring often, for 2 minutes or until smooth. Remove from heat and add lemon juice. Season to taste with hot sauce, soy sauce (if using), and salt. Transfer to a bowl. If dressing is too thick to pour, gradually stir in 1 or 2 tablespoons water.

Add green beans to a saucepan of boiling salted water to cover and cook, uncovered, over high heat for 2 minutes. Add cabbage and cook for 3 more minutes or until vegetables are slightly tender but still crisp. Drain very well.

Add bean sprouts and carrots to cabbage mixture, reserving a little of each for garnish. Add enough dressing to coat mixture lightly. Taste and adjust seasoning. Garnish with tofu, hard-boiled egg quarters, if you like, cucumber sticks, tomatoes (if using), and reserved bean sprouts and carrots. Serve remaining dressing separately.

Makes 4 to 6 servings

LENTILS AND RICE WITH CASHEWS AND VEGETABLES

Lentils and rice are a favorite combination not only in the Mideast, but in India. Cooks from the subcontinent, whether Jewish or of other religions, enliven the pair with interesting spice mixtures. This dish is based on one I tasted at an Indian festival, for which the mixture was studded with diced vegetables. It is enriched not only with sautéed onions, also the favorite partner for lentils in the Mideast, but with roasted cashews.

Cashews are not really nuts, but are seeds of the cashew apple. According to The World's Healthiest Foods Web site (whfoods.com), cashews are heart healthy because much of their fat is the same monounsaturated fat found in olive oil.

Cooks simmer the lentils and rice with whatever vegetables they have on hand—cauliflower, sweet peppers, carrots, tomatoes, potatoes, peas, squash, or eggplant. Some might describe this whole-meal entrée as rice in lentil sauce, because the lentils disintegrate as they cook.

Preparing the stew the authentic South Indian way calls for some unusual seasonings and involves several steps, including toasting and grinding your spices. Here is a simplified version made with easily available ingredients. It's supposed to be spicy, but add the number of hot peppers that suits your taste. Indian cooks generally leave whole spices in the dish. Remove them or remind diners not to eat them. Use enough salt so the dish will not be bland. To make this dish with brown rice, cook the rice in the hot water for 20 minutes before adding the remaining ingredients.

2 to 3 tablespoons vegetable oil

1 large onion, chopped

1 red or green bell pepper, diced

2 to 4 fresh chiles, such as Indian chiles, seeds removed, chopped, or small whole dried chiles, such as chiles japones

1 teaspoon ground coriander

1 teaspoon ground cumin

5 cups water

1 cup orange lentils, picked over and rinsed

1 cup long-grain white rice

1 large carrot, diced

2 pale green Mexican zucchini (also called white or Tatuma squash) or zucchini, diced

¾ cup fresh green beans, cut into 1-inch pieces, or frozen green beans or peas (optional)

Salt and freshly ground black pepper

1 bay leaf

1 cinnamon stick, or pinch of ground cinnamon

Pinch of ground cloves

¼ teaspoon turmeric

¼ to ⅓ cup cashews

Cayenne pepper

2 tablespoons grated coconut, lightly toasted (optional)

2 tablespoons chopped cilantro (optional)

Heat oil in a large saucepan. Add onion and sauté over medium heat, stirring occasionally, for 7 minutes or until softened. Add bell pepper, fresh or dried chiles, coriander, and cumin and sauté for 30 seconds, stirring.

Add water and bring to a boil. Add lentils, rice, carrot, squash, green beans (if using), salt and pepper to taste, bay leaf, cinnamon stick, cloves, and turmeric and return to a boil. Cover and cook over low heat for 20 to 30 minutes or until rice and lentils are very soft. Mixture should be soft and thick but not dry. Add hot water if needed; or, if dish is too soupy, cook uncovered over medium-low heat, stirring often, until thickened. Add half of cashews. Taste for seasoning, adding cayenne if needed. Serve very hot, sprinkled with coconut and cilantro (if using) and remaining cashews.

Makes 4 to 6 servings

PINTO BEAN BURRITOS
WITH GRILLED SALSA AND SOY TURKEY

These burritos make use of one of the best-loved Mexican salsas. It is made entirely on the grill, from four ingredients: tomatoes, onions, hot peppers, and garlic. There is enough of the reddish-brown salsa in this recipe to use twice, but it keeps well and is wonderful to have on hand, as it enlivens just about every food, from grilled chicken to brown rice to steamed vegetables. The charred vegetables give the salsa an appetizing smoky flavor. You can use the same technique to perk up your pasta sauces by substituting grilled tomatoes for the standard peeled tomatoes.

For colorful burritos, use spinach or other vegetable-flavored tortillas, which often have the added benefit of being low in fat. Whole wheat tortillas and those containing soy or oat flour are other nutritious options.

To make these burritos even more quickly, use canned vegetarian or fat-free refried beans. Instead of soy turkey, you can use slices or strips of roasted turkey breast or grilled chicken breast.

1 large white onion, peeled and quartered

1 pound small ripe tomatoes

2 large garlic cloves, peeled

2 fresh chiles, such as jalapeños, preferably red, or serranos, or 2 canned chipotle chiles in adobo sauce

Salt and freshly ground black pepper

One 15-ounce can pinto beans, drained

1 to 2 tablespoons extra virgin olive oil or vegetable oil

1 onion, finely chopped

8 slices of soy turkey or soy salami

4 large tortillas (burrito size), preferably whole grain, vegetable flavored, or low-fat

¼ red or white onion, sliced very thin

1 avocado, sliced thin

Shredded low-fat Cheddar, soy cheese, or rice cheese (optional) (for serving)

Heat a stovetop ridged grill on medium-high heat, or prepare barbecue. Grill vegetables until charred. Onion quarters will need about 8 minutes per side, and tomatoes about 5 minutes per side. Char garlic cloves only about 2 minutes per side. If using fresh chiles, char them until blackened in spots. Remove from grill. Let cool.

Cut cores from tomatoes; there is no need to peel them. Remove seeds and membranes from hot peppers if you would like the salsa to be less hot.

Puree tomatoes, onion, garlic, and one of the chiles in a blender or food processor until smooth. If using canned chiles, remove from adobo sauce before adding to blender. Taste; if you would like a hotter salsa, add second chile to food processor; with canned chiles, you can also add some adobo sauce. Puree again until well blended. Add salt and pepper to taste; salsa should be salted fairly generously. Transfer to a bowl.

Process beans in food processor to a slightly chunky puree. Heat oil in a medium skillet. Add chopped onion and cook over medium-low heat for 5 minutes or until soft and beginning to turn golden. Add bean puree and heat to blend flavors. Taste and add salt if needed. Cover and keep warm.

At serving time, reheat bean puree, set soy turkey on top, and cover so turkey heats gently from the steam. Heat each tortilla briefly on grill or in skillet; or wrap and micro-wave briefly until just warm. Spread with bean puree and add soy turkey and a small spoonful of salsa. Serve red onion slices, avocado, cheese, and more salsa separately.

Makes 4 servings

CATALAN BEAN AND PAREVE SAUSAGE SUPPER STEW

Good olive oil is the key to the fine flavor of the beans in this homey, easy-to-prepare meal-in-one-pan from Catalonia, in northeastern Spain. The oil is used to sauté tomatoes, onions, and garlic to make a preparation called a *sofregit,* which is then blended with the beans—usually white beans or chickpeas. Generally, the sausage is grilled and served on the side, but sometimes it is sliced and heated with the tomatoes and beans. In Catalonia, a rich meat sausage is used, but I prefer to use soy sausages or lean turkey franks.

2 tablespoons extra virgin olive oil
1 large onion, chopped
3 large garlic cloves, chopped
8 to 12 ounces ripe tomatoes, peeled, seeded, and chopped, or one 15-ounce can tomatoes, drained and chopped
Salt and freshly ground black pepper
6 ounces soy or turkey frankfurters or turkey sausage, cut into ½-inch slices
3 cups cooked white beans or chickpeas (28-ounce can)
2 hard-boiled eggs, chopped (optional)
2 to 3 tablespoons chopped parsley

Heat oil in a large skillet. Add onion and cook over medium heat, stirring often, for 7 minutes or until light golden. Add garlic and sauté for 1 minute. Add tomatoes, salt, and pepper and cook gently, uncovered, about 10 minutes or until mixture is thick. Add frankfurters and beans, cover, and cook for 5 to 10 minutes over low heat. Add hard-boiled eggs (if using) and heat through. Taste and adjust seasoning. Stir in parsley.

Makes 4 to 6 main-course servings

I'm always looking for ways to enjoy nutritious greens. One of my favorite Indian recipes is greens with paneer, a cheese that is cut in cubes and simmered with the vegetables. In consistency and appearance, this cheese reminds me of tofu, and to prepare a healthy, pareve version of the dish, I happily use it. Often I add dried and green beans as well, which contribute different textures and flavors.

Use any greens you like for this dish. Indian cooks often use mustard greens on their own or combined with spinach. Now you can buy many of these greens cleaned and chopped, either fresh or frozen.

Serve this dish as a hot entrée with basmati rice, fresh pita bread, or the Indian flatbread called *naan*, which is available at Indian grocery stores and some natural foods markets.

One 12-ounce bunch of mustard greens or chard
¼ pound green beans, cut into 1-inch lengths
2 tablespoons olive oil
1 large onion, chopped
2 teaspoons minced peeled ginger
4 large garlic cloves, chopped
2 or 3 serrano chiles or Indian chiles, minced
1 teaspoon ground coriander
1 teaspoon ground cumin

½ teaspoon turmeric
1½ cups cooked pinto beans or chickpeas (garbanzo beans), or one 15-ounce can pinto beans or chickpeas, drained
One 12- to 14-ounce cake firm tofu, drained of liquid, cut into bite-sized cubes
Salt and freshly ground black pepper
Cayenne pepper (optional)

Rinse greens well and, if they are sandy, soak them in a large bowl of cold water. If using chard, reserve thick stems separately and cut them into ½-inch slices. Coarsely chop leaves.

In a medium saucepan of boiling water, cook green beans and chard stems over medium heat for 2 minutes; green beans will be only partly cooked. Drain vegetables, reserving ⅓ cup of cooking liquid.

Heat 1 to 2 tablespoons oil in a large saucepan. Add onion and sauté over medium heat for 7 minutes or until golden. Add ginger, garlic, and chiles and sauté for ½ minute. Stir in coriander, cumin, turmeric, green bean mixture, pinto beans, and reserved cooking liquid. Bring to a boil.

With pan on low heat, add greens in three batches, covering pan briefly after each addition so they wilt. After adding all of greens, add tofu and simmer, uncovered, for 3 minutes or until green beans are tender. Season to taste with salt, pepper, and cayenne (if using). Serve hot.

Makes 4 to 6 servings

❧ BROCCOLI AND CARROTS WITH EDAMAME

A supernutritious, 7-minute side dish composed of broccoli, carrots, and green soybeans, this is one of our family's favorite vegetable combos. This colorful, warm dish is appealing even in the morning and, indeed, we often eat it for breakfast. People are surprised to hear this, but when we've had overnight guests, they have enjoyed our breakfast broccoli so much, they now make it for breakfast for their families. The vitamin A from the carrots, the healthful cholesterol-lowering fiber of broccoli, and the protein and other beneficial properties of the soy make a great start to the day.

Instead of edamame, we often add tofu to the basic broccoli-carrot medley. We cut firm or medium-firm tofu in cubes and add it for the last minute of cooking so it heats through.

For breakfast we enjoy the medley plain, even without seasoning, but there are many ways to dress it up. The easiest is a light drizzle of extra virgin olive oil or a flavoring sprinkle. Some good ones are Japanese go-masio (toasted sesame seeds with salt) or Middle Eastern za'atar (herbs with sesame seeds), which you can buy in jars. You can quickly put together some gremolata (garlic, herbs, and lemon zest, see page 103) and sprinkle it on top at the last minute, or spoon a little Spicy Salsa (page 364) over the vegetables.

For a more festive dish, turn the combo into a warm salad, on its own or on a bed of greens, and moisten it lightly with Sesame Ginger Dressing or Olive Oil and Lemon Dressing (page 366 and page 365).

2 bunches of broccoli

2 large carrots, sliced diagonally about ¼ inch thick

8 ounces shelled edamame (frozen green soybeans) or firm tofu, cut into 1-inch cubes

Salt and freshly ground black pepper (optional)

3 to 4 teaspoons extra virgin olive oil (optional)

Cut off stem of each broccoli bunch. If peel of stem is tough, cut it off. Trim end, then slice stem about ¼ inch thick. Divide broccoli crown into medium florets.

Boil enough water to nearly cover vegetables in a large saucepan. Add broccoli stems, cover, and cook over medium-high heat for 1 minute. Add carrots and edamame (but not tofu). Cover and return to a boil. Add broccoli florets, pointing stem ends downward so they are in the water.

Cover and return to a boil. Boil over high heat for about 3 minutes, then uncover and boil for 2 or 3 minutes more or until vegetables are crisp-tender; if using tofu, add it during the last minute. Drain well; reserve cooking liquid for soups. Serve vegetables sprinkled, if you like, with salt, pepper, and olive oil.

Makes 4 servings

SAVORY BEAN AND CORN MEDLEY WITH TOMATOES

Combining several types of beans in a single dish is a popular practice among Sephardi Jews. They serve the beans hot or at room temperature, usually with rice. In summertime I include another fast-cooking whole grain instead—fresh corn. Its bright color and flavor complement the beans well. This bean medley simmers in a tomato-onion sauce accented with allspice. If you prefer, use all chickpeas or all pink beans instead of mixing them.

3 to 4 tablespoons extra virgin olive oil
2 large onions, chopped
1/2 to 1 teaspoon ground allspice, or to taste
1 1/2 pounds ripe tomatoes, peeled if desired, diced, or one 28-ounce can tomatoes, drained and diced
Salt and freshly ground black pepper

1 pound green beans, ends removed, broken in half
2 cups fresh or frozen corn kernels
1 1/2 to 2 cups cooked chickpeas (garbanzo beans), or one 15-ounce can chickpeas, drained
1 1/2 to 2 cups cooked pink or red beans, or one 15-ounce can beans, drained
1 tablespoon chopped parsley (optional)

Heat oil in a large, deep, heavy sauté pan. Add onions and sauté over medium heat for 10 minutes or until golden brown. Stir in allspice and tomatoes, add salt and pepper, and bring to a simmer. Cook, uncovered, for about 15 minutes or until sauce is thick.

Add green beans to a saucepan of boiling salted water and boil, uncovered, over high heat for 3 minutes. Add corn and cook for 2 to 3 more minutes or until beans and corn are barely tender. Drain, reserving liquid.

Add 1/2 cup cooking liquid from green beans and corn to tomato sauce. Add chickpeas and pink beans and bring to a simmer. Cover and cook for 5 minutes to blend flavors. Lightly stir in green beans and corn and heat through. Taste, and add more allspice, salt, and pepper, if you like. Serve sprinkled with parsley, if you like.

Makes 4 to 6 servings

ARTICHOKE AND FAVA BEAN STEW

North African and other Sephardi Jews serve artichokes with fava beans at the Passover Seder, but this light dish makes a good appetizer or accompaniment for any festive occasion. Traditionally, it is made with a generous amount of olive oil, but I prefer to set a cruet of extra virgin olive oil on the table and let diners sprinkle a bit on their portion if they wish. Fava beans are more enticing if you peel each bean, but this is time-consuming. See the Note following the recipe for instructions on preparing them.

To save time, you can use frozen fava beans or substitute lima beans, which do not need to be peeled. Baby artichokes cook quickly, but if you're in a hurry, use frozen artichoke hearts or substitute canned ones.

12 baby, 8 small, or 4 medium artichokes
1 lemon
2 tablespoons extra virgin olive oil, plus more for drizzling
4 spring onions, sliced
2 garlic cloves, chopped (optional)
¼ cup dry white wine
1½ cups water

2 fresh thyme sprigs, or ½ teaspoon dried thyme
Salt and freshly ground black pepper
4 to 6 ounces baby carrots or sliced carrots (optional)
1½ to 2 cups fresh shelled or frozen fava beans, cooked and peeled (see Note)
2 tablespoons chopped flat-leaf parsley (optional)

There is no need to trim baby artichokes. With other artichokes, prepare hearts: squeeze juice of ½ lemon into a bowl of cold water. Leave stems on artichokes to use as "handles." Pull off bottom leaves of artichoke. Snap back side leaves to remove tough parts, and trim sides of artichoke so it is smooth. Cut off stem and pare it. Halve artichokes and trim top leaves so they are only ½ inch long. Halve each piece again. Using a spoon, scrape out hairlike choke from each quarter and pull out small, central purple-tipped leaves. Rub each piece with cut lemon; put in lemon water. Continue with remaining artichokes. Wash your hands after handling raw artichokes, or the next foods you touch will get a funny taste.

Heat oil in a sauté pan. Add spring onions and sauté over medium heat for 2 minutes. Add garlic (if using) and artichokes and sauté for 1 to 2 minutes. Add wine, water, thyme, salt, and pepper. Bring to a boil. Cover and cook over low heat for 15 minutes. Add carrots and return to a boil. Cover and simmer, adding a few tablespoons water if necessary, for 6 to 10 minutes or until artichokes and carrots are tender. Remove thyme sprigs. Add fava beans and cook for 2 to 3 minutes to heat through.

If stew is soupy, remove vegetables with a slotted spoon and boil liquid, uncovered, for 2 to 3 minutes to thicken it slightly. Return vegetables to liquid. Taste and adjust seasoning. Add parsley, if you like. Serve hot, warm, or cold, in shallow bowls.

NOTE: To cook fava beans: put them in a saucepan of boiling salted water and cook, uncovered, over high heat for 7 to 10 minutes or until just tender. Remove from heat, drain, and press each bean to remove thick skins, in order to have bright green beans. Or, if leaving skins on, cook a few minutes longer so they will be more tender, and drain well.

Makes 4 servings

Ethiopian Jews know that a good way to transform common vegetables into a lively entrée is to add spice, and they do so with a liberal hand. The fire of the hot peppers is tempered by the sweetness of sautéed onions and ginger and by the warm flavors of paprika, cinnamon, and nutmeg. I enjoyed dishes similar to this one at restaurants in Little Ethiopia in Los Angeles and in Jerusalem.

Traditional cooks sauté the spices in a generous amount of clarified butter, but to turn it into a healthy dish, I use a modest amount of canola oil or olive oil, just enough to moisten the medley. The standard Ethiopian partner for this spicy vegetarian entrée is a thin sourdough flatbread called *injera*, made with healthy teff flour. Other good accompaniments are whole-grain tortillas or lavash, brown rice, or whole wheat couscous, with low-fat plain yogurt on the side to provide protein and calm the chiles' fire.

¾ pound carrots, sliced about ½ inch thick
¾ pound potatoes, peeled and cut into 1-inch dice
Salt
1 pound cauliflower, divided into medium florets
½ pound green beans, ends removed, cut into
    2- or 3-inch pieces
½ pound zucchini, quartered and cut into
    3-inch pieces
2 to 3 tablespoons canola oil or olive oil
1 large onion, halved and sliced thin
3 large garlic cloves, chopped
1 tablespoon minced peeled ginger

1 or 2 jalapeño peppers or other hot chiles, chopped,
    or 1 to 2 teaspoons canned diced roasted
    jalapeño peppers
1 teaspoon paprika
⅛ to ¼ teaspoon cayenne pepper, or to taste
¼ teaspoon ground cinnamon
⅛ teaspoon ground cloves
¼ teaspoon turmeric
Freshly grated nutmeg
½ teaspoon ground cumin (optional)
1 to 2 tablespoons tomato paste or tomato puree
    (optional)

Preheat oven to 350°F. Combine carrots and potatoes in a saucepan. Cover with water and bring to a boil. Add salt and simmer, covered, about 10 minutes or until vegetables are tender. Drain well; reserve cooking liquid for soups.

Add cauliflower to a saucepan of enough boiling salted water to cover florets by about 1 inch and boil, uncovered, over high heat for 2 minutes. Add green beans and boil for 2 minutes. Add zucchini and boil for 1 minute or until vegetables are crisp-tender. Drain in a colander, reserving cooking liquid. Rinse vegetables with cold water and drain well.

Heat oil in a large ovenproof stew pan or sauté pan. Add onion and sauté over medium heat, stirring often, for 10 minutes or until golden brown. Add garlic, ginger, chiles, paprika, cayenne, cinnamon, cloves, turmeric, nutmeg to taste, and cumin (if using) and cook over low heat, stirring, for 1 minute. Remove from heat. Stir in tomato paste (if using) and 2 tablespoons water. Mix with vegetables. Taste and adjust seasoning.

Leave mixture in stew pan or transfer it to a 2-quart casserole. Cover and bake for 20 minutes or until heated through and vegetables are tender enough for your taste. Serve hot.

Makes 4 servings

Vegetable Side Dishes

The importance of vegetables is highlighted in the Torah, when the Children of Israel complained to Moses that they missed the produce of Egypt. Numbers 11:5: "We fondly remember the fish that we could eat in Egypt at no cost, along with the cucumbers, melons, leeks, onions and garlic."

Today's nutritionists would understand their concerns. Vegetables, along with fruit and fish, are considered the foundation of a healthy diet. The easiest way to make meals healthy is to learn to love vegetables and serve them in generous portions. A variety of vegetables of different colors not only makes menus attractive, but also ensures that we benefit from a broad range of nutrients. Red vegetables have different vitamins and other beneficial components from those of green, yellow, and cruciferous (cabbage family) vegetables, so it's a good idea to eat some of each.

Remember to pay special attention to greens. Most people eat spinach, but many supermarket shoppers overlook the other greens, undoubtedly because they don't realize how valuable they are and how simple they are to cook.

Take chard, for example. Its flavor is mild and delicate, with a touch of sweetness in the red-stemmed variety, and its texture is pleasing, with a bit of crispness in the leaves. Chard is beautiful too. Its glossy, dark green leaves are sometimes crinkly and sometimes smooth. The most common kind has white stems, but now there is also a colorful type called "rainbow chard," with yellow and red stems in addition to the usual white. And you don't have to garden in order to enjoy this pretty chard; it enlivens the produce bins of well-stocked supermarkets.

The large leaves of chard, collards, and other greens might seem intimidating, but their size is an advantage. With fewer leaves to rinse, chard demands much less preparation time than an equivalent weight of spinach. And greens cook quickly. Very young chard leaves and mustard greens, like spinach, can even be enjoyed raw.

Cooks have come up with countless ways to take advantage of greens. Sephardi Jews stuff chard leaves, just like cabbage. They also use chard to fill phyllo pastries, either on its own or flavored with cheese. Cooks in southern France turn greens into gratins by baking them with rice, garlic, eggs, and grated cheese instead of making a sauce. A similar dish is made in Sephardi kitchens, with bread crumbs or potato puree rather than rice, and a flavoring of kashkaval and feta cheese.

Mediterranean cooks like tender greens sautéed with olive oil, garlic, and dried hot peppers, or with garlic, cumin, and lemon juice. Such greens often appear on the Moroccan Shabbat table. Another popular preparation is to puree cooked greens and flavor

---

THE TU BISHVAT ALMOND DIET

While Israeli children welcome the holiday of Tu Bishvat by singing about the flowering almond tree—"Hashkedia"—adults should sing the virtues of the almond. This nut packs a potent nutritional punch.

Almonds are the cornerstone of the Portfolio Diet, developed by Dr. David J. A. Jenkins of the University of Toronto as a natural way to lower cholesterol. The other elements of this vegetarian diet are foods rich in soluble fiber, such as apples, broccoli, and oatmeal; soy foods; and plant sterols, found in vegetable oils and nuts and available as supplements.

According to Dr. Steven Pratt and Kathy Matthews, the authors of Superfoods Rx: Fourteen Foods That Will Change Your Life, *"Almonds are the best nut source of vitamin E and a powerful plant source of protein. Almonds also contain riboflavin, iron, potassium and magnesium, and they're a good source of fiber."*

Most people eat almonds because they're delicious. Popular around the world, almonds appear in so many recipes that it's hard to think of a cuisine that does not make use of them. They are usually considered an ingredient for desserts, from Chinese almond cookies to French almond tarts.

But there are countless ways to use almonds to enhance savory dishes as well. Indian cooks use them to thicken sauces and sauté them to garnish fragrant rice dishes. On the menus of Chinese restaurants, you'll often find stir-fried chicken with whole almonds and colorful vegetables. Festive versions of

them with thick yogurt or tahini. Cooks in Nice even use chard in dessert tarts, along with raisins and apples.

There's another good reason to include greens in menus: they are powerhouses of nutrition. Low in calories, greens are rich in beta carotene and vitamin C and many other nutrients. I like to make a point of trying new vegetables that I come across at the market. That's how I discovered Chinese eggplants, long beans, and fresh water chestnuts at Asian markets; orange calabaza squash and green chickpeas at a Mexican market; fresh lima beans in the pod at an outdoor farmers' market; and amazingly sweet purple yams at a Filipino supermarket. Including such new foods makes meals more fun. Long ago jicama became a standard addition to our personal version of Israeli salad after we discovered it at a local supermarket.

Moroccan couscous and Sephardi rice are often embellished with fried or toasted almonds paired with raisins.

It's not surprising that the almond tree is considered the herald of Tu Bishvat, an Israeli holiday. Almonds have had a long history in the lands of the Bible. They are mentioned in the Torah and are thought to have originated in the Mideast. Indeed, cooks in the Mideast have developed numerous ways to enjoy them, from baklava to savory phyllo pastries called burekas.

Burekas? Who puts almonds in burekas? My friend Aviva Maoz does—for a holiday meal, she bakes delicious spiral-shaped burekas with a filling of beef and sautéed almonds.

Aviva creatively uses almonds to highlight all sorts of foods, especially vegetables. I have often made French-style green beans topped with sautéed almonds, but Aviva takes this classic formula one step further. Whether her vegetables are steamed or stir-fried, she often finishes them with a combination of sautéed onions and toasted slivered almonds. Usually she mixes several vegetables for a colorful medley and cooks them lightly so they retain a slightly crisp texture. At potluck dinners with a tempting selection of dishes, her almond-topped vegetables always seem to disappear first. For a winter dinner, she tossed together Brussels sprouts, green beans, water chestnuts, and green soybeans. Another time it was snow peas, sliced mushrooms, carrot strips, and green beans.

The almonds are the secret to making such healthy medleys irresistible, with their good flavor and pleasing crunch. To get even more into the Tu Bishvat spirit, you might like to add a touch of sweetness to your vegetables with a sprinkling of raisins as well.

Most vegetables taste delicious with a just a bit of embellishment, like a drizzle of olive oil or sesame oil or a garnish of chopped toasted almonds. Sometimes one or two spices or herbs are all it takes to perk up a plain cooked vegetable. Cumin lends zest to Yemenite-Spiced Zucchini and Onion Sauté (page 306). Oregano and green onions give a lift to Herbed Eggplant Cubes (page 307). Both are good complements for grilled chicken or for a dairy entrée of pasta topped with diced tomatoes and feta cheese. Fresh ginger enlivens Golden Cauliflower Puree (page 301), which is delicious with chicken, meat, or a meatless meal of tofu and brown basmati rice.

❦

Butternut Squash in Sweet and Spicy Ginger Tomato Sauce

Chinese Long Beans with Garlic and Soy Sauce

Fresh Corn with Cumin Oil

Broccoli and Carrots in Spiced Onion Sauce

Low-Carb Broccoli Kugel

Golden Cauliflower Puree

Sweet-Sour Red Cabbage with Pears and Raisins

Tomato-Braised Cabbage with Garlic

Louisiana Squash and Yam Casserole

Yemenite-Spiced Zucchini and Onion Sauté

Herbed Eggplant Cubes

Easy Eggplant Bharta

Vegetable Medley with Toasted Almonds

Filipino-Mediterranean Vegetable Stew

❦

BUTTERNUT SQUASH IN SWEET AND SPICY GINGER TOMATO SAUCE

Orange-fleshed, hard-shelled squash doesn't have to be loaded with butter and sugar to taste good. Instead match this healthful, vitamin-A rich vegetable with a tasty sauce perked up with fresh ginger, a wonderful flavor accent that's good for you too. Sweeten the sauce with dried blueberries, raisins, or cranberries, and just a hint of honey. The sweetness of this dish makes it ideal for the holiday dinners on Rosh Hashanah, when good tomatoes are in season.

Butternut squash is great in this dish, but you can use another sweet squash like kabocha, delicata, sweet dumpling, Mexican calabaza, or Australian blue squash. If you opt for acorn or banana squash, which is less sweet, you may want to add more dried blueberries or a little more honey. This dish can be prepared 2 or 3 days ahead; it reheats well.

2 pounds butternut or other hard-shelled squash

½ pound tomatoes, peeled (about 2), or one 14-ounce can tomatoes

2 tablespoons canola oil, grapeseed oil, or other vegetable oil

1 large onion, chopped

1 tablespoon minced peeled ginger

2 large garlic cloves, chopped (optional)

⅔ cup water

Salt

¼ to ½ teaspoon freshly ground black pepper

½ teaspoon ground cinnamon, or more to taste

⅓ cup dried blueberries or raisins

2 to 3 teaspoons honey or brown sugar

Dash of freshly grated nutmeg or ground cloves (optional)

Pinch of cayenne pepper (optional)

Peel or cut off squash skin, remove seeds and strings, and cut meat into 1-inch pieces. If using fresh tomatoes, halve and seed them, reserving juice. Drain canned tomatoes, reserving juice. Chop tomatoes.

Heat oil in a large, deep, heavy saucepan or stew pan. Add onion and cook over medium heat until golden, about 7 minutes. Add minced ginger and garlic and cook over low heat for 30 seconds. Add tomatoes and cook, uncovered, for 5 minutes. Add squash, water, salt to taste, ¼ teaspoon pepper, and cinnamon. Stir and bring to a boil. Cover and cook over low heat, occasionally stirring gently, until squash is tender, about 30 minutes. Add blueberries and honey and simmer for 5 minutes to soften the blueberries.

If sauce is too sweet, add 1 to 2 tablespoons of reserved tomato juice. Taste and add nutmeg and cayenne, if you like, and more salt, pepper, cinnamon or honey, if you like. If sauce is too thin, uncover and cook over medium heat until it thickens, 2 to 3 minutes. Serve hot.

Makes 4 to 6 servings

CHINESE LONG BEANS WITH GARLIC AND SOY SAUCE

These striking long beans, often called yard-long beans or asparagus beans, resemble green beans in flavor but are in the black-eyed pea family. You'll find them at Asian markets and at some farmers' markets and supermarkets. Preparing them is easier than other green beans simply because there are fewer ends to remove. You just cut them in convenient-size pieces.

When you eat these green beans at some Chinese restaurants, you might notice that their skin is wrinkled; this indicates that they were deep-fried before being added to a sauce. Some cooks feel that this makes them more tender, but it does add a substantial amount of fat. I find the beans taste good stir-fried in a bit of oil or braised, as in this recipe, or cooked in water like green beans.

In addition to the garlic and soy sauce, this simple dish is flavored with a touch of ginger, green onion, and hoisin sauce. If you like, add a bit of chili paste or hot sauce. Serve the beans with broiled salmon, roast chicken or tofu, and with rice. For a more substantial dish, sauté ½ to 1 pound chicken breast in the oil before adding the beans.

1 tablespoon hoisin sauce	3 large garlic cloves, chopped
⅓ cup water	1 pound Chinese long beans or green beans, rinsed,
1 to 2 tablespoons soy sauce	ends trimmed, cut into 2-inch lengths
1 to 2 tablespoons peanut oil or other vegetable oil	Salt and freshly ground white pepper
2 teaspoons minced peeled ginger	2 tablespoons chopped green onion

Mix hoisin sauce with water and 1 tablespoon soy sauce in a small bowl.

Heat oil in a large skillet or wok over high heat. Add ginger and garlic and stir for 15 seconds. Add beans and sprinkle with salt. Reduce heat to medium-low and cook beans, stirring, for 30 seconds. Add soy sauce mixture. Stir well. Cover and cook, stirring often, for 4 minutes or until beans are crisp-tender. Uncover and boil for 1 minute to evaporate excess liquid. Add green onion and toss for a few minutes over medium heat. Taste and adjust seasoning, adding more soy sauce, salt, and pepper if needed. Serve immediately; if allowed to stand, the beans lose their bright color.

Makes 3 to 4 servings

❖ FRESH CORN WITH CUMIN OIL

Corn is actually a grain, but it is usually treated as a vegetable. Instead of serving it the American way with plain butter, I like to present it with a seasoned oil. There are two reasons for opting for extra virgin olive oil: unlike butter, it has the benefit of monounsaturated rather than mostly saturated fat; in addition, because it is liquid and has a distinctive flavor, a little goes a long way and you can use less total fat than you would if using butter.

With a nod to corn's origin, which historians note is probably Mexico or Central America, I flavor the oil with spices loved by cooks from our neighbor to the south and, incidentally, by Middle Eastern Jews as well—cumin, cilantro, and hot pepper. If you prefer, substitute butter for half the oil, following the variation.

2 to 4 tablespoons extra virgin olive oil
1 teaspoon ground cumin
2 teaspoons minced cilantro or parsley
½ teaspoon fresh lime or lemon juice

Pinch of cayenne pepper or pure chile powder
Salt
6 fresh ears corn

In a small bowl, blend oil with cumin, cilantro, lime juice, cayenne, and salt to taste. Let stand for 1 hour or refrigerate in a covered container up to 1 day to blend flavors. Bring to room temperature before using.

Shuck corn; remove silks. Add corn to a large pot of boiling water and cook it for 5 to 10 minutes or until it's done to your taste. Remove with tongs to a platter or plates. Serve corn hot, with seasoned oil.

Cumin Butter: To substitute butter for half of oil, soften butter and beat it in a small bowl until smooth. Stir in cumin, then slowly stir in oil. Add cilantro, lime juice, cayenne, and salt to taste.

Makes 6 servings

BROCCOLI AND CARROTS IN SPICED ONION SAUCE

Inspired by Indian cuisine, this curry is easy to make and doesn't require complex spice pastes. The spicing is gentle, but you can increase the amount of cayenne if you'd like it fiery. It tastes great with brown basmati rice.

To peel or not to peel? With broccoli stems, like asparagus, it's a matter of personal preference. I generally leave the peel on, in order to benefit from the broccoli's fiber, unless it's very tough. If I find the stem resists being cut, then it's not tender enough and I cut the peel off with my chef's knife. Often the bottom half or third of the stem needs peeling and the rest is fine and can be left unpeeled.

1 pound carrots, sliced diagonally
1 pound broccoli florets, or florets and sliced stems
2 to 3 tablespoons vegetable oil or olive oil
3 large onions, cut into thin slices lengthwise
1 pound zucchini, halved and sliced
Salt
4 large garlic cloves, chopped
2 teaspoons ground coriander
1 teaspoon ground cumin
1 teaspoon ground ginger
⅛ teaspoon cayenne pepper, or to taste
¼ teaspoon turmeric
1 teaspoon paprika
½ cup tomato sauce, homemade, bottled, or canned
3 tablespoons sliced almonds, lightly toasted
   (see page 379)

Cover carrot slices with water in a medium saucepan. Bring to a boil, cover, and cook over medium heat for 6 minutes. Remove carrots with a slotted spoon. Add broccoli and bring to a boil. Cook, uncovered, over high heat for 5 minutes or until crisp-tender. Remove with a slotted spoon, reserving cooking liquid. Rinse broccoli with cold water.

Heat oil in a wide stew pan or very large sauté pan. Add onions. Sauté over medium heat for 10 minutes. Add zucchini and salt and sauté for 3 minutes or until zucchini are crisp-tender.

Add garlic, coriander, cumin, ginger, cayenne, turmeric, and paprika and mix well. Cook over medium heat for 1 minute. Add tomato sauce and ¼ cup reserved cooking liquid. Cook, uncovered, over medium heat for 5 minutes. Add carrots and broccoli and heat through. Taste and adjust seasonings. Serve garnished with toasted sliced almonds.

Makes 6 to 8 servings

✕✕ LOW-CARB BROCCOLI KUGEL

Kugels don't have to be heavy, starchy casseroles. This one is light, yet satisfying and charged with good nutrients from the broccoli. Sautéed onions and garlic complement the broccoli's flavor, and the almond topping gives it a festive finish.

Serve this dairy-free kugel as a Passover or Shabbat side dish. It goes nicely with roast chicken or baked fish. You can also serve it on its own as a meatless entrée. For dairy meals, sprinkle the kugel with 2 or 3 tablespoons grated Parmesan cheese before baking instead of, or in addition to, the almonds.

2 pounds broccoli
Salt
2 to 3 tablespoons vegetable oil or olive oil
1 large onion, chopped
2 large garlic cloves, chopped
2 or 3 large eggs, or 1 to 2 eggs and equivalent
  of 1 egg in egg substitute

1 tablespoon matzo meal
Freshly ground black pepper
4 to 5 tablespoons slivered almonds, coarsely
  chopped
About ½ teaspoon paprika (optional)

Preheat oven to 375°F. Divide broccoli in medium florets. Cut peel from large stems and slice them. Boil broccoli in a large saucepan of boiling salted water for 7 minutes or until very tender. Drain well and cool. Puree in a food processor, leaving a few small chunks. Transfer to a bowl.

Heat 1 to 2 tablespoons oil in medium nonstick skillet. Add onion and sauté over medium-low heat for 7 minutes or until golden brown, adding 1 to 2 tablespoons hot water if pan becomes dry. Add garlic and sauté for 30 seconds.

Add eggs and matzo meal to broccoli mixture and mix well. Lightly stir in onion mixture and any oil in pan. Season well with salt and pepper.

Oil a shallow 8-inch square baking dish. Add broccoli mixture. Sprinkle 1 tablespoon oil over top. Sprinkle with almonds and paprika (if using). Bake in upper third of oven for 40 minutes or until set and very lightly browned on top. Remove from oven and run a knife around edges. To serve, cut carefully in squares. Use a spoon to remove portions.

Makes 4 to 6 servings

I tasted a curried cauliflower puree at the Natural Products Expo in Anaheim, California. Developed for low-carb diets as a replacement for mashed potatoes, it makes use of creamy cauliflower puree with a small amount of cornstarch instead of using the tuber. The puree was available plain or flavored with herbs, cheese, hot pepper, or smoked meat. I find this concept has merit—it helps us to benefit from cauliflower's great nutrition and gives us ideas for coming up with interesting new dishes. I use cauliflower puree for making latkes or patties resembling potato pancakes, or blended with eggs and baked as for mashed potato kugel. Instead of making leek and potato soup, how about a leek-and-cauliflower combination?

When I studied cooking in Paris, we made cauliflower puree with cream and nutmeg, but we also added a little potato. After experimenting, I found that the cauliflower makes a fine puree on its own, although it is not as velvety as the cauliflower-and-potato version. I have been alternating the seasonings, sometimes using Yemenite or Indian spices instead of the French ones. Serve this golden puree with eggs, chicken, or meat, or as an accompaniment for tofu and rice.

1 large or 2 small cauliflowers (total about 3 pounds), divided into medium florets
Salt
1½ to 2 tablespoons olive oil
1 large onion, finely chopped
2 garlic cloves, minced
2 teaspoons minced peeled ginger (optional)
2 teaspoons curry powder
Freshly ground black pepper
Cayenne pepper

Boil cauliflower, uncovered, in a large saucepan of boiling salted water over high heat for 9 to 10 minutes or until stems are very tender when pierced with a sharp knife. Drain thoroughly. Puree in batches in a food processor. If desired, leave a few chunks.

Heat oil in a large, deep skillet. Add onion and cook over medium-low heat, stirring often, for 10 minutes or until tender and light golden. Add garlic and ginger and sauté for 30 seconds, stirring. Add curry powder and sauté 1 minute. Stir in cauliflower puree. Heat until very hot, stirring, and season with salt, pepper, and cayenne to taste. Serve hot.

Makes 6 servings

SWEET-SOUR RED CABBAGE
WITH PEARS AND RAISINS

Although red cabbage is rich in nutrients and inexpensive, it is frequently overlooked at the market because many shoppers don't realize how tasty it can be and how easy it is to prepare. Some are concerned about the cabbage's odor as it cooks. With this easy recipe, there's no need to worry. The vegetable develops a strong smell only from prolonged boiling in water. If it's cooked over low heat in a covered pot, the cabbage will not produce an aggressive flavor or aroma.

To make sweet-and-sour red cabbage, a favorite among German and Russian Jews, I braise the cabbage briefly, so it becomes tender but not flabby and retains a hint of crisp texture, instead of following old-fashioned formulas that call for hours of simmering. As the cabbage gently stews, it loses its harsh, raw taste and acquires a delicate sweetness.

In Europe's cabbage-loving regions, each cook adjusts the proportions of sugar and vinegar to his or her taste. The vinegar acts as a foil for the sugar and keeps the cabbage color bright. Red cabbage cooked without an acid ingredient can turn a weird, unappetizing blue.

In Russia, allspice and cloves are a popular accent, as are celery root and parsley root. Swedish cooks stew red cabbage at length with apples, sugar, and animal fat, then thicken the cooking liquid with potato starch dissolved in vinegar. Europeans serve red cabbage with poached meat, sausages, or roast poultry.

To make an easy, updated sweet-and-sour red cabbage, I sauté an onion until lightly caramelized, so it contributes its natural sweetness to the cabbage. To keep the dish healthy, I use a minimal amount of oil and add a pear or two as well as raisins, so I can use less sugar.

Cabbage is easy to shred with a heavy knife. To save time, you can use a food processor with a shredding disk. This dish keeps well for 3 days in a covered container in the refrigerator. If you like, substitute 1 or 2 finely sliced sweet or tart apples for the pears.

½ large head red cabbage

1 to 1½ tablespoons vegetable oil or olive oil

1 medium onion, chopped

Salt and freshly ground black pepper

½ cup vegetable broth or water, or more if needed

2 Bosc pears, or 1 Bartlett pear, ripe but firm, sliced

3 to 4 tablespoons light raisins

3 to 4 tablespoons vinegar, any kind

1 to 4 tablespoons brown sugar

Pinch of allspice or cloves (optional)

Quarter cabbage, then slice each piece in thin shreds; discard cores.

Heat oil in a large stew pan, add onion and sauté over medium heat for 5 minutes or until light golden. Add cabbage, sprinkle with salt and pepper, and mix well. Add broth and bring to a boil, stirring. Add pear slices. Cover and cook over medium-low heat, stirring occasionally, about 15 minutes or until cabbage is crisp-tender, adding more broth if pan becomes dry.

Add raisins, 3 tablespoons vinegar, and 1 tablespoon brown sugar. Cook, uncovered, over medium heat, stirring often, about 2 minutes to evaporate excess liquid so the cabbage is moist but not soupy. Add allspice. Taste and add more salt, pepper, sugar, or vinegar if needed. You need a fair amount of salt to balance the vinegar and sugar.

Makes 3 to 4 servings

TOMATO-BRAISED CABBAGE WITH GARLIC

Cabbage is a healthy cruciferous vegetable and deserves to appear more often on our plates. A trick I learned in Paris to attenuate the vegetable's strong flavor is to boil it briefly before braising it in a sauce.

For this simple recipe, the cabbage cooks in a garlic- and cumin-flavored tomato sauce. For many years I've found cumin is a great flavor complement for the cabbage, ever since I tasted my Yemenite mother-in-law's cabbage stew. Later I learned from an Egyptian acquaintance in Tel Aviv that cooks in her native country believe that adding cumin to the water for blanching cabbage takes away the vegetable's smell.

Season the cabbage with plenty of black pepper to further enliven its flavor. Serve this fast, easy-to-make dish with roast chicken or, for meatless meals, with beans or tofu and with brown rice. You can prepare it a few days ahead, as its flavor deepens when you reheat it.

1 medium head green cabbage (about 2 pounds), halved and cored
Salt and freshly ground black pepper
1 teaspoon ground cumin

1 to 2 tablespoons extra virgin olive oil
1 large onion, chopped
3 garlic cloves, chopped
1 cup canned diced tomatoes, with their juice

Slice cabbage halves ½ inch thick. Cut each slice into 3 or 4 pieces. In a stew pan, boil 4 cups water or enough to cover cabbage. Add salt and ½ teaspoon cumin, then add cabbage. Cover and cook over high heat, stirring once or twice, for 3 minutes or until cabbage is nearly tender. Drain well, reserving 1 cup cooking liquid.

Heat oil in same pan, add onion and sauté over medium heat for 5 minutes or until softened but not browned. Add garlic, sauté a few seconds, then add cabbage, salt, pepper, and remaining cumin. Stir over low heat for 1 minute. Add tomatoes and ½ cup reserved cabbage cooking liquid. Cover and cook over medium-low heat, stirring often, for 10 minutes or until cabbage is tender, adding more of cabbage cooking liquid by tablespoons if stew becomes too dry. Taste and adjust seasoning. Serve hot.

Makes 4 to 5 servings

Orange-fleshed, vitamin-A rich sweet potatoes and sweet corn gain zing from a tangy tomato-pepper sauce and make this versatile casserole appealing even to people who need a bit of coaxing to eat their vegetables. A sprinkling of green onions gives a lively finish to this spicy Southern-style dish. It makes for a tasty accompaniment to barbecued or baked chicken breasts or a fine vegetarian entrée.

Use any kind of squash you like, from hard-shelled winter squash to summer squash like zucchini.

12 ounces orange-fleshed sweet potatoes (usually labeled yams), peeled

12 ounces summer squash, such as zucchini or pale green Mexican zucchini (also called white or Tatuma squash), halved lengthwise

1 to 2 tablespoons extra virgin olive oil or vegetable oil

1 small onion, chopped

½ green bell pepper, cut into thin strips

1 celery rib, diced small

4 large garlic cloves, chopped

1 bay leaf

1 teaspoon paprika

Salt and freshly ground black pepper

1 cup or one 8-ounce can tomato sauce

2 teaspoons chopped fresh rosemary, or ½ teaspoon chopped dried rosemary

2 teaspoons chopped fresh oregano or ½ teaspoon dried oregano

½ teaspoon hot pepper sauce

2 cups fresh or thawed frozen corn kernels

⅓ cup sliced green onions

Preheat oven to 375°F. Add sweet potatoes to a saucepan of enough boiling water to cover them. Simmer, uncovered, over medium heat for 6 minutes. Add squash and simmer for 4 minutes or until both vegetables are nearly tender but not too soft. Drain, reserving 1 cup cooking liquid. Rinse vegetables with cold water. Cut them into ¾-inch dice.

Heat oil in a medium sauté pan. Add onion, bell pepper, and celery and cook over medium-low heat, stirring, for 7 minutes or until onion begins to brown. Add garlic and cook ½ minute. Add ½ cup of reserved vegetable cooking liquid, bay leaf, paprika, salt, and pepper and bring to a boil. Simmer, uncovered, over medium heat for 3 minutes. Stir in tomato sauce and cook, uncovered, stirring often, for 5 minutes or until vegetables are tender and sauce is thick; if it becomes too thick, stir in a few tablespoons vegetable cooking liquid. Discard bay leaf. Add rosemary, oregano, and hot sauce to taste.

Add squash, corn, and sweet potatoes to sauce and stir gently. Season to taste with salt and pepper. Spoon into a 2-quart casserole. Cover and bake for 20 minutes or until vegetables are tender. Serve sprinkled with green onions.

Makes 4 to 6 servings

Golden-brown onions and a few spices give zucchini an appetizing aroma and a pleasing flavor in this easy-to-make dish. This sauté is convenient whenever you need a quick accompaniment; it makes a lively partner for grilled salmon, chicken breasts, or veggie burgers. It's also good as part of a selection of vegetable dishes to serve with brown rice. For brunch you can add 2 or 3 beaten eggs or egg substitute to this vegetable sauté and scramble them.

Slice the onions lengthwise so they keep a more distinct texture than they would if cut crosswise. To make the dish more colorful, mix green and yellow squashes.

2 tablespoons extra virgin olive oil
2 large onions, halved and sliced lengthwise
Salt and freshly ground black pepper
1½ to 2 pounds zucchini, pale green Mexican
    zucchini (also called white or Tatuma squash),
    or other summer squash, halved lengthwise,
    sliced ⅓ to ½ inch thick

¼ to ½ teaspoon hot red pepper flakes
1 teaspoon ground cumin
¼ teaspoon turmeric

Heat oil in a large sauté pan. Add onions, salt and pepper to taste, and sauté over medium heat for 10 minutes or until golden. Add squash and sprinkle with salt, pepper, pepper flakes, cumin, and turmeric. Sauté, stirring occasionally, for 5 minutes. Pour 2 to 3 tablespoons water into pan near its edge. Cover and cook over medium-low heat for 5 to 10 minutes or until vegetables are done to your taste—either crisp-tender or tender but not mushy. Serve hot or at room temperature.

Makes 4 servings

This basic sauté is a simple, lower-fat alternative to fried eggplant and is one of the fastest ways to prepare the vegetable. I like it as a side dish with grilled chicken, lamb, or beef, or along with edamame (green soybeans) and cooked rice or couscous as a vegetarian entrée. Sometimes I vary the flavor by adding diced tomatoes, garlic, lightly sautéed mushroom slices, or roasted sweet peppers or chiles. On warm days the eggplant cubes are good as a salad, drizzled with a bit of herb vinegar, fresh lemon juice, or light rosemary vinaigrette (see page 183), and garnished with a few olives.

Sephardi cooks often add fried eggplant to meat or poultry stews so they absorb flavor from the sauce. As a healthier alternative, eggplant prepared by this quick sauté technique works wonderfully for those types of dishes. I add the eggplant cubes to such stews for the last few minutes so they retain their texture. You can sauté the eggplant 2 or 3 days ahead and reheat it in a skillet.

1½ to 3 tablespoons extra virgin olive oil
1 eggplant (1 to 1¼ pounds), cut into ¾-inch dice
Salt and freshly ground black pepper
1½ teaspoons chopped fresh oregano or thyme, or ½ teaspoon dried oregano or thyme

½ to 1 teaspoon Aleppo pepper (semihot Middle Eastern red pepper), paprika, or cayenne pepper
1 or 2 green onions, white and green parts, chopped
2 tablespoons chopped flat-leaf parsley or cilantro

Heat 1½ to 2 tablespoons oil in a large, heavy skillet or sauté pan, preferably nonstick. Add eggplant cubes, salt, and pepper and sauté over medium heat, stirring often, for 4 minutes. Sprinkle with oregano and Aleppo pepper to taste. Cover and cook over medium-low heat, stirring often, for 8 minutes or until eggplant is tender. Add green onion. Taste and adjust seasoning; sprinkle with a bit more oil, if desired. Gently stir in parsley before serving.

Makes 3 to 4 servings

Grilling or broiling eggplant is one of the most hassle-free ways to prepare the vegetable. Besides, this cooking technique is fat-free.

Once your eggplant is cooked, this savory specialty of India accented with fresh ginger, garlic, and spices is simple to make. Popular among Jews and others of Indian origin, it has long been one of the dishes I love most. Flavorings vary widely, from a simple mixture of chiles, green onions, and lemon juice to a luscious sauce flavored with ginger, garlic, and cumin.

This scrumptious version is lighter than most and does not contain cream. You can serve it hot or warm with rice or meat dishes as they do in Indian restaurants. In our family we also love it cold as an appetizer with crusty bread or pita. Warm Indian naan bread is great too; you can purchase some from an Indian market.

2 medium eggplants (total 2 to 2½ pounds)

2 to 3 tablespoons vegetable oil or olive oil

1 onion, chopped

4 Thai bird chiles, 3 serrano chiles, or 2 jalapeño peppers or other hot peppers, seeded if you want less heat, minced

2 teaspoons minced peeled ginger

2 large garlic cloves, minced

1½ teaspoons ground coriander

1 teaspoon ground cumin

½ teaspoon turmeric

One 14½-ounce can tomatoes, drained and chopped

Salt

Cayenne pepper (optional)

2 tablespoons chopped cilantro

Prick eggplants a few times with fork. Grill eggplants above medium-hot coals about 45 minutes; or broil for about 35 minutes, turning often, or bake in a roasting pan at 400°F about 1 hour. When done, eggplants' flesh should be tender and eggplants should look collapsed. Cut off stems. Halve eggplants lengthwise; if you have baked them, there may be some liquid inside; drain it off. Scoop out eggplant pulp from inside skin. Chop eggplant pulp fine with a knife; or chop in a food processor with a pulsing motion.

Heat oil in a large sauté pan. Add onion and sauté over medium heat for 7 minutes or until beginning to brown. Add chiles, ginger, and garlic and sauté for 30 seconds, stirring. Stir in coriander, cumin, and turmeric, followed by tomatoes. Bring to a simmer and cook over medium heat for 7 minutes or until thickened.

Add eggplant, salt to taste, and cayenne (if using) and cook, stirring often, for 5 to 10 minutes or until mixture is thick. Taste and adjust seasoning. Serve eggplant hot or at room temperature, spooned into a shallow bowl and sprinkled with cilantro.

Makes 4 to 6 servings

VEGETABLE MEDLEY WITH TOASTED ALMONDS

A sprinkling of toasted almonds does wonders to embellish vegetable sautés, like this colorful combination of zucchini, eggplant, and red bell pepper. If you like, substitute mushrooms for the eggplant. Drained canned water chestnuts or frozen cooked lima beans are also good additions. Serve the vegetables with chicken or spoon them over brown rice or whole wheat linguine.

If you'd like to prepare the dish with less oil, spread the eggplant strips on a baking dish, spray them with oil spray, and bake uncovered at 400°F, stirring a few times, for 15 minutes or until the eggplant is tender.

2 small zucchini or pale green squash (white, Mexican, or clarita squash)
1 small eggplant (about ¾ pound)
4½ to 5 tablespoons extra virgin olive oil
Salt
1 medium or large onion, halved, cut into thin slices
1 large red bell pepper, seeds and ribs discarded, cut into thin strips

Freshly ground black pepper
4 large garlic cloves, minced
2 to 3 teaspoons dried oregano
⅓ to ½ cup slivered almonds, toasted (see page 379)
2 tablespoons chopped flat-leaf parsley

Cut squash into 3 pieces crosswise, then into thin strips lengthwise. Peel eggplant and cut into thin strips.

Heat 2 tablespoons olive oil in a large skillet over medium heat. Add eggplant and sprinkle with salt. Sauté, tossing constantly, for 7 minutes or until just tender. Transfer to a bowl.

Add 2 tablespoons oil to skillet. Heat over medium-low heat. Add onion and cook, stirring often, for 7 minutes or until softened but not brown. Add pepper strips, salt and pepper to taste, and cook, tossing often, for 5 minutes or until onion and peppers are nearly tender. Add squash and eggplant and cook, tossing often, until squash is crisp-tender, about 3 minutes. Transfer vegetables to a shallow bowl or a platter.

Add remaining olive oil to skillet from cooking vegetables and heat over low heat. Add garlic and cook for ½ minute. Add oregano and half of toasted almonds and heat 2 to 3 seconds. Pour mixture over vegetables, add parsley, and toss well. Taste and adjust seasoning. Serve garnished with remaining toasted almonds.

Makes 4 servings

I am constantly searching for interesting ways to vary my vegetable dishes. This stew is an example of how to add Filipino flair to Mediterranean vegetable stews.

The Filipino approach to eggplant is different from the usual Mediterranean methods. When making stews, Filipino cooks often add the eggplant directly to the liquid without sautéing it first. This technique is faster, easier, and makes the dish lower in fat.

When I first tasted this famous Filipino stew, called *pinákbet*, it reminded me of a popular Balkan stew called *guvetch* that is loved in Israel. Both stews may be meatless or might include a little meat or chicken to flavor the sauce. Guvetch combines eggplant, peppers, tomato, onions, and garlic and might also include okra, zucchini, and green beans. The Filipino stew had many similar elements. Instead of green beans, there were Chinese long beans. Instead of zucchini, it included orange calabaza squash and a beautiful but bitter green gourd called bitter melon. Since bitter melon is not for everyone and can be hard to find, you can substitute other soft-shelled squash.

The Filipino stew owes its character to two accents: fresh ginger, as well as a drizzle of fish sauce or a generous dollop of seafood paste. This flavoring is an acquired taste, and several Filipino women told me that when they cook their native dishes to introduce them to Israelis, they omit the fish sauce and substitute soy sauce or salt.

This stew is good over rice as a meatless main course, or as an accompaniment for meat, chicken, or fish. If you like, use a 4-ounce piece of sweet, orange-fleshed squash like butternut, calabaza, or kabocha instead of all or half the zucchini. Some cooks add frozen lima beans to make the stew more substantial. If tomato skins bother you, peel the tomatoes before adding them or use canned tomatoes.

2 tablespoons vegetable oil
1 onion, chopped
2 garlic cloves, chopped
2 teaspoons minced peeled ginger
3 tomatoes, diced
2 ounces fresh or sliced frozen okra
1/3 cup water
1 eggplant, peeled and cut into 1-inch dice
1 to 2 zucchini or pale green Mexican zucchini
    (also called white or Tatuma squash), cut into
    1-inch dice

2 to 3 ounces Chinese long beans or green beans,
    ends trimmed, cut into 2-inch pieces
1 to 2 tablespoons fish sauce or soy sauce, or
    1 to 2 teaspoons anchovy paste, or to taste
    (optional)
Salt (optional) and freshly ground black pepper

Heat oil in a stew pan. Add onion and garlic and sauté for 2 minutes or until onion is translucent. Add ginger and tomatoes and cook, uncovered, over medium heat for 5 minutes.

If using fresh okra, carefully cut off caps. Slice okra or leave it whole, as you like.

Add water to stew and bring to a boil. Add eggplant, zucchini, okra, and beans. Simmer, adding a little hot water if vegetables begin to stick, for 20 minutes or until all vegetables are tender. Add fish sauce (if using), salt if needed, and pepper to taste. Serve hot.

Makes 4 to 6 servings

Grains and Pasta Dishes

It's not surprising that pasta and grains have long been staples of the Jewish kitchen. They are sustaining and inexpensive; and most people enjoy their mild flavors. Ashkenazi Jews are famous for their chicken noodle soup and noodle kugels, both savory and sweet. Among Sephardi Jews, Moroccans are known for their couscous, and Italian Jews use the same forms of pasta as their compatriots.

Rice is the favorite grain of Sephardi Jews, and many eat it every day. Bulgur wheat is popular in their households too. Kasha appears on Ashkenazi tables. In both Ashkenazi and Sephardi homes, barley often appears in the weekly Shabbat overnight stew; Sephardi Jews might use whole wheat berries instead, which have long been a staple in the Mideast.

These wheat berries are delicious and worth getting to know. I first became familiar with them when I lived in Bat Yam, a suburb of Tel Aviv. My next-door neighbor, who was of Moroccan origin, used them in her Shabbat stew, which she called *dafina*. Her dish of beef, beans, and wheat was spicy, but some similar stews are mild in flavor. Other Moroccans, for example, combine whole wheat grains in meat dishes with sweet accents, such as meatballs flavored with raisins and almonds and a honey cumin sauce.

Whole wheat berries also can be made into tasty, nutritious desserts similar to rice pudding. In the eastern Mediterranean, the cooked wheat berries might be flavored with sugar, cinnamon, and some tasty, healthy treats like raisins, toasted walnuts, and, occasionally, pomegranate seeds.

Modern nutritionists back up this time-honored predilection for wheat berries, recommending that we replace refined grains with whole grains. The point is not to avoid carbohydrates altogether, but to choose nutritious ones.

When it comes to choosing whole grains, the most common recommendation—and the

SAUCE YOUR PASTA SENSIBLY

As I stroll among the local farmers' market stands of just-picked vegetables, I fantasize combining them with pasta. When I see lovely wild mushrooms, I visualize them sautéed and tossed with fettuccine, thyme, and garlic, or baked into a moist noodle kugel. The broccoli seems to beg to be matched with sun-dried tomatoes and linguine.

I am not alone in my passion for pasta. A glance at restaurant menus and takeout displays reveals its popularity. In spite of the fad of low-carbohydrate diets, everyone loves spaghetti and its many relatives.

There are good reasons for pasta's popularity. It cooks quickly and is economical. Pasta is delicious with every ingredient, from carrots to caviar, and may be the most versatile of all foods. You can season it with an endless variety of flavorings, from French, Italian, or Israeli cheeses to Indian or Mexican spice mixtures to toasted nuts. Pasta is equally at home with brown sauces, fragrant tomato sauces, pestos, salad dressings, and flavored oils. You can season the sauces with whatever strikes your fancy—from fresh dill to curry blends to sesame oil.

A sauce for pasta should be well seasoned. It may seem too sharp on its own, but will taste just right when mixed with the pasta. If a sauce tastes perfect by itself, it may be bland when combined with the noodles. It is essential to taste again, after you blend the pasta with the sauce.

easiest one to follow—is to purchase different bread. Opt for one labeled "100% whole wheat" or other whole grains, such as the Jewish favorite, rye bread, instead of white bread.

Brown rice is easy to include in menus. Simply substitute it for white rice in your pilafs and other favorite recipes. Brown rice needs the same amount of liquid as white rice; just increase the cooking time from about 15 minutes to about 40 minutes. You can buy short- or long-grain brown rice as well as brown basmati rice. In addition there are other tasty kinds of whole-grain rice, such as red rice and forbidden rice, a black, medium-grain rice from China.

I have friends who always opt for nutritious brown rice when it's on the menu at Chinese or Thai restaurants, and other friends who won't touch it. But I'm glad that members of

For nutrition as well as good taste, the trick is tossing the pasta with the right amount of sauce. There should be just enough to moisten the pasta. It's better to serve extra sauce on the side in case someone wants more than to have a puddle of sauce at the bottom of the pasta bowl.

At the store, you'll see a great variety of pasta shapes. Most people know fettuccine, linguine, and angel-hair pasta, but less familiar shapes that can add interest to menus are cavatappi, or spiral macaroni; cavatelli, small, narrow ripple-edged shells; and farfalle, also known as bow-ties or butterflies. Often you can find fresh pasta, which has a more delicate texture, as well as Asian rice and buckwheat noodles and bean threads. To give your pasta dishes a nutritious boost, choose whole-grain varieties.

For special occasions, even old-fashioned favorites like noodle kugels can be made healthier, with slight adaptation. (See page 128.) To make weekday pasta entrées colorful and nutritious, I like simple dishes graced with fresh vegetables rather than macaroni with long-simmering meat sauces. The resulting entrées are quick, homey, and healthy.

For a fast, lighter dish, I match pasta with briefly cooked spinach or other greens. I sauté the vegetable in olive oil and garlic, then toss it with pasta and perhaps a pinch of a flavorful grating cheese like Parmesan or Gruyère. This is the kind of dish I'm thinking of as I explore outdoor markets, whether it's Jerusalem's Mahaneh Yehudah or the weekly organic market of Santa Monica, California.

my family like the taste of both brown and white rice so that I have more options of different flavors, textures, and colors when I plan menus.

Because brown rice takes longer to cook than white, I like to cook enough for two or three meals. To reheat it, I simply spoon the cooked rice into a casserole, cover it, and put it into the microwave, where it reheats quickly and beautifully.

Another way to save time is to simmer quick-cooking vegetables along with the rice, creating a rice-and-vegetable casserole to serve as a side dish or a vegetarian main course. I love brown rice with onions and mushrooms, or with a colorful combination of tomatoes and diced squash.

Corn is another familiar grain that's simple to incorporate in menus. When serving it on the cob, instead of using butter, you can moisten it lightly with seasoned olive oil.

BARLEY'S NUTRITIONAL BOOST

*T*here is some controversy over where barley originated. Many say it came from the Middle East or Ethiopia. After all, barley is mentioned in the Torah as one of the Seven Species of the Promised Land. Around the Mediterranean and the Mideast, barley was once much more widely used than it is today. It was used for soups, stews, and desserts resembling rice pudding. Ancient Egyptians used it to make beer, and both they and the Greeks made barley into bread. Barley bread is still baked in Crete and Tunisia.

I had always associated this grain with Ashkenazi cooking, probably because my mother put it in her cholent. But it turns out that Mexicans like it too. I find it among the Latin American ingredients at Mexican markets. It's used in a refreshing beverage called **agua de cebada**, or barley water. I've also found barley in Chinese breakfast cereals and in Korean grain mixtures served as accompaniments.

Barley is tender, creamy, and easy to love, and deserves to appear on the table more often. Nutritionists encourage us to use barley for its special benefits. It is a very good source of fiber and, like oatmeal, is considered helpful in lowering cholesterol. In addition, barley contains phosphorus, copper, and manganese.

Many of us are familiar with mushroom barley soup, a Russian–Ashkenazi specialty that has become an Israeli favorite; but there are many other soups featuring barley. Armenians make chickpea soup with barley and fried onions. According to Claudia M. Caruana, author of **Taste of Malta**, cooks on that island prepare a savory spinach soup with barley, lamb, onion, and garlic sautéed in olive oil, carrots, and dill. Chaldeans also combine greens and barley, cooking them as a chard and barley stew with tomatoes, green peppers, and onions.

(See page 298.) Of course, you can add corn kernels to all sorts of soups, stews, and salads. Consider it the grain element of that meal.

It's fun to experiment with other grains as well. When you're making salads, stuffings, or casseroles that call for cooked rice, you can substitute an equal volume of cooked barley, quinoa, millet, wheat berries, or bulgur wheat. Even oatmeal has uses beyond breakfast. I like it instead of flour for thickening vegetable soups (see pages 194–195). When I make matzo balls, I sometimes substitute oat bran for about a quarter of the matzo meal in the recipe.

Pasta also has a place in the healthy diet. It's a great partner for vegetables, which can

BULGUR BEYOND TABBOULEH

If you go to a mizrahi, or Middle Eastern restaurant, in Jerusalem, you're likely to find tabbouleh on the menu. When made properly, this fresh, colorful, light Lebanese salad of parsley, mint, and tomatoes contains a small amount of bulgur wheat, so the salad is a bit more substantial than the usual Israeli salad.

You can utilize bulgur wheat in plenty of other ways. A staple of Sephardi and Middle Eastern cooking, this versatile grain is available in many American supermarkets, as well as in kosher, Middle Eastern, and natural foods markets. Since it's tasty, satisfying, and simple to prepare, it's worth getting to know.

Bulgur is precooked wheat, so it can be prepared quickly. I see bulgur as one of the world's first convenience foods; it has been a staple in the Mideast since ancient times. To make bulgur, the wheat kernels are steamed, dried, and cracked in small pieces. I always valued the selection available at Israel's outdoor markets, like Jerusalem's Mahaneh Yehudah and Tel Aviv's Hatikvah. In Middle Eastern groceries in the United States, you'll also find bulgur in several sizes. Purists insist that fine bulgur is best for salads, medium size for pilafs, and large grains for soups. But you can use whatever kind you have for these purposes; substituting a different size will simply result in a slight variation in texture. Bulgur is sometimes called "cracked wheat," but cracked wheat can be raw and takes longer to cook than bulgur.

For preparing side dishes, think of bulgur as a wheat form of rice and use it in the same recipes. Indeed, Greeks sometimes dub bulgur wheat "rice of the poor." Like rice, bulgur can be boiled, but it's more interesting when prepared as a pilaf: it is first sautéed in a little oil, then moistened with double its volume in hot water or broth. The mixture is then simmered in a covered saucepan over low heat. Because the bulgur is already cooked and needs only to be rehydrated, it takes a few minutes less than rice.

I love bulgur pilaf embellished with a festive topping of toasted almonds or pine nuts and a few raisins. It's also great combined with sautéed onions, peppers, eggplant, mushrooms, squash of all types, broccoli, or tomatoes. Combine it with lentils, chickpeas, or other beans for a meatless entrée. For seasoning, Mediterranean flavors like garlic, mint, cilantro, basil, cumin, ground coriander seed, allspice, and cinnamon are good partners for the grain.

be cooked and tossed with the pasta and a little olive oil, making a satisfying plant-based meal. To boost the nutrition of such dishes, use pasta made of whole wheat, brown rice, or soy, instead of white flour pasta. If you're preparing couscous, you might enjoy the nutty taste of whole wheat couscous.

BENEFICIAL BUCKWHEAT

*T*he first time I tried kasha, or buckwheat groats, its flavor was too earthy for my taste. Then I learned from kasha mavens that the key to making delicious kasha is to combine it with a generous amount of well-browned onions. The flavor of kasha grows on you; after a few more tastings, I became fond of it.

You'll find kasha, a favorite ingredient in the culinary repertoire of Jews from Russia and Poland, at many supermarkets, as well as in kosher and Eastern European grocery stores. Kasha is best known as a filling for popular pastries, especially knishes and piroshki, but is also used in kreplach, a sort of ravioli.

As a side dish, kasha usually accompanies beef or chicken. A traditional Ashkenazi recipe calls for pairing kasha with pasta bow-ties or with egg noodles. The mild flavor of the pasta is a good foil for the robust taste of the kasha. I also like to combine kasha with sautéed sliced mushrooms for a vegetarian entrée. For dairy dinners you can soften the assertive flavor of kasha by topping it with a dollop of yogurt.

In some families a bowl of cooked kasha is served for spooning into chicken soup; see Chicken Soup with Kasha, Bow Ties, and Carrots (page 144). Several of my mother's friends enjoy kasha as a breakfast cereal, with milk.

In the kitchen, kasha is treated as a grain, although buckwheat is the fruit of a leafy plant related to sorrel rather than a true grain. Unlike raw buckwheat kernels, kasha is roasted. It comes in three sizes—fine, medium, and whole granules. Buckwheat is also made into flour and makes tasty blintzes. (See Buckwheat Blintzes with Goat Cheese and Ratatouille, page 118.)

Like white rice, kasha cooks quickly—in about 15 minutes. From a nutrition standpoint, kasha gives you as much protein as rice and more fiber for a lower "price" in calories, and it contains magnesium, iron, and folate.

Hawaiian Brown Rice with Smoked Chicken

Sephardi Rice with Beef and Cabbage

Rice Pilaf with Caramelized Onions and Mushrooms

Bulgur Wheat with Garlic

Ten-Minute Bulgur Skillet Supper with Turkey and Beans

Baked Barley with Chard and Garlic Pesto

Biblical Baked Barley with Almonds, Raisins, and Mint

Pasta Spirals with Sautéed Spinach

Two-Way Pasta with Lima Beans, Basil, and Tomatoes

Speedy Spiral Pasta with Smoked Turkey and Tomatoes

Penne Bolognese with a Bonus

Saffron-Spiced Spaghetti Sauce with Yellow Split Peas

❧ HAWAIIAN BROWN RICE WITH SMOKED CHICKEN

A tasty Hawaiian breakfast specialty I enjoyed in Honolulu—fried rice embellished with a variety of smoked and cured meats—gave me the idea for this dish. The rice was flavored with green onions and soy sauce and was topped with a fried egg.

For me this entrée is too substantial for breakfast, but it's great for lunch. To make it healthier, I skip the frying and add a drizzle of oil for richness, and I use lean meats like smoked chicken or turkey breast. For pareve options I like soy chicken, veggie pepperoni, or meatless salami. You can make it with any kind of whole-grain rice, including quick-cooking brown rice. I add plenty of vegetables too; they enhance the entrée's nutrition and color, and their flavors and textures make it more interesting to eat. Instead of the fried egg, I top the rice with quartered warm hard-boiled eggs.

1½ to 2 tablespoons vegetable oil

1 red bell pepper, finely diced (about
⅜-inch dice)

1 green bell pepper, finely diced

6 ounces mushrooms, quartered

2 teaspoons minced peeled ginger

4 green onions, white and green parts chopped
separately

2 garlic cloves, chopped

2 to 3 cups thin strips of smoked chicken, turkey, or
soy chicken

3 cups cooked brown rice (see page 362)

1 tablespoon soy sauce

Salt and freshly ground black pepper

Cayenne pepper (optional)

2 to 3 teaspoons toasted sesame oil

2 or 3 warm hard-boiled eggs, quartered
(optional)

Heat oil in a large skillet. Add red and green peppers, and sauté over medium heat, stirring often, for 7 minutes or until nearly tender. Add mushrooms and sauté for 2 minutes. Add ginger and white part of green onions and cook for 1 minute. Remove from heat and stir in garlic and chicken. Add cooked rice and mix lightly.

Add soy sauce, salt, black pepper, and cayenne (if using). Reserve a little of green part of green onions for garnish and add rest to rice mixture. Taste and adjust seasoning. Either cover and heat through, occasionally stirring lightly, or microwave in a covered dish until hot. Drizzle with sesame oil and mix lightly. Serve sprinkled with reserved green onions and topped with eggs, if you like.

Makes 5 to 6 servings

Cabbage tends to be associated with Ashkenazi cooking, but Mediterranean Jews have a healthy culinary custom of cooking rice with greens such as spinach, chard, or cabbage. Often cooks flavor these casseroles with tomatoes and ground meat and spice them with cinnamon, nutmeg, or allspice. Although white rice is the traditional choice, I like the nutty taste and nutritional boost of brown rice. To make this dish with white rice, cook the rice only 10 minutes before adding the cabbage.

For a pareve/vegetarian dish, omit the meat or substitute soy ground "meat" or 6 to 8 ounces of chopped mushrooms, and use vegetable broth. This easy casserole makes a casual family supper entrée for wintertime. Serve Diced Vegetable Salad with Pepitas and Papaya (page 182) on the side.

2½ to 3 tablespoons olive oil

2 onions, chopped

12 ounces extra-lean ground beef, ground turkey, or
soy ground "meat"

½ teaspoon ground cinnamon

Freshly grated nutmeg (optional)

½ small head cabbage (about ½ pound), shredded
(4 to 5 cups)

Salt and freshly ground black pepper

One 14-ounce can diced tomatoes, with their liquid

3¼ to 3½ cups hot beef, chicken, or vegetable broth
or water

1½ cups long-grain brown rice

1 tablespoon chopped flat-leaf parsley (optional)

Heat 1½ to 2 tablespoons oil in a deep sauté pan. Add onions and sauté over medium heat for 7 minutes or until softened. Add meat, cinnamon, and nutmeg and sauté, stirring to separate meat into small pieces, until it changes color. Add cabbage, salt, and pepper and sauté for 3 minutes, stirring often. Add tomatoes and ¼ cup broth and simmer for 10 minutes or until meat and cabbage are tender, adding a few tablespoons broth from time to time if mixture becomes too thick.

Meanwhile, heat 1 tablespoon oil in a stew pan. Add rice and cook over medium-low heat, stirring, for 3 minutes or until it is evenly coated and lightly toasted. Add 3 cups broth, salt, and pepper. Stir once and bring to a boil. Cover and cook over low heat, without stirring, for 25 minutes.

Add cabbage mixture to pan of rice, without stirring. Bring to a simmer. Add a few tablespoons broth or water if mixture is dry. Cover and cook over low heat for 10 minutes or until rice is tender. Let stand, covered, for 5 minutes. Fluff rice with fork, mixing gently with remaining ingredients. Taste and adjust seasoning, adding more nutmeg, if you like. Serve hot, sprinkled with parsley (if using).

Makes about 6 servings

RICE PILAF WITH CARAMELIZED ONIONS AND MUSHROOMS

Rice with mushrooms has been a popular partner for the Shabbat chicken in my family since I was a child, but this way of preparing it came about by accident. I sautéed my onions over heat that was too high and they browned to such a deep caramel color that they nearly burned. To avoid giving the rice a muddy brown hue, I cooked it separately and folded in the onions, together with mushrooms sautéed with paprika, at the end. The result was delicious.

In contrast to classic pilaf, which calls for sautéing the onions very lightly so they remain white and provide a delicate flavor, this rice had a pronounced taste of caramelized onions. Keeping the onions separate until the end gives each bit of onion more of a sautéed texture, instead of a simmered one.

Use either white or brown rice to make this simple but savory pilaf. If using brown rice, add the optional parsley so the dish will be more colorful. To keep the fat content low, cover the pan while sautéing the onions.

3 to 3½ tablespoons vegetable oil or olive oil
2 onions, chopped
8 to 12 ounces mushrooms, halved and cut into
   thick slices
Salt and freshly ground black pepper
1 teaspoon sweet paprika

Pinch of hot paprika or cayenne pepper
2 cups long-grain white or brown rice
4 cups hot vegetable broth, vegetable cooking liquid,
   or water
2 tablespoons chopped flat-leaf parsley (optional)

Heat 1 tablespoon oil in a large sauté pan or wide casserole. Add onions and sauté over medium-high heat, stirring often, for 2 minutes. Cover and cook over medium heat, stirring often, for 5 minutes or until deeply browned; if pan becomes dry, add ½ tablespoon oil or 1 to 2 tablespoons water and continue browning. Remove from pan.

Add 1 tablespoon oil to pan and heat it. Add mushrooms, salt, and pepper and sauté over medium-high heat, stirring, for 2 minutes. Add sweet and hot paprikas and sauté for 1 to 2 more minutes or until mushrooms are tender. Remove from pan.

Add remaining oil to pan and heat it. Add rice and sauté over medium-low heat, stirring, for 2 minutes or until it changes color slightly and smells toasted. Add hot vegetable broth, 1½ teaspoons salt, and a pinch of pepper. Stir once with a fork and cover. Cook over low heat, without stirring, taking 15 minutes for white rice or 40 minutes for brown rice. Taste rice; if not yet tender, simmer 2 more minutes. Add more salt and pepper if needed. Cover and let stand for 5 minutes.

Gently fluff rice with a fork. Lightly stir in sautéed onions and mushrooms. Taste and adjust seasoning. Cover and let stand for 5 more minutes. Stir in parsley, if you like. Serve hot.

Makes 8 servings

❧ BULGUR WHEAT WITH GARLIC

When you need a quick, healthy side dish, this one is a good choice. You can throw it together in a flash, and you have a whole-grain accompaniment that is ready to eat in minutes. Because bulgur is made from wheat that has been boiled before being cracked and dried, it cooks very quickly.

For a fast flavor boost, I add chopped garlic and ground ginger. The garlic adds plenty of punch because it is cooked briefly. If your meal is fairly rich, you can steam the bulgur in broth for a fat-free dish. At other times, you might like to enrich it with a bit of olive oil.

The fluffy bulgur grains are a pleasing partner for roast chicken. The bulgur tastes great with the chicken juices, but be sure to thoroughly skim the fat before using them.

1 cup bulgur wheat, medium or small
2 cups vegetable or chicken broth or water
Salt and freshly ground black pepper

3 large garlic cloves, minced
½ teaspoon ground ginger, or more to taste
1 tablespoon extra virgin olive oil (optional)

Put bulgur in a heavy saucepan and stir over medium-low heat for 1 minute to lightly toast the grains. Add stock, salt, and pepper and bring to a boil. Add garlic, cover, and cook over low heat for 10 minutes. Add ginger, stir lightly, cover, and cook for 5 more minutes or until water is absorbed and bulgur has softened to your taste. Taste and adjust seasoning. Fluff with a fork, adding olive oil, if you like. Serve hot.

Makes 4 servings

TEN-MINUTE BULGUR SKILLET SUPPER WITH TURKEY AND BEANS

Israeli cooks take full advantage of bulgur wheat's short cooking time and ease of preparation, which makes it convenient for a variety of one-pot dishes. For this easy, versatile dish flavored with herbs and accented with sautéed peppers, you can use any roasted, grilled, poached, or smoked poultry or meat that you have on hand. Turkey pastrami or lean chicken franks are other tasty options. For a pareve/vegan dish, use mushrooms, spicy tofu franks, diced firm tofu, or soy ground "meat."

1 to 2 tablespoons extra virgin olive oil
1 green or red bell pepper, or ½ green and
    ½ red pepper, cut into 1-inch dice
1⅓ cups bulgur wheat
Salt and freshly ground black pepper
2⅔ cups hot water
One 15-ounce can red, white, or pinto beans,
    drained

2 cups shredded roast turkey or chicken, or
    1 cup thin strips smoked turkey
1 teaspoon paprika
½ teaspoon dried thyme
Cayenne pepper
2 tablespoons chopped cilantro or flat-leaf parsley
    or shredded fresh basil

Heat oil in a sauté pan. Add green pepper and sauté over high heat for 2 minutes. Add bulgur wheat and a little salt and pepper and stir briefly over low heat. Add hot water and bring to a boil. Cover and cook over low heat for 8 minutes. Add beans, turkey, paprika, and thyme. Cover and cook over low heat for 2 minutes or until meat and beans are heated through. Add cayenne to taste and cilantro. Taste and adjust seasoning. Serve hot.

Makes 4 servings

❧ BAKED BARLEY WITH CHARD AND GARLIC PESTO

To make barley dishes lively, be generous with vegetables and flavorings. This barley casserole is dotted with green beans and red bell pepper, and is flavored with a pestolike chard sautéed with garlic, coriander, and mint. It makes a hearty accompaniment for roast chicken or for vegetarian burgers; or, when made with vegetable broth, it can be served as a meatless entrée topped simply with plain yogurt.

3 tablespoons extra virgin olive oil

1 large onion, sliced

1 red bell pepper, cut into strips

1 cup medium pearl barley, rinsed and drained

3 cups hot vegetable or chicken broth or water, or more if needed

Salt and freshly ground black pepper

1½ cups cooked green beans, cut into 1-inch pieces

6 large garlic cloves, chopped

2 cups coarsely chopped Swiss chard leaves

1 teaspoon ground coriander

1 tablespoon chopped mint, or 1 teaspoon dried leaf mint, crumbled

Cayenne pepper

Preheat oven to 350°F. Heat 2 tablespoons oil in a large skillet. Add onion and sauté over medium heat for 7 minutes or until softened. Add red bell pepper to skillet and sauté for 5 minutes or until onion begins to turn golden. Stir in barley and sauté for 1 minute. Remove from heat.

Oil a 2-quart casserole. Transfer barley and vegetable mixture to casserole, reserving skillet. Pour hot broth over barley mixture. Season with salt and pepper. Cover and bake, stirring 3 or 4 times, for 1¼ hours or until barley is tender. Lightly stir in cooked green beans.

Heat remaining oil in skillet. Add garlic and sauté for 15 seconds. Add chard and sauté over medium heat, stirring, for 3 minutes. Stir in coriander and mint. Puree mixture in a food processor. With a fork, gently blend chard puree into barley. If mixture is too thick, stir in a few tablespoons broth or hot water. Adjust seasoning, adding cayenne to taste. Serve hot.

Makes 4 to 6 servings

BIBLICAL BAKED BARLEY
WITH ALMONDS, RAISINS, AND MINT

This hearty side dish matches barley with other foods that were available in the land of Israel during the biblical period. The ingredients also happen to be healthy—barley, almonds, raisins, and onions have healthy fiber, while onions are also a good source of vitamin C, disease-fighting antioxidants, and chromium, which helps cells respond to insulin. Almonds enrich the dish in two ways—ground and baked with the barley, and toasted and sprinkled on top as garnish.

For Shabbat or Sukkot, this festive accompaniment is a good partner for baked chicken or fish or for beef stews. Since this hearty dish is enriched with olive oil, it's also appropriate for honoring the Hanukkah miracle. For a light meal, you can serve the baked barley as an entrée with Baby Greens with Toasted Walnuts, Figs, and Light Rosemary Vinaigrette (page 183) or with Turkish Carrots with Walnuts and Yogurt Garlic Dressing (page 188).

⅓ to ½ cup sliced almonds

1 to 2 tablespoons extra virgin olive oil

1 large onion, chopped

2 large garlic cloves, chopped

1 cup medium pearl barley

3 cups vegetable broth

Salt and freshly ground black pepper

2 teaspoons chopped fresh mint, or
   1 teaspoon dried mint

1 teaspoon dried oregano

¼ cup raisins or currants

2 tablespoons chopped parsley (optional)

Preheat oven to 350°F. Toast 3 tablespoons almonds on a baking sheet in oven for 5 minutes. Transfer to a plate and set aside for garnish. Grind remaining almonds in a small food processor or nut grinder.

Heat oil in a skillet. Add onion and sauté over medium heat for 5 minutes. Add garlic and barley and sauté for 1 minute, stirring.

Lightly oil a 2-quart casserole. Transfer barley mixture to casserole. Add broth, salt, pepper, dried mint (but not fresh mint), oregano, raisins, ground almonds, and 1 tablespoon parsley, if you like. Cover and bake, stirring 3 or 4 times, for 1¼ hours or until barley is tender. Fluff with a fork before serving. Taste and adjust seasoning. Serve topped with remaining parsley, fresh mint, and toasted sliced almonds.

Makes 5 to 6 servings

✥ PASTA SPIRALS WITH SAUTÉED SPINACH

In spite of the low-carbohydrate fad, everyone loves spaghetti and its relatives. And there are plenty of ways to make pasta healthy, like this quick, easy dish of whole-grain pasta seasoned with a sauce of spinach, garlic, and olive oil. To make it even faster, you can use frozen spinach or other greens. Diced fresh tomatoes tossed with the pasta at the last minute add a lively touch. If you'd like cheese, pick a pungent one so you won't need much, such as Bulgarian brined sheep's milk cheese or grated Israeli kashkaval, or, for a pareve meal, soy or other nondairy cheese.

When I was growing up, this kind of light, fast pasta dish was one of our favorites for Saturday night, after a copious Shabbat lunch. This vegetable-sauced pasta is also good for Sukkot, the harvest holiday, or for Shavuot, when dairy dishes dominate the menu.

2 to 3 tablespoons extra virgin olive oil
*1 bunch of spinach (about ¾ pound), rinsed
    thoroughly, stems removed, leaves chopped*
Salt and freshly ground black pepper
1 tablespoon butter (optional)
2 large garlic cloves, minced

*8 ounces spiral pasta (about 3 cups), preferably
    soy or whole grain*
2 firm ripe tomatoes, diced
*½ cup crumbled Bulgarian sheep's milk cheese or
    feta cheese, or grated kashkaval, Gruyère,
    or soy cheese*

Heat 2 tablespoons oil in a very large skillet or shallow stew pan over low heat. Add spinach and sprinkle with salt and pepper. Cover and cook, stirring often, for 2 minutes or until just tender; add 1 to 2 tablespoons water if pan becomes dry. Transfer to a plate. Add 1 tablespoon butter or remaining oil to skillet and heat over low heat. Add garlic and sauté for 1 minute. Remove from heat. Return spinach to pan and mix well.

Add pasta to a large pot of boiling salted water and cook, uncovered, over high heat, stirring occasionally, for 8 minutes or until tender but firm to the bite. Drain, reserving about ¼ cup pasta cooking liquid. Transfer pasta to skillet with spinach and toss over low heat, adding a little pasta cooking liquid if mixture is too thick. Add tomatoes and toss gently. Add cheese and toss. Taste and adjust seasoning. Serve immediately.

Makes 3 servings

❧ TWO-WAY PASTA WITH
LIMA BEANS, BASIL, AND TOMATOES

Serve this colorful, easy-to-make pasta dish hot as a meatless main course or a partner for fish or chicken, or cool as a refreshing but nourishing salad for summertime buffets. You don't need to make a separate sauce; fruity extra virgin olive oil, along with the fresh basil and a little salt and pepper, are all you need to complement the pasta and the vegetables. When I serve it as a salad, I add a squeeze of fresh lemon or lime juice.

Lima beans contribute healthy vegetarian protein, but you can replace them with edamame or fresh fava beans, and the dish will still have a bright green color. To boost the nutrition even more, use whole wheat or soy pasta.

One 10-ounce package frozen baby lima beans
Salt
8 ounces medium pasta shells (about 3 cups), cooked, drained, and rinsed
2 large ripe tomatoes, cut into ½-inch dice
2 to 3 tablespoons extra virgin olive oil
⅓ cup finely chopped red onion

2 tablespoons chopped fresh basil leaves, or 2 teaspoons dried basil
Freshly ground black pepper
¼ cup sliced black olives (optional)
1 to 2 tablespoons strained fresh lemon juice (optional)

Add lima beans to a medium saucepan containing enough boiling water to cover them generously and cook, uncovered, over medium-high heat until just tender, about 7 minutes. Drain well.

Combine lima beans, pasta, and tomatoes in a large bowl and toss lightly.

In a small bowl, mix olive oil with onion, basil, salt, and pepper. Add to salad and toss until ingredients are coated. Add olives and lemon juice, if you like. Taste and adjust seasoning. Serve warm or at room temperature.

Makes 2 to 3 main-course or 4 side-dish servings

❊ SPEEDY SPIRAL PASTA
WITH SMOKED TURKEY AND TOMATOES

Garlic, olive oil, and oregano flavor this easy pasta entrée, which is convenient for serving during the holiday of Sukkot for a midweek meal in the sukkah. The sauce needs no cooking; you can warm it briefly in the microwave if you want to serve the pasta hot. Use smoked turkey slices, baked deli turkey, or home-cooked chicken or turkey. For a healthier dish, use whole wheat pasta. If you like, cook 1 cup frozen green beans or mixed vegetables with the pasta. To complete the meal, serve a green salad topped with toasted almonds.

2 to 4 tablespoons extra virgin olive oil
1 tablespoon wine vinegar (optional)
1 small garlic clove, minced
Salt and freshly ground black pepper
1 teaspoon dried oregano, crumbled
8 ounces ripe tomatoes, diced

1½ cups (6 ounces) thin strips of thin-sliced
  smoked turkey
8 to 9 ounces pasta spirals or shells, preferably
  whole grain
1 tablespoon chopped green onion or parsley

In a large bowl, combine 2 tablespoons oil, vinegar (if using), garlic, salt, pepper, and oregano. Add tomatoes and turkey and mix well.

Cook pasta, uncovered, in a large pot of boiling salted water over high heat, stirring occasionally, for 8 minutes or until tender but firm to the bite. Meanwhile, cover tomato mixture and microwave for 45 seconds to 1 minute or until just warm.

Drain pasta and add to tomato mixture. Mix well. Taste, adjust seasoning, and add more oil if needed. Sprinkle with green onion and serve hot, warm, or at room temperature.

Makes 4 servings

PENNE BOLOGNESE WITH A BONUS

At a restaurant with a "create your own pasta" feature on the menu, where diners could design their own dish from a selection of pastas, toppings, and sauces, I chose whole wheat penne (quill-shaped pasta) with spinach and toasted pine nuts. My husband suggested embellishing it with a masterpiece of Italian sauce making—Bolognese sauce. The dish was delicious and I was determined to make a healthy version.

To make my Bolognese sauce beefy but still healthy, I use a trick I learned long ago during my college years in Israel. For half the meat I use "cheaters' beef" made of soy. In those days the soy granules were frequently used by frugal Israeli cooks because meat was very expensive. To make meatballs or meat loaf, people mixed an equal part of this soy "meat" with ground beef, thus keeping the meaty taste.

You can use either soy ground "meat," which is available in log-shaped packages like ground beef, or buy dry packaged granules of TVP (textured vegetable protein), which you soak in water according to the package directions. Both have a texture similar to that of ground beef.

If you use all soy and omit the beef, you can add a few halved small mozzarella balls; put them in for the last minute or two, so the cheese begins to soften but keeps its enticing moist texture. Add sautéed mushroom chunks for another tasty variation.

2 to 3 tablespoons extra virgin olive oil

1 onion, minced

1 carrot, chopped

1 celery rib, chopped

6 ounces extra-lean ground beef

6 ounces soy "ground beef"—fresh or reconstituted dry granules

1 garlic clove, minced (optional)

Ground cloves or freshly grated nutmeg

Salt and freshly ground black pepper

¼ cup dry red wine

½ cup beef or chicken broth (optional)

One 14-ounce can tomatoes, drained and pureed in a food processor, or ⅓ cup tomato sauce

12 ounces to 1 pound fresh spinach, stems removed, leaves rinsed well, or 6 to 8 ounces frozen spinach, thawed

1 pound penne (diagonal-cut macaroni), preferably whole wheat

2 tablespoons pine nuts, lightly toasted

Heat 1 tablespoon oil in a heavy, medium saucepan. Add onion, carrot, and celery and cook over medium heat, stirring, for 10 minutes or until onion is soft but not brown; add 1 to 2 tablespoons water if pan becomes dry. Add ground beef and sauté over medium heat, crumbling with a fork, until it changes color. Add soy "meat," garlic, ground cloves to taste, and salt and pepper. Add wine and bring to a boil, stirring. Add broth, if desired, and return to a boil. Cover and cook over low heat, stirring from time to time, for 20 minutes, adding water if pan becomes dry. Add pureed tomatoes and cook, stirring often, for 10 minutes or until well flavored.

Boil a large pot of water, add fresh spinach, and return to a boil. Remove with a slotted spoon. Return water to a boil; add salt, then pasta. Cook, uncovered, over high heat, stirring occasionally, for 9 minutes or until tender but firm to the bite. Meanwhile, reheat sauce in a covered saucepan over medium-low heat.

Drain pasta and transfer to a large heated bowl. Add 1 to 2 tablespoons olive oil and toss with pasta. Add sauce and toss. Add spinach and toss lightly. Taste and adjust seasoning. Serve sprinkled with pine nuts.

Makes 4 main-course or 6 to 8 first-course servings

SAFFRON-SPICED SPAGHETTI SAUCE WITH YELLOW SPLIT PEAS

Persian cooks make sauces from yellow split peas by simmering them with diced meat, tomatoes, and sometimes with eggplant. By doing this they make good use of a small amount of beef or lamb, complementing it with the healthy protein of the legume. I use ground meat rather than diced meat so the sauce will cook faster. For a vegetarian version, you can omit the meat or use soy ground "meat." Unlike green split peas, the yellow ones usually hold their shape, and so the sauce is composed of pretty yellow disks.

Usually Persians serve the split pea sauce with basmati rice, but I also like it as spaghetti sauce, with whole wheat or other whole-grain or high-fiber spaghetti. You can also serve it with Persian toasted noodles, which resemble tan linguine, brown basmati rice, or whole wheat pita.

1 cup yellow split peas, sorted and rinsed (or green split peas, see Note)

3 cups water

1½ tablespoons vegetable oil or olive oil

1 large onion, halved and chopped

4 to 6 ounces lean ground lamb or beef

1 fairly small eggplant (about ¾ pound), diced small (about ½ inch)

Salt and freshly ground black pepper

½ teaspoon ground cinnamon

⅛ to ¼ teaspoon saffron threads, or ½ teaspoon turmeric

One 14-ounce can diced tomatoes, with their liquid

2 tablespoons tomato paste

1 to 2 tablespoons lemon juice, or to taste

1 tablespoon minced flat-leaf parsley

Combine split peas and water in a large saucepan and bring to a boil. Cover and simmer for 20 minutes or until peas are just tender, adding water if mixture becomes too thick.

Heat oil in a large, deep skillet. Add onion and sauté over medium heat for 5 minutes or until softened but not browned. Add lamb and sauté over medium heat, stirring often to crumble meat, for 5 minutes or until lamb changes color. Add eggplant, salt and pepper to taste, and mix well. Cover and continue cooking, stirring occasionally, for 5 minutes or until eggplant begins to soften. Add cinnamon, saffron, and tomatoes. Cover and cook for 15 minutes.

Mix tomato paste with ¼ cup water and add to meat sauce. Combine with split peas (either in saucepan or in skillet). Simmer for 5 to 10 minutes or until eggplant is tender and peas are well flavored; add a few tablespoons water if sauce is too thick. Stir in lemon juice. Taste and adjust seasoning. Serve hot, topped with parsley.

NOTE: If you are using green split peas instead of yellow ones, cook them in 4 cups water for 1 to 1¼ hours or until tender, adding water as needed.

Makes 4 to 5 servings

Desserts

According to Jewish tradition, when you eat a new fruit or one that has just come into season, you say a blessing to express your joy and thanks. What a perfect way to emphasize the pleasure of eating a fruit, the healthiest of desserts.

Another useful custom that I learned from my mother is to reserve eating a piece of cake mainly for Shabbat and holidays. I try to follow her example, as it helps prevent me from eating sweets too often.

Some fruit is so delicious that, with little or no embellishment, it satisfies the craving for dessert. Which fruit it is depends on personal taste. For my mother, it was fresh, sweet blueberries at the peak of their season. For my husband and me, the raspberries from our backyard vines and the fresh figs from our tree have long been at the top of our list. My editor at the *Jerusalem Post*, Liat Collins, told me that when she visited Oman in the Persian Gulf, she noticed they used dates for everything. "When we left," she said, "I bought dates instead of chocolates!"

Fruit can also be made into tasty desserts that are still beneficial from the standpoint of nutrition. Of course, you can make beautiful fruit salads, like Holiday of Love Fruit Salad (page 336). Puree fresh strawberries with yogurt and a little syrup or honey, and you'll have a healthy, cooling fruit soup. In hot weather make a luscious fruit shake from mangoes or peaches with yogurt, or a refreshing sorbet, like Ginger-Scented Plum Sorbet.

You can use whole grains to make satisfying, creamy sweet finales to a meal, as in Pareve Corn and Rice Pudding. Nuts are a healthful ingredient to turn into desserts, such as Hazelnut Macaroons for Passover (page 109) and Macadamia Orange Cake with Red Berry Sauce (page 108).

The good news for the sweet side of the menu is that chocolate is good for you! Dark chocolate is a great source of disease-fighting substances called antioxidants and substances similar to the heart-healthy compounds in green tea. Of course, it should be eaten in moderation because of its high calorie content. For a special treat, make it into Light and Creamy Chocolate Mousse with Grand Marnier (page 342).

TOO MANY STRAWBERRIES? TURN THEM INTO SOUP!

When I lived in a suburb of Tel Aviv, I loved to stop at Hakarmel market on my way home from work or from my classes at Tel Aviv University. It was such a pleasure to find so much fresh produce. When strawberries were in season, I always overbought. Those berries were so aromatic, beautiful, and enticing! Besides, many strawberry sellers wouldn't let me buy a small amount. I quickly learned that they spoiled rapidly, especially if left in the plastic bag that the vendor scooped them into.

Before refrigerating them, I tried to spread them out in a single layer on a tray, so they wouldn't crush each other. Although we eagerly savored them plain, with leben (a mild yogurt), in fruit salad, and on ice cream, I had trouble using them up fast enough, until my neighbor taught me how to make fruit soup, a popular dessert in Israel.

Strawberry soup is easy to make, refreshing, and perfect for late spring. You can sweeten fruit soup and enjoy it for dessert or leave it fairly tangy and serve it as a first course. Sweet berry soups are favorites in Eastern Europe, especially in Poland and Russia. Some people puree raw strawberries or raspberries and mix them with sugar, water, and sometimes white or rosé wine or lemon juice. Others cook the berries with the same ingredients, and then thicken the soup lightly with potato starch, cornstarch, or bread crumbs. Raw berries keep a fresher flavor and more of their perfume, but those cooked and thickened with starch give the soup a satisfying body. I like to combine both techniques, cooking some of the berries and leaving the rest raw.

Nearly as popular as berries for soup are cherries, apricots, plums, apples, and in winter, dried fruit. Some fruit soups, especially those made with blueberries, blackberries, or apples, call for spices like cinnamon, cloves, or cardamom, and might be sweetened with honey. In some homes the soups are served hot, but generally they are preferred cold.

Fruit soups can be clear, made only of the fruit in its sweet poaching liquid; or they can be made creamy. Polish strawberry soup is often enriched with sour cream, but to make mine lighter I use yogurt. It complements the berries nicely.

Holiday of Love Fruit Salad

Mango Yogurt Cooler

Svelte Isabelle's Peaches

Carrot Compote in Cinnamon Clove Syrup

Ginger-Scented Plum Sorbet

Sesame Sundae with Halvah, Date Syrup, and Fresh Figs

Light and Creamy Chocolate Mousse with Grand Marnier

Light Peach Trifle

Strawberry Shortcake in Seconds

Apple Cinnamon Tart

Double Pear Cake

Pareve Strawberry Crepes

Spirited Challah Kugel with Almonds and Fruit

Pareve Corn and Rice Pudding

HOLIDAY OF LOVE FRUIT SALAD

Tu B'Av is a minor biblical holiday that occurs in July or August (it means the fifteenth day of the month of Av). According to the Talmud, on this day young women danced in the vineyards so the men could see whom they liked. Some in Israel are reviving this holiday, as a sort of Jewish Valentine's Day.

Fresh figs are the perfect fruit for the holiday of love, given the fig tree's role in the story of Adam and Eve. (Indeed, some scholars say the fruit of temptation was the fig, not the apple!) Combine them in a colorful salad with wine, honey, and other foods associated with romance, such as grapes, bananas, and berries. Be sure all the fruit is perfectly ripe.

2 to 3 tablespoons white or red wine
1 tablespoon honey, or to taste
1 cup fresh figs, quartered lengthwise
½ cup raspberries

½ cup blueberries or grapes (optional)
3 ripe apricots, or 1 banana, peach, pear, or
   Asian pear

In a bowl mix wine and honey. Add figs, raspberries, and blueberries (if using). Slice apricots or other fruit and add. Mix very gently. Taste and add more wine or honey if desired. Serve cool.

Makes 2 servings

MANGO YOGURT COOLER

When making this refreshing, Indian style fruit and yogurt cooler called *lassi*, you can replace the mango with 4 sliced fresh peaches or nectarines (about 1 1/2 cups), 1 or 2 bananas, or 10 to 16 ounces frozen peaches, berries, or other frozen fruit. If using fresh peaches, increase the honey to 5 tablespoons, or to taste. If you opt for frozen fruit in syrup, use the syrup as the drink's sweetener and omit the honey. To make a pareve lassi, substitute 1 cup soy yogurt and 1 cup soy milk. If you like, serve the drink over ice cubes.

1 large or 2 medium mangoes (1 1/4 to 1 1/2 pounds), or 10 to 16 ounces frozen mango, thawed but still cold, or 1 to 1 1/4 cups canned mango pulp

2 cups nonfat plain or low-fat plain yogurt, or 1 cup plain yogurt and 1 cup milk
1 cup ice-cold water
2 to 3 tablespoons honey or sugar, or to taste

If using a fresh mango, hold it with one end pointing toward you. Cut downward on either side of flat pit, as near to pit as possible, cutting mango into two near-halves; a ring of mango meat will adhere to pit. On each mango half, score mango meat in cubes in a criss-cross pattern without piercing skin, then press from skin side upward; cubes of mango can then be removed easily with a spoon. Cut remaining mango meat from around pit and cut off peel from these pieces.

In a blender puree mango with yogurt, water, and honey until smooth and frothy. Taste and add more yogurt, water, or honey, according to desired consistency and sweetness. Serve in glasses.

Makes 4 servings

❧ SVELTE ISABELLE'S PEACHES

In France, peach desserts are generally served with a separate sauce. Take French chef Escoffier's famous creation, Peach Melba, which comes with a raspberry sauce and vanilla ice cream. Similarly, Pêches Eugénie, named for the wife of Napoleon III of France, is made of peaches, wild strawberries, and kirsch and accompanied by a champagne sabayon sauce.

The traditional Pêches Isabelle, also created by Escoffier, is a dessert of peaches macerated in sweetened red wine and served with Chantilly cream.

This version of the dessert is not only much lower in fat than the old-fashioned one; it is also much easier to prepare. Simply serve the peaches with a creamy peach sauce made from low-fat peach yogurt.

After you have served the peaches, if any of the wine syrup is left, you can reuse it to prepare more peaches in wine. If you make this dessert with nectarines instead of peaches, you don't need to peel them.

6 ripe peaches
¾ cup sugar
2 cups dry red wine, such as Cabernet Sauvignon
Four 6-ounce containers peach yogurt—low-fat,
    nonfat, or light

1 teaspoon pure vanilla extract
1 to 2 tablespoons low-fat or nonfat milk

If peaches are very ripe, peel them carefully with a vegetable peeler, holding them over a deep glass serving dish to catch juice that escapes. If this proves difficult, scald them in boiling water for ½ minute; drain, rinse, and peel with a knife. Cut peaches into quarters and put them in the glass serving dish.

Stir sugar into wine until dissolved. Pour mixture over peaches. If peaches are not covered with liquid, add enough water to cover them. Cover and refrigerate for 2 hours.

To make peach sauce, stir peach yogurt lightly in a bowl. Stir in vanilla and enough milk to make sauce pourable. Serve peaches cold, in their wine. Serve sauce separately.

Makes 6 servings

CARROT COMPOTE IN CINNAMON CLOVE SYRUP

Moroccan Jews make preserves and jams from vegetables as well as fruit. This refreshing dessert is in the spirit of such recipes, but instead of making jam or preserves, I poach the carrots in a much lighter syrup, scented with cinnamon, cloves, and lemon. If you like, add dried cherries or dried cranberries along with or instead of the raisins. Instead of sugar, you can use natural sweeteners like agave nectar or brown rice syrup; they are available at natural foods stores.

Using carrots as dessert is not so surprising; after all, carrot cake is one of the most popular American treats. You can also serve these carrots as a sweet side dish or a sweet appetizer soup, with lime or lemon wedges.

1½ pounds carrots, sliced about ¼ inch thick
3 cups water
Pinch of salt
1 cinnamon stick, or ¾ teaspoon ground cinnamon
2 whole cloves, or pinch of ground cloves

¼ cup sugar
¼ cup honey or additional sugar
1½ to 2 tablespoons fresh lemon or lime juice
½ cup raisins

Combine carrots, water, and salt in a heavy saucepan with cinnamon stick and whole cloves, but not with ground spices. Bring to a boil. Cover and simmer over medium-low heat for 7 minutes.

Add sugar, honey, ground cinnamon, and ground cloves to pan. Stir gently to blend in sugar and bring to a simmer. Cover and cook over medium-low heat for 5 minutes or until carrots are tender and well flavored. Add lemon juice and raisins.

Let carrots stand in syrup for at least 4 hours to absorb flavors; or refrigerate in a covered container until ready to serve. Serve cold as dessert or as an appetizer soup or warm as a side dish. Serve carrots in small dessert dishes with some of their syrup.

Makes 4 to 6 servings

Sorbets are fat-free, pareve, and easy to make. The syrup is the key to their seductive smoothness and sweetness. There's nothing complicated about making it. You bring sugar and water to a boil and cook it for 1 minute. For a more complex flavor, you can first infuse the syrup with vanilla beans, cinnamon sticks, fresh ginger or candied ginger, lemon or orange zest, fresh mint or, for a more unusual note, rosemary, thyme, or tarragon. Lemon juice is a good addition when fruit lack acidity.

Plums are high in disease-fighting antioxidants, and so it's good to include them on the menu often. Red-fleshed plums give this sorbet a lovely color. If you prefer, substitute a vanilla bean for the ginger, or red wine for half the water. You can serve the sorbet sprinkled with plum brandy.

1½ cups sugar
1 cup water

3 to 5 tablespoons sliced candied ginger
3 pounds ripe plums, preferably red–fleshed, halved

Combine sugar, water, and 3 tablespoons candied ginger in a heavy saucepan. Cook over low heat, stirring gently, until sugar dissolves. Bring to a boil over high heat. Add plums. Cover and cook plums over low heat about 12 minutes or until tender when pierced with a sharp knife. Cool in syrup. Refrigerate for 30 minutes.

Remove plums from poaching syrup; reserve syrup, removing ginger slices. Remove any pits from plums. Puree plums with 1¼ cups poaching syrup in a food processor or blender. For a smoother sorbet, strain mixture into a bowl, pressing gently on pulp in strainer; with rubber spatula, scrape remaining puree from underside of strainer.

Stir mixture until smooth. Taste; if you would like a more prominent ginger flavor, mince 1 to 2 tablespoons reserved candied ginger and stir into mixture. Add more syrup if needed; mixture should taste a little too sweet at this point because sweetness of sorbet will be less apparent when it is frozen.

Chill medium metal bowl and airtight container in freezer. Transfer sorbet mixture to ice cream machine and process according to manufacturer's instructions until mixture has consistency of soft ice cream; it should not be runny but will not become very firm. Transfer sorbet as quickly as possible to chilled bowl; sorbet melts very quickly. Cover tightly and freeze until ready to serve.

To keep sorbet longer than 3 hours, transfer it when firm to airtight container and cover tightly. When serving sorbet, if it is frozen solid, soften it by pulsing briefly in food processor, and serve immediately. If you like, garnish with more candied ginger.

Makes 3 to 4 cups, or 6 to 8 servings

SESAME SUNDAE
WITH HALVAH, DATE SYRUP, AND FRESH FIGS

Date syrup, like carob syrup, resembles chocolate syrup in consistency. Some say that this syrup is actually the "honey" referred to in the Torah as one of the Seven Species. You'll find it in Israeli markets as *silan*. It's great partnered with a popular Middle Eastern treat: halvah. This wonderful sesame sweet is traditionally served on its own like candy, but is increasingly used in modern Israeli desserts. Choose good-quality halvah. I prefer the classic type made without the addition of hydrogenated fat. For this sundae you can use pistachio, vanilla, chocolate, or marbled halvah, and match it with any fruit you like.

4 ounces sesame halvah, plain or pistachio
4 fresh figs, quartered
1 orange, peeled and cut into segments
1 banana, sliced
1 pint light vanilla ice cream or frozen yogurt

¼ to ½ cup date, carob, chocolate, or strawberry syrup
2 teaspoons toasted sesame seeds or toasted slivered almonds (see pages 380 and 379)

Put halvah in a bowl and use a spoon to divide it in small chunks of ½ to 1 teaspoon each; don't worry if it crumbles. Mix quartered figs, orange segments, and banana slices in another bowl.

At serving time, scoop ice cream into 4 dessert dishes or sundae glasses. Spoon fruit and halvah around edges of dish, and pour a little date syrup over ice cream. Sprinkle with sesame seeds. Serve immediately, with more syrup on the side.

Makes 4 servings

LIGHT AND CREAMY CHOCOLATE MOUSSE WITH GRAND MARNIER

When research came out that dark chocolate is healthy, the news traveled fast. Nearly everyone was happy to learn that dark chocolate is high in important disease-fighting antioxidants. Of course, if you're using it in recipes, you don't want to negate its healthy qualities by adding saturated or trans fats.

This recipe gains its richness from the chocolate, and needs no egg yolks or whipped cream. You can make it pareve but still creamy by melting the chocolate in soy milk or other nondairy milk.

7 ounces fine-quality semisweet or bittersweet
   chocolate, chopped
½ cup low-fat milk or soy milk
5 large egg whites
2 tablespoons sugar

1 tablespoon Grand Marnier
2 teaspoons grated orange zest
4 or 5 chocolate-coated nuts, or small pieces
   chocolate-coated or candied orange peel, or
   candied violets (optional)

Melt chocolate in milk in a medium bowl set above hot water over low heat. Stir until smooth. Remove from water; cool for 3 minutes.

In a large dry bowl, whip egg whites to soft peaks. Gradually beat in sugar; whip at high speed until whites are stiff and shiny but not dry.

Stir Grand Marnier and orange zest into chocolate. Fold in about one-quarter of whites until blended. Spoon mixture over remaining whites; fold gently just until blended. Divide among 4 or 5 small ramekins. Refrigerate for 3 hours or up to 1 day; if keeping for longer than 3 hours, cover after mousse has set.

Serve garnished with chocolate-coated nuts, if you like.

Makes 4 to 5 servings

The British originated the trifle, a delicious dessert of sherry-soaked cake layered with custard and fruit or jam. It comes in many variations, some substituting other spirits or fruit juice for the sherry, others using whipped cream instead of custard, still others using both. Although it is luxurious, it can be made into a fairly nutritious dessert.

Sponge cake is the traditional cake for trifle, but macaroons are popular choices and angel food cake works well too. The fruit layer can be jam, preserves, canned or frozen fruit, or fresh soft fruit. Trifle is a good way to utilize leftover sweets of all sorts, and perhaps this homey nature is behind its name.

The custard for trifle is usually a pastry cream resembling an éclair filling—a sweet creamy sauce thickened with cornstarch or flour. This rich-tasting version features a light vanilla custard, blended with vanilla yogurt and layered with sherry-soaked ladyfingers, fresh peaches, and apricot preserves. For the healthiest choices, use low-fat or nonfat milk and yogurt to make the custard. To make the dessert pareve, substitute soy milk for the milk and soy yogurt for the dairy yogurt. Use a wide-bottomed glass bowl or glass soufflé dish so the layers are visible.

To peel the peaches, scald them for 1 minute in boiling water, then transfer them briefly to a bowl of cold water. If you'd rather skip this step, substitute nectarines. Instead of half the peaches, you can also substitute pitted halved cherries, raspberries, or blueberries.

2 tablespoons cornstarch

1½ cups milk

1 large egg

1 large egg yolk (optional)

3 tablespoons sugar, or to taste

1 teaspoon pure vanilla extract

About 3½ ounces ladyfingers

½ cup sherry or ¼ cup kirsch (clear cherry brandy)

½ cup vanilla yogurt

⅓ cup apricot preserves

2 cups peeled, sliced peaches

6 to 8 peach slices, strawberries, or fresh cherries, stems trimmed short

Mix cornstarch with 2 tablespoons milk in a small cup. Heat remaining milk in a small, heavy saucepan until bubbles form around edge of pan. Whisk egg and yolk (if using) in a medium bowl. Add sugar; whisk until blended. Whisk in dissolved cornstarch. Gradually whisk in hot milk. Return mixture to saucepan. Cook over medium-low heat, whisking constantly, for 3 minutes or until mixture thickens slightly and reaches 160°F on an instant-read thermometer or a candy thermometer. Do not boil. Remove from heat. Stir 1 minute. Let cool, stirring occasionally. Whisk in vanilla. Cover and refrigerate for 1 to 2 hours.

Put enough ladyfingers in a 1½-quart glass bowl or deep baking dish to make one layer. Brush ¼ cup sherry or 2 tablespoons kirsch evenly over them. Stir custard until smooth. Stir in yogurt and more sugar if desired. Pour ¾ cup custard mixture over ladyfingers in bowl. Cover and refrigerate for 1 to 2 hours to firm custard slightly.

Heat preserves until melted in a small saucepan over low heat, stirring occasionally. Strain if you like. Arrange remaining ladyfingers in one layer on custard in bowl. Brush with remaining sherry or kirsch. Scatter 2 cups fresh peaches on top. Spoon preserves evenly over them. Carefully spoon remaining custard on top. Cover and refrigerate for 2 hours. Serve garnished with fruit.

Makes 6 to 8 servings

This technique is good when you want to use up leftover cakes before Passover, or whenever you need a fast, healthy dessert.

Any kind of cake will work in this dessert, and since the cake is cut in thin strips, a little goes a long way. Opt for lower-calorie cakes, such as angel food, vanilla, or chocolate sponge cake or ladyfingers. Even sliced breakfast "health" muffins, such as bran or banana-walnut, make good shortcakes.

Instead of the usual high-fat whipped cream of most strawberry shortcakes, the mixture of vanilla yogurt and low-fat sour cream makes a light and tasty topping. If you prefer, use only vanilla yogurt or only low-fat sour cream. If you use noncaloric sweeteners, to reduce the sugar content, substitute one such as sucralose for half the sugar.

You can make this incredibly easy dessert with other berries and many other fruit. Peaches, bananas, mangoes, or tender ripe pears are good choices, or indeed any soft fruit. If you have poached or canned fruit in syrup on hand, use a little of the syrup to moisten the cake. If you like, sprinkle the cake lightly with fruit-flavored spirits, such as Grand Marnier or kirsch.

1 to 1½ cups fresh strawberries, rinsed, hulled, and
  sliced lengthwise
2 to 3 tablespoons sugar
½ cup low-fat or nonfat vanilla yogurt

½ cup low-fat sour cream
½ to 1 teaspoon pure vanilla extract
8 thin small slices of cake without frosting, cut into
  strips

Sprinkle strawberry slices evenly with 1 tablespoon sugar, or more to taste. In a bowl mix yogurt with sour cream, remaining sugar, and vanilla. Divide cake strips among 4 plates or shallow dessert dishes. Top cake with most of the berries. Spoon ¼ cup sour cream mixture onto center of each dessert, partially covering berries and cake. Arrange remaining berry slices decoratively on top, or around dollop of sour cream. Serve cold.

Makes 4 servings

✠ APPLE CINNAMON TART

The French often refer to fruit tarts with a yeast-dough base as country tarts, because this type of dough gives them a rustic appearance. The delicious result is like a breakfast yeast cake crowned with fruit. This one is topped with sautéed apple slices and a buttery cinnamon-sugar topping. It's great as a Sukkot dessert or for breakfast on Shabbat.

Make the dough by any of the methods below. The food processor is fastest; the dough is ready in less than 3 minutes!

YEAST CAKE DOUGH

One ¼-ounce package yeast, or 2½ teaspoons
  active dry yeast, or a ⅗-ounce cake fresh yeast
¾ cup warm water (105°F to 115°F)
1 tablespoon sugar
1½ cups whole wheat flour
1½ cups all-purpose flour
1 teaspoon salt
2 large eggs
⅓ cup vegetable oil

APPLE CINNAMON TOPPING

1 pound sweet apples, such as Fuji, Gala, or
  Golden Delicious
2 tablespoons vegetable oil
5 tablespoons sugar
1 teaspoon ground cinnamon
2 tablespoons cold unsalted butter

Sprinkle dried yeast or crumble fresh yeast over ¼ cup warm water in a small bowl and add 1 teaspoon sugar; if using fresh yeast, stir to blend. Let yeast mixture stand for 10 minutes. Oil a medium or large glass bowl.

To make dough in a food processor: combine both types of flour, salt, and 2 teaspoons sugar in a large food processor with a dough blade or metal blade. Process briefly to blend. Add eggs. With machine running, quickly pour in yeast mixture and remaining ½ cup water. Process for 1 minute to knead dough. Add oil and process until it is absorbed. The dough will be soft and sticky. (To use a mixer or make the dough by hand, see Notes.)

On a lightly floured surface, shape dough in a rough ball. Transfer it to oiled bowl and turn it over to oil its surface. Cover with plastic wrap and let rise in a warm, draft-free place for 1 hour or until nearly double in volume.

Lightly grease two baking sheets. Divide dough in 2 equal parts. Place each on a baking sheet and pat with lightly floured hands to a 10-inch circle, with a 1-inch rim slightly higher than center.

To make topping: peel apples and slice thin. Heat oil in a large skillet. Add apples and sauté over medium heat for 5 minutes or until nearly tender. Sprinkle with 3 tablespoons sugar and toss over low heat until coated.

Mix remaining 2 tablespoons sugar with cinnamon. Arrange apple slices in an even layer over dough. Cut chilled butter into very thin slices, about ⅛ inch thick, and scatter them over apples. Sprinkle with cinnamon-sugar mixture. Let cakes rise for 15 minutes. Meanwhile, position rack in center of oven and preheat to 425°F.

Bake for 20 minutes or until dough browns and apples are tender. Serve warm or at room temperature. Serve tart on day it was baked; or freeze tart and reheat it in a low oven (not a microwave) before serving.

NOTES: To make dough in a mixer: sift both types of flour into bowl of a sturdy mixer with a dough hook. Make a large well in center of flour, and add in yeast mixture, remaining ½ cup water, eggs, oil, 2 teaspoons sugar, and salt. Mix at medium-low speed, pushing flour in gradually and occasionally scraping dough down from bowl and hook, until ingredients form a soft dough. Mix at medium speed to knead dough for 7 minutes or until it almost cleans bowl's sides and is smooth and elastic.

To make dough by hand: sift both types of flour into a large bowl. Make a large well in center and add in yeast mixture, remaining ½ cup water, eggs, oil, 2 teaspoons sugar, and salt. Mix ingredients in well. Stir in flour, first with a wooden spoon and then with your hands. Transfer dough to a lightly floured work surface and knead it until smooth and springy, lightly flouring it if necessary.

Makes 2 tarts, 4 to 6 servings each

❧ DOUBLE PEAR CAKE

Fresh and dried pears in a flavorful honey-lemon batter make this cake an enticing sweet. Soaking the dried pears in pear brandy adds extra pizzazz. Low in saturated fat and cholesterol, the cake is enhanced in both taste and nutrition by a small amount of walnuts. To further increase the cake's nutritional value, you can make it with olive oil. Light olive oil is a good choice; or use a mixture of vegetable oil and olive oil. Along with the oil and honey, applesauce helps to keep the cake moist. Another advantage of this cake—it is pareve and very good for Shabbat or Rosh Hashanah. If you like, serve it lightly dusted with powdered sugar and accompanied by additional slices of fresh and dried pears.

5 dried pear halves, finely chopped
1 tablespoon pear brandy, rum, or any fruit liqueur
¾ cup sugar
1 teaspoon ground cinnamon
1½ cups all-purpose flour
1¼ teaspoons baking powder
¼ teaspoon baking soda
2 small ripe juicy pears (total ¾ pound)

2 large eggs
⅓ cup honey
6 tablespoons vegetable oil
¼ cup applesauce
1 teaspoon finely grated lemon zest
2 tablespoons lemon juice
1 tablespoon water
3 to 4 tablespoons chopped walnuts

Combine dried pears and brandy in a small jar. Cover tightly and let stand for 4 hours or overnight.

Preheat oven to 350°F. Lightly oil an 8-inch square pan, line it with foil and lightly oil and flour foil. Mix 1 tablespoon sugar with cinnamon. Sift flour, baking powder, and baking soda. Pare, halve, core, and slice fresh pears thin, under ¼ inch thick; set aside. In a mixer beat eggs with remaining sugar on medium speed for 3 minutes or until light. Add honey, oil, applesauce, and lemon zest and beat to blend. In a small cup, mix lemon juice and water. With mixer on low speed, add flour mixture and lemon juice alternately in 3 batches. Blend in dried pears with any brandy left in jar. Add walnuts; blend on low.

Spoon about a third of cake batter into pan. Smooth with rubber spatula. Arrange about half of pear slices on batter in one layer without letting them touch sides of pan and sprinkle with 2 teaspoons sugar-cinnamon mixture. Carefully spoon another third of batter over pears without moving them and spread it smooth. Arrange another layer of pears and sprinkle with remaining sugar-cinnamon mixture. Carefully spoon remaining batter over pears. Gently spread it smooth. Pears may peek through in spots.

Bake about 40 minutes or until cake is done; a cake tester inserted in cake's center should come out dry. Cool cake in pan on a rack about 30 minutes. Run a metal spatula carefully around cake and turn out onto rack. Let cool before serving.

Makes 9 to 10 servings

When you want a dairy-free strawberry sweet that's more substantial than fruit salad, these crepes fit the bill. For nutritious crepes, you can use whole wheat flour and soy milk. To make the crepes lower in fat and cholesterol, make the batter with egg whites instead of all whole eggs. The result is tasty, healthy, and pareve.

The flavor of strawberries is more vivid when they are raw. For a simple filling, you could mix sliced berries with a little sugar, fold them inside the crepes, and serve them at room temperature. This might be welcome on a hot summer day, but it would feel like fruit salad inside a crepe.

A thicker, cooked filling is more satisfying. However, cooked strawberries don't have enough body to stand on their own as a filling. And if you thicken the cooked berries with cornstarch or flour, the filling would be heavy and sticky.

The solution is to mix the fresh berries with a cooked fruit. Apples are a good choice, as they cook to a thick compote that gives the filling a denser texture but doesn't overwhelm the taste of the berries, the way prunes would.

Stirring a little strawberry jam or preserves into the filling further boosts the berry flavor. Serve the crepes with a liberal amount of sliced and pureed raw berries, and the dessert will be bright and fragrant, like strawberry fields in springtime.

¼ cup all-purpose flour

¼ cup whole wheat flour or additional all-purpose flour

½ teaspoon salt

3 tablespoons plus ½ teaspoon sugar, or to taste

2 large eggs, or 1 egg and 1 egg white

¾ to 1 cup soy milk or water

4 tablespoons vegetable oil, plus a few teaspoons for pan

1 pound tender apples, such as Golden Delicious, peeled and sliced thin

2 tablespoons strawberry jam or preserves

½ cup halved sliced strawberries

Red Berry Sauce (page 372)

Sift together both types of flour, salt, and ½ teaspoon sugar. In a blender combine eggs, ¾ cup soy milk, and flour mixture. Blend on high speed for 1 minute or until batter is smooth. Strain batter if it is lumpy. Cover and refrigerate about 1 hour or up to 1 day.

Stir batter well. Gradually whisk in 2 tablespoons oil. Batter should have consistency of whipping cream. If it is too thick, gradually whisk in water, about 1 teaspoon at a time.

Heat a crepe pan or skillet with a 6-inch base, preferably nonstick, over medium-high heat. Sprinkle with a few drops of water; when pan is hot enough, water should sizzle immediately. Brush pan lightly with oil. Remove pan from heat and quickly add 2 tablespoons batter to one edge, tilting and swirling pan until base is covered with a thin layer of batter. Immediately pour any excess batter back into bowl.

Return pan to medium-high heat. Loosen edges of crepe with a metal spatula, discarding any pieces clinging to sides of pan. Cook until bottom browns lightly. Slide spatula under crepe and turn carefully. Cook until second side browns lightly in spots. Slide crepe onto a plate. Reheat pan a few seconds. Continue making crepes, stirring batter occasionally. If first crepes are too thick, whisk a teaspoon of water into batter. Adjust heat and add more oil to pan if necessary.

Heat 2 tablespoons oil in a large skillet. Add apples and sauté over medium-high heat for 2 minutes. Cover and cook over low heat for 10 minutes or until apples are tender. Add 3 tablespoons sugar and cook over medium-high heat, stirring, until mixture thickens. Remove from heat and stir in strawberry jam and sliced strawberries and cook over low heat for 2 minutes. Taste and add more sugar if needed.

Gently spread 1 tablespoon filling on each crepe and roll it up lightly or fold it in four. If you like, put filled crepes in an oiled baking dish and keep them warm, loosely covered, in a low oven (about 300°F). Serve with sauce.

NOTE: To make crepes ahead, pile them on a plate as they are done. You can keep them, covered tightly, for 3 days in refrigerator; or you can freeze them.

Makes about 4 servings

SPIRITED CHALLAH KUGEL
WITH ALMONDS AND FRUIT

Traditional Jewish cooks make sweet kugel not only from noodles, but also from rice and from challah. This one is partly inspired by New Orleans–style bread puddings, which are often served with a rich whiskey sauce. Instead of making a high-calorie sauce, here's a trick I learned in France to add spirits: I soak raisins or dried cranberries in whiskey or rum and stir them into the kugel mixture. If you like, you can double the raisins and whiskey, and stir the mixture into warm applesauce, for a lively accompaniment to the kugel. To make the kugel seem creamy, I soak the challah in low-fat milk or, for a pareve version, soy milk. Use whole wheat challah or other whole wheat bread for the best nutrition.

⅓ cup raisins or dried cranberries, rinsed with hot
    water
2 tablespoons whiskey or rum
4 ounces (4 thick slices) stale challah, preferably
    whole wheat, crust removed
1¼ cups low-fat milk or soy milk
6 tablespoons sugar
1 teaspoon ground cinnamon

¾ pound ripe pears or sweet apples, such as Golden
    Delicious or Gala
2 eggs, separated
1 teaspoon grated lemon zest
⅓ cup chopped almonds
2 tablespoons butter or healthy margarine, cut into
    small pieces, or vegetable oil

Combine raisins and whiskey in a jar; cover and let stand for 30 minutes. Preheat oven to 400°F. Grease a 5-cup baking dish. Cut bread into cubes and put them in a medium bowl. Bring milk to a simmer in a small saucepan and pour it over bread. Let stand a few minutes so bread absorbs milk.

Mix 1 tablespoon sugar with ½ teaspoon cinnamon. Peel and core pears or apples. Slice very thin.

Mash bread with a fork. Stir in 3 tablespoons sugar. Add remaining ½ teaspoon cinnamon, egg yolks, lemon zest, pears, almonds, and raisins, with their whiskey. Mix well.

Beat egg whites to soft peaks. Beat in remaining 2 tablespoons sugar and whip until stiff and shiny. Fold whites, in 2 portions, into bread mixture. Transfer to baking dish. Sprinkle with reserved sugar-cinnamon mixture. Scatter butter pieces or drizzle oil on top.

Bake for 40 to 50 minutes or until a toothpick inserted in center comes out dry. Serve hot or warm.

Makes 6 servings

PAREVE CORN AND RICE PUDDING

When I sampled Filipino ginataang mais, a creamy corn and rice pudding with coconut milk, my first spoonful took me back to Paris. I thought of my friend Somchit Singchalee, a Thai chef who taught my husband and me how to make luscious warm coconut-milk desserts with such ingredients as tapioca and taro root (a pota-tolike tuber).

We discovered that Filipinos have a whole category of similar warm coconut-milk desserts, including some with supersweet purple yams and tropical fruit. We also discovered such enticing desserts at a Viet-namese eatery.

Notwithstanding coconut's saturated fat, some nutritionists feel that it has redeeming qualities. While these opinions go against the advice of mainstream health professionals, most agree that once in a while, it's okay to indulge in luscious foods like butter, cream, and coconut milk.

Instead of using all coconut milk, I cook the rice in soy milk or rice milk and add just a little coconut milk. If you like, omit the coconut milk and garnish the finished pudding with a sprinkling of lightly toasted shredded coconut or chopped nuts. Another way to introduce coconut flavor without added fat is to stir a few drops of coconut extract into the finished pudding.

You can vary the proportions and the type of rice, and this dessert will still be delicious. I use risotto rice, which is easier to find in most supermarkets than Asian sticky rice; but any short-grain or medium-grain rice works well. If you want to use brown rice, cook it for 30 minutes in the first step of the recipe. Instead of sugar, you can add evaporated cane juice or beige-colored natural sugar, which is less refined than white sugar.

¾ cup rice, preferably short-grain rice
2½ to 3 cups soy milk
Pinch of salt
½ cup canned coconut milk, preferably light, or
    additional soy milk
1 cup frozen or canned corn

⅓ cup sugar, or half sugar and half noncaloric
    sweetener
Coconut extract to taste (optional, if not using
    coconut milk)
Toasted grated coconut or toasted slivered almonds
    (optional)

Bring 6 cups water to a boil in a large, heavy saucepan and add rice. Boil, uncovered, for 7 minutes; drain well.

Bring 2½ cups soy milk to a boil in same saucepan. Add rice and salt. Return to a simmer. Stir in coconut milk. Cook, uncovered, over medium-low heat, stirring often, for 10 minutes. Add corn and bring to a simmer, stirring. Cook for 5 to 7 minutes or until rice and corn are very soft and absorb the milk. If they absorb the milk before becoming soft, gradually add a few more tablespoons soy milk or water and continue to cook. Pudding should be creamy, not soupy and not dry.

Stir in sugar and cook over low heat for 1 minute, stirring; if using sweetener that is sensitive to heat, add it off heat. Taste and add more sugar if needed and coconut extract, if using. Serve warm, sprinkled, if you like, with toasted coconut.

Makes 4 servings

Basics

✿

These recipes and techniques are useful for a variety of dishes. Some preparations, like chicken broth, tomato sauce, vinaigrette, and hummus, can be bought ready-made but are much fresher and better when they are homemade.

Use this chapter as a reference when you need to refresh your memory for such techniques as cooking beans, toasting nuts, and peeling tomatoes.

A BRIEF OVERVIEW OF KEEPING KOSHER

*A*ll the recipes in this book are kosher. Keeping kosher is a way of life. Kashrut, the laws regarding keeping kosher, involves shopping for the right foods, combining them properly in menus and recipes, and using the right dishes and utensils to prepare them. Keeping kosher is not difficult once you're familiar with a few rules.

In a kosher menu, meat foods and dairy foods must be kept completely separate. Meals are categorized according to whether they include meat or dairy. "Fleishig" meals in Yiddish or "bsari" in Hebrew are those that include meat, and "milkchig" (Yiddish) or "halavi" (Hebrew) meals contain dairy products. The third category is "pareve" (Yiddish) meals, or "stami" (Hebrew), which has neither meat nor milk products. Pareve, or neutral foods, can be served in any kind of meal. These include eggs, vegetables, fruits, grains, and oils. Fish is also pareve, but should not be served on the same plate as meat.

After eating meat, many Orthodox Jews wait for 6 hours before eating dairy foods. Meat and dairy must be cooked and served using separate pans, dishes, and utensils. On Passover, separate Passover meat and dairy pans, dishes, and utensils must be used.

This is why many people insist on buying only prepared foods that have been certified as kosher. Even an ingredient like canned vegetables, in theory, might have been processed in a pan used to prepare meat, if it doesn't have the assurance that the food is kosher. For the same reason, many buy bread only at a kosher bakery or with a kosher label, to be sure the same machines were not used to mix dough containing lard.

Kosher labels have symbols to make them easy to recognize. The best-known one is O-U, the seal of approval of the Union of Orthodox Jewish Congregations. Some products are labeled with K for Kosher. There also are many local kosher symbols.

MEAT AND POULTRY

Kosher animals are those that have split hooves and chew their cud. Beef, veal, lamb, and goat are kosher animals. Only meat cuts from the forequarter of the animal are kosher. Poultry—chicken, turkey, ducks, geese, and Cornish hens—is also kosher.

To be kosher, the animals and birds must be slaughtered by a kosher butcher according to specific rules. The meat and poultry must then be salted or "kashered" with coarse kosher salt, to remove as much blood as possible. This is usually done by the butcher or packager.

You can purchase kosher meat and poultry at kosher butcher shops or kosher markets, or in packages with certified kosher labels at supermarkets.

Because kosher meat and poultry have been salted, they taste like meat that has been brined. How salty the meat tastes often depends on the size or shape of the piece of meat. Before roasting or grilling it, you don't need to season it with salt. If you're using it in a soup or stew, you can salt it lightly and once it's cooked, taste before adding any more. Some people soak kosher meat and poultry in water for 30 minutes to reduce its sodium content.

Meat is cooked until well done in the kosher kitchen, and never rare, because of the Torah's prohibition against eating blood.

DAIRY FOODS

Many hard cheeses are made with an animal product called rennet, which helps the milk to coagulate. Kosher cheeses must be made without it. Instead, vegetable or microbial rennet is used.

Soft dairy products, such as yogurt, cannot contain nonkosher gelatin, which is made with animal bones. If gelatin is used, it must be kosher gelatin, which is vegetable based.

Kosher dairy foods are found at kosher markets, natural foods stores, and many supermarkets.

FISH

Kosher fish have scales and fins. They include most of the familiar fish at the market, like salmon, halibut, and trout, but not monkfish or shark. Fish do not require salting or any special treatment to become kosher, and can be cooked any way.

EGGS

Eggs that have blood spots are not kosher and must be discarded. When making batters, you first break each egg into a separate dish in order to check it, and then add it to the batter.

PRODUCE

All fresh vegetables and fruits are kosher. They must be rinsed carefully and inspected to be sure they contain no bugs.

RECIPES

Light and Easy Eggplant Dip

Healthy Hummus

Basic Brown Rice Pilaf

Easy Green Chile Garlic Relish—Zehug

Spicy Salsa, Israeli Style

Olive Oil and Lemon Dressing

Sesame Ginger Dressing

Tomato Sauce

Speedy Brown Sauce

Chicken Broth or Stock

Vegetable Broth

Quick Fish Stock

Red Berry Sauce

Spiced Chocolate Wine Glaze

Turkish Lemon Syrup

❦

TECHNIQUES

BROILED EGGPLANT SLICES

BROILED PEPPERS AND CHILES

PEELED TOMATOES

SEEDED TOMATOES

COOKED BEANS

TOASTED ALMONDS

TOASTED PINE NUTS

TOASTED HAZELNUTS

TOASTED WALNUTS AND PECANS

TOASTED SESAME SEEDS

❦

❊ LIGHT AND EASY EGGPLANT DIP

Use this dip as an appetizer with whole wheat pita or healthy crackers, or as a spread for sandwiches such as Three-Way Submarines (page 225).

The first paragraph of the recipe is the basic method for baking, broiling, or grilling whole eggplants.

One 1- to 1¼-pound eggplant, or 3 or 4 Japanese eggplants

1 minced garlic clove

2 to 3 tablespoons light mayonnaise, or 2 tablespoons tahini paste, or 1 to 2 tablespoons extra virgin olive oil

Salt and freshly ground black pepper

1 tablespoon lemon juice, or to taste

Pierce eggplant a few times with a fork. Bake large eggplant whole on a foil-lined baking sheet at 400°F for 1 hour, turning once; or broil or grill it for 40 to 50 minutes, turning occasionally, until very tender. If using Japanese eggplants, bake for about 25 minutes, or broil for about 15 minutes. Cool eggplant slightly, remove cap, halve eggplant, and scoop out its meat with a spoon.

Chop eggplant fine with a knife or pulse it in a food processor, taking care not to overprocess it so it won't liquefy. Transfer eggplant to a bowl. Add minced garlic, mayonnaise, and salt, pepper, and lemon juice to taste. If using tahini, stir in 1 to 2 tablespoons water if dip is too thick.

Makes 3 to 4 servings

At natural foods stores and many supermarkets you'll find hummus in a dizzying array of flavors, from chipotle to sun-dried tomato to olive to black bean; but hummus mavens prefer it plain, and it's better and fresher when homemade. It's healthier too, because you can adjust the fat and salt contents to your needs. Many of the packaged varieties are dense and high in fat and calories.

Spread healthy hummus on bread as a snack or when making a submarine (page 225) or other sandwich, or serve it as a dip, sprinkled lightly with extra virgin olive oil, minced flat-leaf parsley, and ground hot or sweet red pepper.

Stir the tahini paste before using it; often the thinner, oily part is on top and the more solid part sinks to the bottom. If you don't have tahini paste on hand, you can substitute 1½ or 2 tablespoons olive oil; in this case you'll need only about 1 or 2 tablespoons water. If your chickpeas are home-cooked rather than canned, use the cooking liquid instead of the water in the recipe.

1 large garlic clove, peeled
One 15-ounce can chickpeas (garbanzo beans),
    drained and rinsed, or 1½ cups cooked
    chickpeas (page 378), drained, liquid reserved
1½ to 2 tablespoons tahini (sesame paste)
2 tablespoons strained fresh lemon juice, or more
    to taste

¼ to ½ teaspoon ground cumin
About ¼ cup water
Salt
Cayenne pepper

Mince garlic in a food processor. Add chickpeas and process to chop. Add tahini, lemon juice, cumin, and 2 tablespoons water or chickpea cooking liquid and puree until finely blended. Add more water by tablespoons if mixture is too thick; it should have consistency of a smooth spread. Season with salt and cayenne to taste.

Makes about 4 servings

I usually prepare brown rice as a simple pilaf because I like the flavor the grains acquire from being very lightly sautéed before they are moistened with liquid. When I lived in Israel, I adopted this popular way to prepare rice, and I have used it ever since.

It's worth preparing enough pilaf for at least two meals because brown rice is a healthy whole grain that is good to have on hand. Refrigerate or freeze the extra portions, then reheat them in a covered dish in the microwave when you need them.

Whether to add salt is up to you and depends on how you intend to use the rice. You can prepare it without salt, like Chinese steamed rice, in case you'll be serving it with sauces that already include salty ingredients.

If you want plain cooked brown rice, omit the oil and the step of sautéing (see Note).

2 to 3 teaspoons vegetable oil or olive oil
2 cups long-grain or short-grain brown rice
4 cups hot vegetable or chicken broth, vegetable
   cooking liquid, or water

Freshly ground black pepper
Salt (optional)

Heat oil in a large sauté pan or wide casserole. Add rice and sauté over medium-low heat, stirring, for 2 minutes or until it changes color slightly and smells slightly toasted. Add hot vegetable broth and a pinch of pepper. If using broth that contains salt, do not add salt at this point. If using unsalted broth or water, you can add 1 to 1½ teaspoons salt, or leave the rice salt-free, if, you prefer. Stir once with a fork and cover.

Cook over low heat, without stirring, for 40 minutes. Taste rice; if not yet tender, simmer 2 more minutes or until just tender. Let stand, covered, for 10 minutes.

Gently fluff rice with a fork. Season to taste. Serve hot; or cool to use in recipes.

NOTE: Plain Cooked Brown Rice: combine rice and unheated liquid and bring to a boil. Cover and cook over low heat. Continue with rest of recipe.

Makes 8 servings

Yemenite relish, or zehug, is basically made of two healthy ingredients—chiles and garlic, used raw. Zehug comes in two colors—bright green and brick red, depending on the chiles used. Its taste can be fiery from tiny dried chiles and plenty of black pepper and other spices.

This fresh-tasting, bright green version is one of the easiest ways to make the relish. It needs only four ingredients: chiles, garlic, cilantro, and salt. With jalapeño peppers, I find it delicious and not overwhelmingly pungent, but you could use hotter chiles if you prefer.

The Yemenites serve it as an accompaniment for soup; people usually spread it on bread and eat it with the soup. I like to stir it into Vegetable Soup with Smoked Turkey and Fresh Green Hot Sauce (page 211) for extra zing, as a sort of lean and spicy kind of pesto. Indeed, you could use it like pesto and mix it with pasta and a little oil. It's also a tasty addition to Israeli diced salad of cucumbers, tomatoes, and onion.

Since this relish is so quick and easy to prepare, I make it in small quantities as needed so the flavor stays fresh. I leave the seeds and membranes in the jalapeño peppers so they give their heat to the relish, but you can remove them for a milder effect. Since the cilantro stems give plenty of flavor, don't bother picking off only the leaves to use in the relish. If you don't like cilantro, substitute flat-leaf parsley or omit it.

2 jalapeño peppers, quartered
4 garlic cloves, peeled
½ cup cilantro sprigs, including stems, cut into pieces

2 to 4 teaspoons water
Pinch of salt

This relish is easiest to make in a mini-food processor. Combine jalapeño peppers, garlic, cilantro, 2 teaspoons water, and salt in processor. Process ingredients to a smooth puree, stopping a few times to push mixture down so ingredients are ground evenly. Add a little more water if necessary.

NOTE: If you're not used to handling hot peppers or your skin is sensitive, wear gloves. If not using gloves, wash your hands well after handling the peppers. Wash the knife and cutting board also.

Makes ⅓ to ½ cup, 4 to 6 servings

❧ SPICY SALSA, ISRAELI STYLE

Like Mexicans, many Israelis like a hot pepper relish with their meals. For this fresh Mediterranean-style, medium-hot salsa, I use tomatoes, jalapeño peppers, and green onions. Unlike typical Mexican salsa, it includes lemon juice and a little olive oil, and parsley instead of cilantro. It's good with all sorts of foods, from broiled eggplant (page 360) to hard-boiled eggs, and even makes a change-of-pace accompaniment for gefilte fish!

2 to 3 medium jalapeño peppers or 4 serrano peppers
⅓ cup flat-leaf parsley sprigs
1 pound ripe tomatoes, finely diced

2 green onions, chopped
1 to 2 tablespoons lemon juice
1 tablespoon extra virgin olive oil
Salt and freshly ground black pepper

Core jalapeño peppers and remove seeds and ribs if you want them to be less hot. Put jalapeño peppers in a small food processor and chop finely. Add parsley and chop finely. Transfer to a medium bowl. Add tomatoes, green onions, lemon juice, and oil. Season to taste with salt and pepper. Refrigerate salsa in a covered container until ready to serve. Serve cold.

Makes about 2 cups, about 8 servings

❧ OLIVE OIL AND LEMON DRESSING

This is a basic Mediterranean dressing, used in salads and with cooked greens and vegetables. If you use a fruity extra virgin olive oil or substitute an aromatic nut oil, it will be very flavorful and a little will go a long way. The simple dressing is good as is, or you can add minced fresh garlic, or chopped fresh or dried herbs to taste, or Dijon mustard for its flavor and to thicken the dressing.

To turn it into vinaigrette, substitute vinegar for all or half the lemon juice. French wine vinegar will give the sharpest result, Asian rice vinegar the mildest. Tarragon or other herb-scented vinegar, balsamic vinegar, and raspberry vinegar are good too. Classic French vinaigrette calls for three times as much oil as vinegar, but for most salads, the proportions here taste fine.

2 tablespoons strained fresh lemon juice
Salt and freshly ground black pepper

4 tablespoons extra virgin olive oil

Combine ingredients in a bowl and beat with a whisk or fork until blended. Taste and adjust seasoning.

Makes ⅓ cup dressing

❈ SESAME GINGER DRESSING

This dressing is good on vegetables, noodles, chicken, fish, and tofu. Try it with Broccoli and Carrots with Edamame (page 284).

1 tablespoon sesame seeds
3 tablespoons rice vinegar
1 to 2 tablespoons sugar, or to taste
1 tablespoon Asian (toasted) sesame oil

2 tablespoons soy sauce
½ to 1 teaspoon grated ginger
Ground black or white pepper or cayenne pepper
    (optional)

Toast sesame seeds in a small skillet over medium heat, shaking pan often, about 2 minutes or until golden brown. Transfer immediately to a plate and let cool.

Whisk vinegar, 1 tablespoon sugar, and oil in a medium bowl. Whisk in soy sauce and ginger, and add pepper to taste. Whisk in sesame seeds. Taste and whisk in more sugar if desired.

Makes about ⅓ cup

Israeli cooks know that tomato sauce is a good partner for most foods, from pasta to rice to meat to eggs to vegetables. Although you can use bottled or canned tomato sauce, when tomatoes are at the peak of their season, it's worth making your own. You can flavor the sauce with sautéed onion, garlic, or both.

Tomatoes have gained new interest among nutritionists because they are high in lycopene, a pigment that can help protect the body from certain cancers. It's a good idea to use a little oil in the sauce, not only from the standpoint of flavor, but also because lycopene works better in the presence of fat. When the sauce is ready, you may like to add a teaspoon or two of sugar or lemon juice, depending on whether the tomatoes were tart or sweet, and according to personal taste.

1½ to 2 tablespoons extra virgin olive oil
1 onion, finely chopped (optional)
2 to 4 large garlic cloves, minced (optional)
2½ pounds ripe tomatoes, peeled, seeded, and chopped, or two 28-ounce cans tomatoes, drained and chopped

1 large thyme sprig, or ½ teaspoon dried thyme
1 bay leaf
Salt and freshly ground black pepper
½ teaspoon dried oregano (optional)
1 tablespoon tomato paste (optional)

Heat oil in a large sauté pan, stew pan, or shallow saucepan. Add onion and sauté over medium heat for 7 minutes or until soft but not browned. Stir in garlic, if desired, and sauté for ½ minute. Stir in tomatoes, thyme, bay leaf, salt, pepper, and oregano, if you like. Cook, uncovered, over medium-high heat, stirring often, for 10 to 15 minutes or until tomatoes are soft and sauce is thick. Discard thyme sprig and bay leaf. If you would like a deeper color, stir in tomato paste and simmer for 5 more minutes. For a smoother sauce, puree sauce in a food processor. Taste and adjust seasoning.

Makes about 2 cups

You can make this sauce base ahead and keep it for 2 days in the refrigerator or, if you like, prepare a double or triple quantity and keep it in the freezer for up to several months. All that is needed to turn it quickly into a tasty sauce for meat or chicken is a splash of Madeira, port, or fruit juice and a little salt and pepper.

An even faster, low-fat option is Two-Minute Sauce Base (see below). If you have flavorful broth, the sauce will taste good, although it's not a classic brown sauce because it doesn't contain sautéed foods to turn it brown.

1½ teaspoons olive oil or vegetable oil
½ onion, diced
½ carrot, diced
1½ cups chicken or beef broth, thoroughly skimmed
   of fat
1 celery rib, diced (optional)
1 fresh thyme sprig, or ½ teaspoon dried thyme

1 bay leaf
6 parsley stems (optional)
1½ teaspoons potato starch, arrowroot, or
   cornstarch
2 tablespoons cold water
2 teaspoons tomato paste (optional)

Heat oil in a heavy, medium saucepan. Add onion and carrot and sauté over medium-high heat, stirring often, for 5 minutes or until browned, reducing heat if necessary. Add broth, celery (if using), thyme, bay leaf, and parsley (if using). Bring to a boil. Simmer, uncovered, over medium-low heat for 10 minutes. Strain into a bowl, pressing on vegetables. If possible, let cool for 30 minutes. Skim excess fat. Return broth to saucepan.

In a small bowl, whisk potato starch and water to a smooth paste. Whisk in tomato paste, if desired. Bring broth to a simmer. Gradually pour in tomato mixture, whisking. Return to a boil, whisking. Simmer for 1 or 2 minutes or until thickened.

Two-Minute Sauce Base: Omit oil, onion, carrot, celery, bay leaf, and parsley. Combine broth with dried thyme in saucepan. Thicken mixture with potato starch and water slurry (and tomato paste, if you like), following directions in second paragraph.

Makes about 1 cup

✺ CHICKEN BROTH OR STOCK

Soups and stews are much more delicious when made with homemade broth or stock. Besides, you can control the amount of salt; often packaged broth is salty.

Technically, broth is made from chicken pieces or whole chickens, and stock is made from bones, wing tips, trimmings, and giblets. Although you can use pieces with skin and then skim off the fat from the broth at the end, it takes time and patience to do this thoroughly. I prefer to use skinless chicken legs or thighs to avoid having a fatty broth, and then I have the meat for making into salads or casseroles or for adding to soups. I use pieces on the bone, as they produce a more flavorful broth than boneless chicken. In many markets you can ask the butcher to remove the skin.

When making stock, be sure to remove any blobs of fat from the chicken backs and gizzards. You can keep stock or broth for 2 or 3 days in the refrigerator; or you can freeze it.

3 pounds chicken legs or thighs, skin removed, or
    chicken bones, backs, necks, and giblets (except
    livers)
2 onions, quartered
2 carrots, quartered

2 celery ribs, with leaves
Dark green parts of 2 leeks, cleaned (optional)
4 fresh thyme sprigs
2 bay leaves
About 5 quarts water

Combine chicken, onions, carrots, celery, leeks (if using), thyme, and bay leaves in a large pot. Add enough water to cover ingredients. Bring to a boil, skimming froth.

Reduce heat to low so that stock bubbles very gently. Partially cover and cook, skimming foam and fat occasionally, for 1 hour if using chicken legs or thighs, or for 2 hours if using bones. Strain stock into large bowls. If not using immediately, cool to lukewarm. Refrigerate until cold. Thoroughly skim fat off top.

Turkey Stock: Substitute bones and scraps from a roast turkey for chicken pieces. Cook stock for 2 to 3 hours.

Makes 3 to 3½ quarts

❧ VEGETABLE BROTH

Like chicken broth, vegetable broth tastes better when homemade and you have the advantage of being able to control the salt. You can make it from whole vegetables or trimmings of mild and sweet vegetables like the ends of onions, carrots, zucchini, and green beans and the dark green parts of leeks. Asparagus bases and shiitake mushroom stems also add good flavor.

The easiest way to have vegetable broth on hand is to save the cooking liquid from vegetables. I often make simple vegetable dishes like Creamy Broccoli Soup Without the Cream (page 202), and keep the broth in a jar to use for soups or stews or for cooking grains. Vegetable broth can be kept in the refrigerator for 2 or 3 days; or you can freeze it.

3 onions, coarsely chopped
2 carrots, sliced
2 celery ribs, sliced
Dark green parts of 2 leeks, rinsed thoroughly
(optional)
1 bay leaf
2 fresh thyme sprigs

2 garlic cloves, peeled and crushed
5 parsley stems (optional)
½ teaspoon peppercorns
½ to 1 cup shiitake or other mushroom stems
(optional)
About 6 cups water

Combine ingredients in a large saucepan, adding enough water to cover them. Bring to a boil. Cover and cook over low heat for 1 hour. Strain broth, pressing on ingredients in strainer; then discard them. Cool promptly, and refrigerate or freeze until ready to use.

Makes about 1 quart

❧ QUICK FISH STOCK

To give fish soups and sauces a fresh, natural seafood flavor, use homemade fish stock. This time-honored trick of simmering fish bones briefly in water to give their essence to sauces is one I learned long ago at cooking school in Paris.

Whenever you buy whole fish and have it filleted, it's a good idea to cook the bones in water for a few minutes to make a quick stock. You can also make it from fish pieces for chowder or bony pieces labeled fish collars, which are sold at many markets. If you have parsley stems from which you've already used the leaves, add them for extra flavor. Keep the delicate broth in the freezer.

1 pound fish heads, tails, and bones
1 quart water
1 bay leaf

1 fresh thyme sprig, or ½ teaspoon dried thyme
6 parsley stems (optional)
1 onion, sliced (optional)

Rinse fish heads and bones thoroughly and put them in a medium saucepan. Add water, bay leaf, thyme, parsley, and onion (if using). Bring to a boil. Cover and simmer over low heat for 20 minutes. Strain stock. Cool promptly, and refrigerate or freeze until ready to use.

Makes about 3½ cups

⚹⚹ RED BERRY SAUCE

Serve this luscious, orange-scented raspberry and strawberry sauce with nut cakes, cheesecakes, fruit salads, poached fruit, and frozen yogurt.

1½ cups fresh strawberries, rinsed and hulled
About ½ cup powdered sugar, sifted
3 cups (about 12 ounces) fresh raspberries, or one
   10- to 12-ounce package frozen unsweetened
   or lightly sweetened raspberries, thawed

2 tablespoons fresh orange juice, or to taste
¼ cup brown rice syrup, honey, maple syrup, or
   brown sugar
½ teaspoon grated orange zest

Puree strawberries in a food processor or blender with 1 tablespoon powdered sugar. Transfer to a bowl.

Add raspberries and orange juice to food processor and puree them. Add ⅓ cup powdered sugar. Process until very smooth.

Spoon half of raspberry puree into a strainer. Strain sauce into a bowl, pressing on pulp in strainer; use a rubber spatula to scrape mixture from underside of strainer. Continue straining remaining raspberry puree. Stir in syrup, strawberry puree, and orange zest.

Stir sauce before serving. Taste and add another 1 to 2 tablespoons powdered sugar or more orange juice if desired. Serve cold.

Makes about 8 servings

❈ SPICED CHOCOLATE WINE GLAZE

This rich, shiny glaze lends a festive note to cakes, brownies, and cookies and is based on two healthy ingredients—chocolate and red wine, and just a touch of butter (or margarine for a pareve glaze). Try it on Almond Applesauce Cake with Chocolate Chips and Honey (page 21), Macadamia Orange Cake (page 108), or Passover Chocolate Cinnamon Brownies with Almonds (page 107). After spreading the glaze, you can sprinkle the cake with ¼ cup toasted slivered or sliced almonds or other chopped toasted nuts.

¼ cup brown or granulated sugar
½ teaspoon ground cinnamon
⅓ cup dry red wine
4 ounces bittersweet or semisweet chocolate,
    chopped

2 tablespoons vegetable oil
2 tablespoons unsalted butter or margarine, chilled,
    cut into pieces

In a small saucepan, whisk sugar with cinnamon and wine until blended. Bring to a boil over medium-high heat, whisking. Simmer over low heat for 2 minutes, whisking occasionally. Add chocolate and oil and stir over very low heat until melted. Off heat, stir in butter until blended in. Refrigerate, stirring occasionally, about 45 minutes or until spreadable.

Stir glaze until smooth. Spread over cake, brownies, or cookies. Refrigerate for about 30 minutes or until glaze sets.

Makes enough for a 9-inch square cake

❧ TURKISH LEMON SYRUP

Instead of serving their pastries with honey and cinnamon (see Honey Cinnamon Hanukkah Pastry Balls, page 69), some Turkish and Greek cooks prepare a lemon syrup. If you like, you can flavor it with a little grated lemon rind as well as the juice. You can sweeten it with honey, which is more healthful than sugar, or use all sugar, according to your taste.

When serving it with pastry balls, you can spoon a little syrup over each one or, for a sweeter taste, dip the pastries in the syrup. This syrup is also good with simple sponge cakes and for moistening fruit salad. For an offbeat dessert that I learned at a vegetarian Vietnamese restaurant, you can flavor the syrup with 1 or 2 slices of fresh ginger instead of lemon and drizzle a little over portions of very soft tofu.

½ cup sugar
½ cup honey or additional sugar
¾ cup water

1 tablespoon fresh lemon juice
1 to 2 teaspoons grated lemon zest (optional)

Combine sugar, honey, and water in a small, heavy saucepan and cook over medium-low heat, stirring constantly, until sugar dissolves. Bring to a boil and simmer without stirring for 3 minutes or until syrup is clear. Add lemon juice and simmer for 1 to 2 minutes. Remove from heat and add lemon zest, if you like. Let cool.

Makes about ¾ cup

BROILED EGGPLANT SLICES

Broiling eggplant slices is an easier, healthier way to prepare them than frying. You can use the slices in recipes that call for fried eggplant, or serve them as an accompaniment or appetizer with Easy Green Chile Garlic Relish (page 363) or homemade Tomato Sauce (page 367).

1 medium eggplant (about 1 pound), or 1 pound Japanese, Chinese, or small Italian eggplants

2 to 3 teaspoons extra virgin olive oil
Salt and freshly ground black pepper

Slice eggplant about ¼ inch thick. Arrange slices on a foil–lined baking sheet or broiler pan. Brush lightly with oil and sprinkle with salt and pepper. Broil for 5 to 6 minutes. Turn over and broil about 7 minutes or until tender. Serve hot, warm, or at room temperature.

Makes 3 to 4 servings

Vitamin A–rich peppers, especially red ones, are one of the healthiest vegetables. Many nutrition experts consider them a superfood. Serve broiled peeled peppers plain as an appetizer, use them in sauces, or turn them into dips like Balkan Pepper Dip (page 158).

The easiest way to peel peppers and chiles is to broil them first. For easy cleanup I often put them on a foil-lined broiler rack. You can also grill them on the barbecue or on a stovetop grill. If you're roasting a chicken or other food at 400°F to 450°F, you can roast the peppers at the same time.

Do not rinse the grilled peppers to help remove the skins and seeds. This would sap their flavor.

Preheat broiler with rack 2 to 4 inches from heat source, or far enough so that peppers can just fit; or heat grill. Broil or grill peppers until their skins are blistered and charred in spots, but do not let them burn. If you don't want peppers to soften too much, grill them until only slightly charred but still firm. The approximate cooking times are:

Bell peppers: 15 to 20 minutes

Anaheim (California, green, or mild) chiles: 10 to 12 minutes

Poblano (pasilla), jalapeño, serrano, or other small chiles: 5 minutes

During broiling, turn peppers occasionally with tongs so another side faces heat source—bell peppers every 4 to 5 minutes, Anaheim chiles every 3 minutes, small chiles every minute.

Transfer peppers to a bowl and cover bowl; or put them in a paper or plastic bag and close bag. Let stand for 10 minutes. Peel peppers, using paring knife. If your skin is sensitive, wear gloves when handling hot chiles.

Halve peppers; be careful because they may have hot juice inside. Discard seeds and ribs, and pat dry. Do not rinse. Seeds can be easily scraped off with a knife.

❧ PEELED TOMATOES

Prepare a bowl of cold water. Cut green cores from tomatoes, turn each tomato over and, with point of paring knife, slit skin on bottom of tomato in an ✕ shape.

Put a few tomatoes in a saucepan of enough boiling water to cover them generously. Boil tomatoes for 10 to 15 seconds or until their skin begins to pull away from their flesh. Immediately remove tomatoes from water with a slotted spoon and put them in a bowl of cold water. Leave for a few seconds so they cool.

Remove tomatoes from water and peel their skins with aid of a paring knife. Continue with remaining tomatoes.

❧ SEEDED TOMATOES

You can seed peeled or unpeeled tomatoes.

Cut tomatoes in half horizontally. Hold each tomato half over a bowl, cut side down. Squeeze tomato to remove most of seeds and juice; some seeds may remain.

❧ COOKED BEANS

There is no need to soak dried beans or chickpeas before cooking them. Since their cooking time is long, it's a good idea to prepare a double or triple batch and keep them in the freezer. The bean cooking liquid is good for soups and stews.

1 pound (2¼ to 2½ cups) dried white, red, pink,
    peruano, or black beans, soybeans, or chickpeas
    (garbanzo beans)

7 cups water, or more if needed
Pinch of salt

Put beans in a large pot and add 7 cups water or enough to cover generously. Bring to a boil. Cover and simmer over low heat until tender, 1¼ to 1½ hours for most beans, 1½ to 2 hours for chickpeas, or 2 to 3 hours for soybeans, adding hot water occasionally to keep them covered with water. If you like, add a little salt to cooking liquid after beans have cooked for 1 hour. If cooking beans ahead, refrigerate them in their cooking liquid.

Makes 5 to 7 cups cooked beans, about 6 servings

❧ TOASTED ALMONDS

A few almonds make a healthy snack, and they taste even better when toasted. Use them also to embellish desserts, such as Almond Applesauce Cake (page 21) frosted with Spiced Chocolate Wine Glaze (page 373), or sprinkled on salads, cooked vegetables, grain, and pasta dishes.

Preheat oven to 350°F; for a small amount of almonds, you can use a toaster oven. Put whole, slivered, or sliced almonds on a baking sheet. Toast, shaking baking sheet once or twice, until almonds are aromatic; blanched ones should turn from cream colored to light tan. Watch them carefully so they don't burn.

For whole almonds: allow about 7 minutes

For slivered almonds: allow 4 to 5 minutes

For sliced almonds: allow 2 to 3 minutes

As soon as almonds are ready, transfer them to a plate so they won't continue to brown from the heat of the baking dish.

Toasted Pine Nuts: Follow directions above for sliced almonds.

❧ TOASTED HAZELNUTS

Unlike other nuts, hazelnuts are peeled after they are toasted.

Preheat oven to 350°F. Put hazelnuts on a baking sheet. Toast hazelnuts, shaking baking sheet once or twice, about 8 minutes or until their skins begin to split. Transfer to a strainer. While nuts are hot, remove most of skins by rubbing nuts energetically with a towel against a strainer.

TOASTED WALNUTS AND PECANS

Preheat oven to 350°F; for a small amount of nuts, you can use a toaster oven. Put nuts on a baking sheet. Toast, shaking baking sheet once or twice, for 5 minutes or until nuts are aromatic and turn a very slightly darker shade of brown than when they are raw.

As soon as nuts are ready, transfer them to a plate so they won't continue to brown from heat of baking dish.

TOASTED SESAME SEEDS

Preheat oven or toaster oven to 350°F. Put sesame seeds on a small baking sheet and toast, shaking pan or stirring seeds occasionally, until golden brown, about 5 minutes. Transfer immediately to a plate.

To toast a few tablespoons of seeds in a skillet, put seeds in a small, heavy skillet over medium-low heat. Toast them, shaking pan often, for 4 minutes or until golden brown. Transfer immediately to a plate.

Index

※

About the Author

Faye Levy is well known to lovers of good cooking. The *New York Times* profiled her in 1987 in an article about her entitled "Modest Beginnings for an Expert Chef."

Jewish cooking aficionados are familiar with Levy as the author of four other Jewish cookbooks. *Faye Levy's International Jewish Cookbook* was published in 1991 to rave reviews. The *New York Times* deemed her book *1,000 Jewish Recipes* "a culinary Bible," and the *Los Angeles Times* referred to it as "the Jewish joy of cooking." Faye also wrote *The Low-Fat Jewish Cookbook* and *Jewish Cooking for Dummies*.

Faye's recipes and food articles are prominently featured every week in Judaism's holiest city—in the *Jerusalem Post*, for which Faye has been writing the main cooking column for eighteen years. She also writes a weekly "Cooking Class" column for the paper's new *Weekend* magazine.

For the last eighteen years Faye has also been a nationally syndicated cooking columnist for the Los Angeles Times Syndicate (now Tribune Media Services), focusing on healthful, easy, savory dishes. For four years she was the culinary columnist of Israel's foremost women's magazine, *At*, and for six years she wrote the prestigious column "The Basics" for *Bon Appétit* magazine. She has written on such delicious Jewish matters as "Sephardic Seder" *for Gourmet* and "Challah" for *Bon Appétit*, as well as Jewish holiday cooking articles for the *Los Angeles Times* and other newspapers around the United States.

Faye has lived and learned about Jewish cooking in the capitals of the countries with the world's largest Jewish populations—the United States, Israel, and France. She is fluent in the languages of these lands and proficient in their culinary cultures and she has the unique achievement of writing cookbooks in English, Hebrew, and French.

Born and raised in our nation's capital in a strictly kosher Orthodox home, Faye received her Jewish education at the Hebrew Academy of Washington, D.C.; as an adult she was honored with the Academy's "Eishet Hayil" or Woman of Valor award. She attended college at the Hebrew University in Jerusalem and Tel Aviv University, where she graduated magna cum laude in sociology and anthropology.

Faye trained to become a professional chef at the renowned Parisian cooking school École de Cuisine La Varenne. She spent five additional years at the school, authoring the school's first cookbook, designing the curriculum, and researching and drafting the recipes for La Varenne's award-winning cookbooks. This exceptional experience gave her a priceless perspective for an American cook.

Nutritious cooking has always interested Faye. At La Varenne she planned the menus and helped develop the recipes for the class on "cuisine minceur," or slimming French cooking, at a time when few people thought that French food and healthy food could go together. In addition to *The Low-Fat Jewish Cookbook,* Faye is the author of two other low-fat cookbooks, *30 Low-Fat Meals in 30 Minutes* and its vegetarian sequel, *30 Low-Fat Vegetarian Meals in 30 Minutes.*

Healthful cooking was a primary theme in Faye Levy's *International Vegetable Cookbook,* for which she won the James Beard Cookbook Award in 1994 for the best book of the year in the category of fruits, vegetables, and grains, and in her recent book, *Feast from the Mideast,* which *Publishers Weekly* called "an important volume rich in content and knowledge."

Faye also won awards from the International Association of Culinary Professionals for her books *Vegetable Creations, Chocolate Sensations,* and *Classic Cooking Techniques.*

Faye cooked on such TV programs as *Good Morning America* and *Good Morning Israel* and demonstrated how to cook a four-course Passover menu on the PBS show "Seasoning." Faye loves teaching and imparting to her students her enthusiasm and joy in discovering new tastes and ingredients and in experimenting in the kitchen. Faye and her husband and writing partner, Yakir Levy, enjoy cooking, dining, and learning in their home in Woodland Hills, California, and during their culinary pilgrimages around the country and across the globe.